Gamuts & Pearls in MRI

Second Edition

Stephen J. Pomeranz

Director of Advanced Imaging
Director of Magnetic Resonance Imaging
Director of Nuclear Medicine
Director of Metabolic Imaging
The Christ Hospital
Cincinnati, Ohio

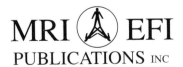

MRI EFI
PUBLICATIONS INC

Cincinnati, Ohio

Managing Editor and Design Coordinator: Diana R. Vester
Copy Editor: Christopher Clyde
Production and Manufacturing: Don Beville and Phil Councill

Library of Congress Cataloging-in-Publication Data

Pomeranz, Stephen J.
        Gamuts & Pearls in MRI 2nd

CIP 93-80444
ISBN 1-882576-04-7

Printing and Manufacturing by:
Cadmus Fine Books
2901 Byrd Hill Road Box 26459
Richmond, Virginia 23261
1-800-899-8833

Dedication

To my devoted wife, companion and best friend, Penny, and our six little Indians, Christy, Corbin, Taylor, Jory, Kellen and Cody.

Preface

It has been over three years since the first edition of Gamuts and Pearls in MRI was published. During that time, MR, particularly clinical MR, has evolved a great deal.

This text is not meant to be encyclopedic, but rather to be used as a handy reference by the clinical interpreter for problems which arise in everyday MR practice.

Issues of interest may not just be directly related to MR findings but can also include important clinical tenets, relevant anatomy and critical differential diagnoses to clarify findings and reports. These will assist indirectly in common MR diagnosis.

As you can see, the text has doubled in size since the first edition. We have attempted to include more anatomy, more information in the orthopedic axis where MR has been growing steadily, and more in-depth differential diagnostic lists. The increase in text volume reflects not only a greater number of differential diagnoses but also more diagramatic information and an increased number of relevant clinical pearls relating to diseases commonly approached with MRI. Frequently utilized classification systems relevant to MR practice are also included in this text.

It is my hope that this book will be most useful for questions arising in clinical interpretation, particularly when MR differential diagnoses are at issue. As MR continues to grow, so too will this text, and it is not unlikely that Gamuts and Pearls in MRI will again double in size by the year 2000.

Acknowledgements

This text was carefully and lovingly prepared by the chief editor and design coordinator, Diana Vester. The copy editing was astutely carried out by Christopher Clyde, and I am deeply grateful to both of them. The manuscript was proofread by my friends and colleagues Daniel Bodor, MD; Kendall Goldschmidt, MD; and Peter Moorton, DO. I would also like to extend my appreciation to our production manager in Virginia, Don Beville, for his assistance. This book could not have been completed without the continued support and assistance of my loving wife, Penny.

About This Text

This text is divided by anatomic headings, subcategorized (e.g., brain into posterior fossa, etc.; musculoskeletal into joints) and then listed with titles encompassing anatomy, pathology, pitfalls and variations. Related topics are arranged consecutively within sections, as are corresponding text and diagrams. This format along with the extensive table of contents (both comprehensive and specific for each section) should provide ease of reference for the topic or entity of interest. Most of the text emphasizes imaging and clinical material relevant to MR; technical information regarding imaging can be found in the final chapter, which includes optimal and proven guidelines for scanning. While it is not the nature of a gamuts text to be an exhaustive exploration of topics, we feel this collection of listings is both concise and thorough, clinically relevant and user-friendly, and we hope you find it useful.

CATEGORY A: THE BRAIN

CATEGORY A: THE BRAIN

Page

CATEGORY A: THE BRAIN

Page

CATEGORY A: THE BRAIN

Page

CATEGORY A: THE BRAIN

CATEGORY B: THE SPINE

CATEGORY C: HEAD & NECK

CATEGORY F: THE KNEE

Page

CATEGORY F: THE KNEE

CATEGORY G: FOOT & ANKLE

Page

CATEGORY H: THE SHOULDER

Page

CATEGORY J: HAND, WRIST & ELBOW

Page

CATEGORY K: ABDOMEN & BODY

Page

CATEGORY L: IMAGES & PREDICAMENTS

Section 1: Contraindications

Section 2: Contrast

CATEGORY A: THE BRAIN

Page

CATEGORY A: THE BRAIN

Section 1: Signal Intensities   Page

A-1 Intracranial Signal: Hyperintense T1 & T2

Common

1. Chronic or late subacute hematoma or clot (mid or high field)
2. Flow (first echo slice entry phenomenon, second echo rephasing)
3. Aneurysm with chronic clot or flow phenomenon
4. Cholesterol cyst or granuloma
5. Craniopharyngioma
6. Rathke's cyst
7. Posterior pituitary bright spot (normal variant)
8. Cavernous malformation
9. Post-hemorrhagic calcification
10. Mucocele

Uncommon

1. Dermoid tumor
2. Teratoma
3. Hemorrhagic lipoma
4. Xanthogranuloma
5. Xanthoastrocytoma
6. Atypical epidermoid

A-2   **Intracranial Signal: Hyperintense T1, Hypointense T2**

Common

1.   Subacute hematoma or clot (mid or high field)
2.   Flow (first echo slice entry phenomenon)
3.   Melanoma metastases
4.   Hemorrhagic metastases (choriocarcinoma, neuroblastoma, embryonal cell carcinoma, thyroid carcinoma, renal cell carcinoma, malignant melanoma)
5.   Lipoma
6.   Pantopaque

Uncommon

1.   Colloid cyst
2.   Calcified xanthogranuloma
3.   Aneurysm (with clot or slice entry)
4.   Craniopharyngioma

**A-3   Intracranial Signal: Hypo- to Isointense T1, Hypointense T2
(1.5 T)**

Common

1.   Acute hematoma
2.   Flow (first echo flow void, second echo rephasing)
3.   Aneurysm with flow phenomenon or acute clot
4.   Calcification (nontraumatic, nonhemorrhagic)
5.   Brain iron
6.   Neoplasm with acute hemorrhage or extensive calcification
7.   Meningioma
8.   Metastases (colon, prostate, osteogenic sarcoma, breast)

Uncommon

1.   Colloid cyst
2.   Melanoma

Rare

1.   Chloroma

A-4   **Intracranial Signal: Isointense T1 & T2**

Common

1. Hyperacute hematoma (transition to acute hematoma [1.5 T])
2. Acute hematoma (mid field [0.5 T])
3. Subacute hematoma (high field)
4. Flow (combinations of flow void adding to flow-related hyperintensity)
5. Aneurysm with flow phenomenon
6. Meningioma
7. Brain iron (low field)
8. Isointense metastases (colon, prostate, osteogenic sarcoma, breast)
9. Hamartoma

Uncommon

1. Colloid cyst

Rare

1. Medulloblastoma or adult cerebellar sarcoma
2. Lymphoma
3. Tuberculoma
4. Chloroma

A-5 **Intracranial Signal: Homogeneous Water Signal, Very Hypointense T1, Very Hyperintense T2**

Common

1. Cystic encephalomalacia
2. Porencephalic cyst
3. Arachnoid cyst
4. Nonependymal-lined cyst
5. Blake's pouch or mega cisterna magna
6. Pineal cyst (normal variant)
7. Intraventricular neuroepithelial cyst (normal variant)
8. Xanthogranulomatous cyst (of choroid plexus, normal variant)
9. Remote hematoma

Uncommon

1. Trapped ventricle (fourth)
2. Trapped temporal horn
2. Dandy-Walker malformation
3. Meningocele
4. Pseudomeningocele (dural leak)

Rare

1. Seroma (postsurgical)
2. Trapped lateral ventricle

A-6   Intracranial Signal: Iso- to Hypointense T1, Hyperintense T2

Common

1. Glial neoplasms
2. Metastatic neoplasia
3. Infarction, nonhemorrhagic
4. Lymphoma (primary or secondary)
5. Cerebritis, encephalitis
6. Meningioma (especially angioblastic or fibrovascular)
7. Neuroma
8. Pituitary macroadenoma
9. Acute hematoma (low field)

Uncommon

1. Tuberculoma
2. Pinealoma
3. Pineoblastoma
4. Chordoma
5. Choroid plexus papilloma
6. Medulloblastoma
7. Radiation necrosis
8. Gliosis/scar
9. Hamartoma
10. Ependymoma
11. Subependymoma
12. Craniopharyngioma
13. Active granuloma
14. Hyperacute hematoma
15. Aneurysm (with flow or clot)
16. Epidermoid

A-7   Intracranial Signal: Inhomogeneous Water Signal, Hypointense T1, Hyperintense T2

Common

1. Abscess
2. Aneurysm (with clot)
3. Complex porencephalic cyst
4. Complex arachnoid cyst
5. Complex nonependymal-lined colloid cyst
6. Cystic or radiated metastases (oat cell carcinoma, squamous cell carcinoma, ovarian carcinoma, colon carcinoma, renal cell carcinoma, craniopharyngioma)
7. Acute hemorrhage (low field)
8. Mucocele
9. Cystic astrocytoma
10. Hemangioblastoma

Uncommon

1. Epidermoid
2. Hyperacute hemorrhage (high and low field)

Rare

1. Amyloidoma
2. Cysticercosis

A-8   Gyriform Cortical-Subcortical Hypointense T2 Signal (High Field)

Common

1. Acute hemorrhagic cortical infarction
2. Subacute hemorrhagic cortical infarction (early)
3. Luxury flow effect in bland cortical infarct

Uncommon

1. Superficial siderosis (remote subarachnoid hemorrhage)
2. Acute subarachnoid hemorrhage (high field)
3. Meningitis (flow phenomenon in subcortical U-fibers)

A-9   Gyriform Cortical-Subcortical T1 Hyperintense Signal

Common

1. Chronic hemorrhagic cortical infarction
2. Subacute hemorrhagic cortical infarction (late)
3. Subacute or chronic subarachnoid hemorrhage
4. Contrast enhancement of subacute cortical infarct

Uncommon

1. Contrast enhancement of leptomeningeal/dural neoplasm or inflammation
2. Dural or cortical AVM (slice-entry or even-echo rephasing)

A-10   Gyriform Peripheral T2 Hyperintensity with Parenchymal Lesions

Common
1. Deep white matter and peripheral cortical infarction

Uncommon
1. Parenchymal metastases with cerebral carcinomatosis
2. Lymphoma
3. Primary intracranial neoplasm with subarachnoid or leptomeningeal tumor seed (ependymoma, medulloblastoma, oligodendroglioma, glioblastoma, ependymoblastoma)
4. Viral meningoencephalitis
5. Cryptococcoma with cryptococcal meningitis
6. Autoimmune vasculocerebritis

Rare
1. Tuberculosis
2. Neurosarcoidosis
3. Syphilis
4. Other fungal meningoencephalitis (blastomycosis, aspergillosis, etc.)

A-11   Black Signal

1.   Flow
2.   Air or gas
3.   Hemosiderin (T2 dependent)
4.   Iron, copper or metal
5.   Bone
6.   Calcium
7.   Superparamagnetic contrast agents
8.   Ligaments, tendons, fascia
9.   Magnetic susceptibility

A-12   Hypointense Rings

1.   Hemosiderin ring: Chronic hematoma
2.   Susceptibility rim artifact: Glial or astrocytic neoplasm
3.   Pseudocapsule of dura, cerebrospinal fluid, cleft, desmoplasia, vessels: Meningioma
4.   Fibrous rim: Abscess, neurocysticercosis, meningioma

A-13   Parenchymal Lesions (Hypointense T1, Hyperintense T2)*

Long T1 and T2 Relaxation, Nonenhancing, No Mass Effect
1. Anoxia
2. Gliosis (infection, infarction, trauma)
3. Low grade astrocytic neoplasm
4. Demyelinative plaque
5. Shear injury
6. Tuberous sclerosis

Long T1 and T2 Relaxation, Enhancing, No Mass Effect
1. Flow
2. Low grade infection
3. Multiple sclerosis or demyelinative plaque
4. Normal vessel or vein
5. Small astrocytic neoplasm
6. Small or early metastasis
7. Small vascular anomaly
8. Vasculocerebritis
9. Meningoencephalitis
10. Late acute or subacute infarction

Long T1 and T2 Relaxation, Nonenhancing, Mass Effect
1. Late acute or early subacute infarction
2. Contusion
3. Cryptococcoma
4. Hyperacute hemorrhage
5. Low grade glioma

A-13   **Parenchymal Lesions (Hypointense T1, Hyperintense T2) (Cont'd)**

Long T1 and T2 Relaxation, Enhancing, Mass Effect

1.   Abscess
2.   Cerebritis
3.   Ganglion cell tumors (rare)
4.   High grade astrocytic neoplasms
5.   Metastasis
6.   Lymphoma (primary or metastatic)
7.   Primitive neuroectodermal tumor
8.   Radiation necrosis
9.   Tumefactive multiple sclerosis

* Adapted from Reeder MM, Bradley WG. Reeder and Felson's Gamuts in Radiology: Comprehensive Lists of Roentgen Differential Diagnosis, p 613. New York, Springer-Verlag, 1993.

A-14   Periventricular Lesions*

Dark on T1, Bright on T2, Subependymal, Nonenhancing

Smooth

1. Centrally tracking vasogenic edema
2. Interstitial edema
3. Ischemic gliosis/demyelination
4. Normal caudate body
5. Subependymal demyelination after interstitial edema

Lumpy

1. Hamartomas of tuberous sclerosis
2. Heterotopic gray matter

Dark on T1, Bright on T2, Subependymal, Enhancing

Smooth

1. Subependymal tumor spread
2. Ventriculitis/ependymitis

Lumpy

1. Giant cell astrocytoma (tuberous sclerosis)
2. Subependymal tumor spread

Subependymal Tumor Spread

1. Breast metastasis
2. Ependymoma
3. Glioblastoma
4. Lung metastasis
5. Lymphoma
6. Medulloblastoma
7. Melanoma metastasis

A-14   Periventricular Lesions (Cont'd)

Dark on T1, Bright on T2, No Mass Effect, Nonenhancing

Patient Under 40: Common

1.   HIV encephalitis

2.   Migraine

3.   Multiple sclerosis

4.   Systemic lupus erythematosus

Patient Under 40: Uncommon

1.   Lyme disease

2.   Periventricular leukomalacia

3.   Postviral leukoencephalopathy (acute disseminated encephalomyelitis)

Patient Over 40

1.   Deep white matter ischemia/infarction

2.   Multiple sclerosis

3.   Normal (ependymitis granularis)

4.   Post-irradiation

Nonspecific with Respect to Age

1.   Diffuse necrotizing leukoencephalopathy (DNL)

2.   Hamartomas of tuberous sclerosis

3.   Heterotopic gray matter

4.   Neurofibromatosis

5.   Normal late myelinating fibers (thalamoparietal tracts)

6.   Shear injury

Dark on T1, Bright on T2, No Mass Effect, Enhancing

1.   Early metastatic disease

2.   Early toxoplasmosis

3.   Leukodystrophies (enhancing active border [rare])

4.   Subacute infarction

A-14   Periventricular Lesions (Cont'd)

Periventricular Hyperintensity in Patients with AIDS
1. Cytomegalovirus
2. HIV encephalitis
3. Kaposi's sarcoma
4. Lymphoma
5. Progressive multifocal leukoencephalopathy
6. Toxoplasmosis
7. Vasculitis secondary to vasophilic infection

Leukodystrophies
Macrocephaly (in infant)
1. Alexander's disease (anterior, sparing of internal capsule, enhances with gadolinium)
2. Canavan's disease (peripheral to central, early involvement of subcortical U-fibers)

Normocephaly
1. Adrenoleukodystrophy (posterior, male, enhances with gadolinium)
2. Krabbe's disease (central to peripheral, nonenhancing)
3. Metachromatic leukodystrophy (central to peripheral, nonenhancing)
4. Pelizaeus-Merzbacher's disease (males, central to peripheral, nonenhancing, brain stem atrophy)

Dark on T1, Bright on T2, Mass Effect, Nonenhancing
1. Hamartoma of tuberous sclerosis or neurofibromatosis
2. Infarction from vasculitis
3. Postviral leukoencephalopathy (ADEM)
4. Sickle cell infarcts
5. Visual pathway glioma (neurofibromatosis)

A-14   Periventricular Lesions (Cont'd)

Dark on T1, Bright on T2, Mass Effect, Enhancing

1.   Abscess (e.g., CMV, toxoplasmosis)
2.   Degenerated visual pathway glioma (neurofibromatosis)
3.   Giant cell astrocytoma (tuberous sclerosis)
4.   Intraventricular drop metastasis (e.g., from glioblastoma)
5.   Lymphoma
6.   Metastatic disease
7.   Tumefactive multiple sclerosis

* Modified from Reeder MM, Bradley WG. Reeder and Felson's Gamuts in Radiology: Comprehensive Lists of Roentgen Differential Diagnosis, p 615-616. New York, Springer-Verlag, 1993.

A-15   Intraventricular Masses*

Hypointense T1, Hyperintense T2, Nonenhancing

1. Arachnoid cyst
2. Cysticercosis
3. Colloid cyst (3rd ventricle)
4. Cystic craniopharyngioma
5. Cystic meningioma
6. Dandy-Walker cyst (4th ventricle)
7. Epidermoid (4th ventricle)
8. Neuroepithelial cyst, intraventricular type
9. Neuroepithelial cyst (xanthogranuloma of the choroid plexus)

CSF Signal Mass

1. Arachnoid cyst
2. Cysticercosis
3. Dandy-Walker cyst or variant (4th ventricle)
4. Mega cisterna magna (pseudocyst)
5. Trapped ventricle (pseudomass)

Hypointense T1 & T2, Enhancing

1. Acute hematoma
2. Calcified giant cell astrocytoma
3. Calcified glomus of choroid plexus
4. Dense or calcified metastases (prostate, colon, osteogenic sarcoma)
5. Heavily calcified meningioma
6. Hemorrhagic ventricular metastases

A-15   Intraventricular Masses (Cont'd)

Hyperintense T1, Hypointense T2

1. Colloid cyst
2. CSF flow
3. Dermoid
4. Early subacute hemorrhage
5. Intraventricular craniopharyngioma (heavily calcified)
6. Lipoma
7. Pantopaque
8. Xanthogranuloma of the choroid plexus

Hyperintense T1 & T2

1. Dermoid
2. Flow
3. Intraventricular craniopharyngioma (3rd ventricle)
4. Late subacute hemorrhage

* Modified from Reeder MM, Bradley WG. Reeder and Felson's Gamuts in Radiology: Comprehensive Lists of Roentgen Differential Diagnosis, p 626-627. New York, Springer-Verlag, 1993.

A-16 Peri- & Intraventricular Masses (Lateral Ventricles)

Isointense T1, Iso- or Hypointense T2

1. Meningioma: Enhances
2. Metastases: Colon, prostate, osteogenic sarcoma, melanoma; uncommon, enhances
3. Medulloblastoma[a]
4. Subependymal calcifications[a]
5. Acute hematoma
6. Exophytic brain stem glioma[a]

Hypo- or Isointense T1, Hyperintense T2

1. Meningioma
2. Metastases:[b] Breast, lung, melanoma (esp. amelanotic), choriocarcinoma
3. Ependymoma:[a] Heterogeneous, may hemorrhage, enhances
4. Subependymoma: Homogeneous
5. Exophytic brain stem glioma:[a] Variable enhancement
6. Choroid plexus papilloma: Hydrocephalus, enhances
7. Lymphoma:[b] Enhances
8. Metastatic seed implants: Germinoma, ependymoma, glioblastoma or glial sarcoma, medulloblastoma, lymphoma

Hypointense T1, Hyperintense T2 (Water-like)

1. Epidermoid: Proteinaceous water signal, inhomogeneous
2. Xanthogranuloma of the choroid plexus glomera: Nonenhancing
3. Ventricular neuroepithelial cyst: Thin-walled, nonenhancing
4. Cysticercosis: Isointense nodule present

Hypointense T1, Hypointense T2

1. Choroid plexus calcification[c]
2. Vascular malformation: Linear, gyriform[c]
3. CSF flow void[c]

A-16   Peri- & Intraventricular Masses (Lateral Ventricles) (Cont'd)

Hyperintense T1, Hypointense T2

1.   Lipoma[c]
2.   Subacute hematoma (early)
3.   Melanoma metastases
4.   Pantopaque[b]

Hyperintense T1, Hyperintense T2

1.   Chronic hematoma
2.   Melanoma metastases[a]
3.   Dermoid

a Common in children
b Common in adults
c Common in both

A-17   Peri- & Intraventricular Masses (Third Ventricle)

Isointense T1, Iso- or Hypointense T2

1.   Meningioma: Common, enhances
2.   Metastases: Colon, prostate, osteogenic sarcoma, melanoma; uncommon, enhances
3.   Hamartoma
4.   Subependymal calcifications
5.   Giant cell astrocytoma
6.   Colloid cyst: Anterosuperior third ventricle
7.   Acute hematoma

Hypo- or Isointense T1, Hyperintense T2

1.   Meningioma
2.   Metastases:[b] Breast, lung, melanoma (esp. amelanotic), choriocarcinoma
3.   Ependymoma: Heterogeneous, enhances
4.   Subependymoma: Homogeneous
5.   Exophytic hypothalamic glioma:[a] Variable enhancement
6.   Exophytic optic chiasm glioma[a]
7.   Choroid plexus papilloma: Hydrocephalus, enhances

Hypointense T1, Hyperintense T2 (Water-like)

1.   Xanthogranuloma of the choroid plexus glomera: Nonenhancing
2.   Ventricular neuroepithelial cyst: Thin-walled, nonenhancing
3.   Cavum septum pellucidum and vergae[c]
4.   Colloid cyst:[b] Anterosuperior third ventricle, second most common signal pattern for this mass

A-17   Peri- & Intraventricular Masses (Third Ventricle) (Cont'd)

Hypointense T1, Hypointense T2

1. Choroid plexus calcification: Common
2. Vascular malformation: Linear, gyriform
3. CSF flow void:[c] (especially NPH and aqueductal narrowing)
4. Vein of Galen aneurysm: Posterior third ventricle

Hyperintense T1, Hypointense T2

1. Colloid cyst:[b] Anterosuperior third ventricle, most common signal pattern for this mass
2. Lipoma[c]
3. Craniopharyngioma (calcified)[c]
4. Early subacute hematoma
5. Melanoma metastases

Hyperintense T1, Hyperintense T2

1. Colloid cyst
2. Chronic hematoma
3. Melanoma metastases
4. Dermoid
5. Craniopharyngioma

a Common in children
b Common in adults
c Common in both

A-18   Intraventricular Masses (Fourth Ventricle)*

Common

1. Ependymoma: Mixed T1 intensity and T2 hyperintensity
2. Medulloblastoma: Intermediate T1, mild hyperintense T2

Uncommon or Rare

1. Choroid plexus papilloma: Mild hypointense T1, hyperintense T2
2. Arachnoid cyst: Very hypointense T1 and hyperintense T2, homogeneous
3. Epidermoid: Hypointense T1, hyperintense T2
4. Vascular malformation: Variable flow void and T2 hypointensity
5. Exophytic brain stem/pontine glioma: Isointense T1, mild hyperintense T2
6. Metastatic disease

* The normal cerebellar vermian nodulus should not be confused with a tumor and is isointense with normal gray matter.

A-19   Subcortical Lesions*

Dark on T1, Bright on T2, No Mass Effect, Nonenhancing
1. Embolic infarction
2. Progressive multifocal leukoencephalopathy (PML)
3. Shear injury (nonhemorrhagic)

Dark on T1, Bright on T2, No Mass Effect, Enhancing
1. Leptomeningeal carcinomatosis
2. Lymphoma
3. Meningitis (bacterial, occasional fungal and viral)
4. Sarcoid

Dark on T1, Bright on T2, Mass Effect, Nonenhancing
1. Heterotopic gray matter
2. Low grade glioma
3. Progressive multifocal leukoencephalopathy (PML)

Dark on T1, Bright on T2, Mass Effect, Enhancing
1. Abscess
2. Emboli
3. Metastases
4. Multiple sclerosis
5. Sarcoid

* Modified from Reeder MM, Bradley WG. Reeder and Felson's Gamuts in Radiology: Comprehensive
   Lists of Roentgen Differential Diagnosis, p 617. New York, Springer-Verlag, 1993.

A-20   Cortical Lesions*

Hypointense T1, Hyperintense T2, No Mass Effect, Nonenhancing

1. Postinfarct
2. Postbleed
3. Postinfection
4. Postoperative defect/encephalomalacia
5. Post-trauma

Hypointense T1, Bright T2, No Mass Effect, Enhancing

1. Leptomeningeal carcinomatosis
2. Lymphoma
3. Meningitis
4. Subacute infarct
5. Vasculocerebritis, autoimmune

Hypointense T1, Hyperintense T2, Mass Effect, Nonenhancing

1. Acute infarct
2. Low grade glioma

Hypointense T1, Hyperintense T2, Mass Effect, Enhancing

1. Acute infarct (vascular enhancement secondary to stasis, pial collaterals)
2. Leptomeningeal metastases
3. Subacute infarct (gyral enhancement)
4. Vasculocerebritis, autoimmune

* Modified from Reeder MM, Bradley WG. Reeder and Felson's Gamuts in Radiology: Comprehensive Lists of Roentgen Differential Diagnosis, p 613. New York, Springer-Verlag, 1993.

A-21   Subarachnoid Space*

Isointense to Brain

1. Acute subarachnoid hemorrhage (protein effect)
2. CSF flow (flow-related enhancement, even echo rephasing/gradient moment nulling)
3. Meningitis

Hyperintense to Brain on T1 & Proton Density

1. CSF flow (flow-related enhancement)
2. Dermoid or ruptured dermoid (chemical meningitis)
3. Lipoma (e.g., cerebellopontine angle)
4. Pantopaque
5. Subacute subarachnoid thrombus (methemoglobin)
6. White epidermoid (rare)

Isointense to CSF

1. Arachnoid cyst (middle fossa, in posterior fossa, associated with acoustic neuroma, interhemispheric, suprasellar, post-trauma/infection)
2. Cysticercosis (basilar racemose form)

Signal Void

1. Normal CSF flow
2. Normal flow in artery
3. Juxta-arterial CSF dephasing
4. Postoperative metallic (clip) artifact

* Modified from Reeder MM, Bradley WG. Reeder and Felson's Gamuts in Radiology: Comprehensive Lists of Roentgen Differential Diagnosis, p 627. New York, Springer-Verlag, 1993.

A-22   Bilateral Putaminal Symmetric T2 Hyperintensity

Common

1. Bilateral putaminal (lenticulostriate artery) infarctions
2. Microvascular arteriopathy or état criblé

Uncommon

1. Alcohol toxicity (Wernicke-Korsakoff syndrome)
2. Carbon monoxide poisoning
3. Cyanide poisoning
4. Ethylene glycol poisoning
5. Olivopontocerebellar degeneration
6. Wilson's disease
7. Aminoacidurias
8. Hallervorden-Spatz disease
9. Cytoplasmically inherited striatonigral degeneration
10. Methanol poisoning
11. Mucopolysaccharoidosis
12. Leigh's disease
13. MELAS syndrome
14. MERRF syndrome
15. Subacute sclerosing panencephalitis
16. Kearns-Sayre syndrome

A-23   Bilateral Putaminal Symmetric T1 Hyperintensity

Common

1. Microcalcification
2. Microvascular arteriopathy

Uncommon

1. Portosystemic encephalopathy
2. Hyperalimentation
3. Aluminum toxicity
4. Bilateral basal ganglia hemorrhage

Rare

1. Wilson's disease

A-24   Brain Stem Lesions *

Hypointense T1, Hyperintense T2, No Mass Effect*

Nonenhancing

1. CSF flow artifact
2. Infarct/ischemic gliosis
3. Lupus
4. Multiple sclerosis
5. Progressive multifocal leukoencephalopathy (PML)
6. Shear injury (posterolateral upper brain stem)
7. Small low grade glioma
8. Wallerian degeneration (e.g., secondary to stroke or adrenoleukodystrophy)

Enhancing

1. Acute multiple sclerosis
2. Small tumor (primary or metastasis)

A-24   Brain Stem Lesions (Cont'd)

Hypointense T1, Hyperintense T2, Mass Effect

Nonenhancing

1. Early brain stem encephalitis, especially rhombencephalitis (herpetic)
2. Low grade glioma
3. Ramsay Hunt syndrome (retrograde spread of varicella virus)

Enhancing

1. Abscess
2. Acute central pontine myelinolysis
3. Acute tumefactive multiple sclerosis
5. Behçet's encephalitis
6. Brain stem encephalitis
7. Brain stem glioma
8. Ependymoblastoma (rare)
9. Ependymoma
10. Lymphoma
11. Metastasis
12. Perineural spread of squamous cell carcinoma
13. Primitive neuroectodermal tumor (PNET)

* Modified from Reeder MM, Bradley WG. Reeder and Felson's Gamuts in Radiology: Comprehensive Lists of Roentgen Differential Diagnosis, p 619. New York, Springer-Verlag, 1993.

CATEGORY A: THE BRAIN

Section 2: Vascular, Hydrocephalus, Atrophy, Neurodegenerative

Page

A-25   Classification of Cerebral Angiitis[*]

Degenerative Causes of Arteriopathy and Arteritis

1.   Arteriosclerosis: Hyaline, hyperplastic, and arteriolar necrosis
2.   Arteriosclerosis: Atheromatosis and atherothrombosis
3.   Calcifying sclerosis of the tunica media (Mönckeberg)

Necrosing Arteritis

1.   Arteritis with obliteration of the supra-aortic trunks (Takayasu)
2.   Temporal arteritis

Infectious Viral or Bacterial Arteritis

1.   Viral meningoencephalitis
2.   Purulent meningitis
3.   Tuberculous meningitis
4.   Syphilitic meningitis

Arteritis Caused by Collagen Disease

1.   Polyarteritis nodosa
2.   Arteritis of lupus erythematosus
3.   Arteritis of hypersensitivity
4.   Arteritis of rheumatoid disease
5.   Granulomatous allergic arteritis
6.   Granulomatous arteritis of Wegener

A-25   Classification of Cerebral Angiitis (Cont'd)

Miscellaneous

1.   Thromboangiitis obliterans (Buerger)
2.   Thrombotic microangiopathy (Moschcowitz)
3.   Neoplastic angiitis
4.   Arteritis caused by radiation
5.   Arteritis caused by chemical agents
6.   Mycotic or infectious arteritis
7.   Sarcoidosis of Boeck

* Soleus-Llenas J, Pons-Tortella E. Cerebral Angiitis. Neuroradiology 15:1, 1978.

A-26   Bland Infarct Dating

1. Hyperacute (< 24 hours): Hyperintense T2, isointense T1 and N(h)*

2. Acute (1-5 days): Hyperintense T2 and N(h), iso- or hypointense T1, peak mass effect 3-5 days, enhancement on T1 may begin 2-5 days

3. Subacute (5-14 days): Hyperintense T2, N(h), hypointense T1, mass effect wanes, enhancement persists for weeks and peaks 7-14 days

4. Chronic (> 14 days): Hyperintense T2, hypointense N(h) and T1, negative mass effect, enhancement wanes > 2-4 weeks

* N(h) is a proton density or spin density image, usually the first echo of a multiecho sequence.

A-27   Hemorrhagic Infarct Dating

1. Hyperacute (< 6 hours): Hypointense T1, hyperintense T2

2. Acute (< 3 days): Hypointense T1, hypointense T2

3. Subacute (< 10-14 days): hyperintense T1, variable T2 hypointensity and hyperintensity (edema)

4. Chronic (10-14 days to weeks): Hyperintense T1 and T2

5. Remote (months to years): Hypointense T1, hyperintense T2 with circumferential T2 hemosiderin rim

A-28   Luxury Perfusion Sign of Cortical Infarction (Bland)

T2 cortical gyriform signal hyperintensity with subcortical T2 gyriform hyperintensity (flow phenomenon)

A-29   Causes of Brain Infarction

Arterial Occlusive Disease
1.   Atherosclerotic occlusion
2.   Embolism
3.   Hemodynamic ischemia
4.   Arteriosclerosis (lacunar disease)
5.   Vasculitis
6.   Moyamoya disease
7.   Arterial dissection

Anoxic Ischemia
1.   Hypotension
2.   Hypoxemia
3.   Carbon monoxide

Venous Thrombosis
1.   Compression from mass
2.   Hypercoagulability
3.   Idiopathic

A-30   **Vascular White Matter Disease Versus MS**

1. MS plaques are linear or ovoid in shape and oriented at right angles to the ventricular system

2. Ring enhancement with multiple sclerosis, rare with infarct

3. MS may involve the temporal lobe white matter while vascular disease usually spares the temporal lobe

4. Hemorrhage in multiple sclerosis is rare, not unusual with infarct

5. MS plaques are hyperintense relative to gray matter on spin density

6. Corpus callosum is involved in MS, spared with infarct

7. Frequent middle cerebellar peduncle involvement in MS, uncommon with infarct

8. Brain stem involvement in MS is patchy rather than confluent & symmetric in microvascular disease

9. Posterolateral spinal cord lesions with enhancement in MS but rare in vascular disease

A-31   Cerebrovascular Accident in the Young Adult

1. Atherosclerosis (patients with high risk factors): 20%
    a. Smoking
    b. Hypertension
    c. Hypercholesterolemia
    d. Juvenile onset diabetes mellitus
2. Thromboembolism: 20%
    a. Cardiac disease
        i.   Rheumatic heart
        ii. Prosthetic valve
        iii. Endocarditis
        iv. Mitral valve prolapse
        v.   Atrial fibrillation
        vi. Left atrial myxoma
    b. Fat embolism (associated with long bone fractures)
    c. Paradoxical embolism
        i.   ASD
        ii. Osler-Weber-Rendu
        iii. Patent foramen ovale
        iv. Pulmonary AVM
3. Vasculopathy: 10%
    a. Inflammatory
        i.   Takayasu
        ii. Infection (TB, syphilis, herpes zoster, fungus disease, HIV)
        iii. Amphetamine abuse
        iv. Herpes zoster ophthalmicus
        v.   Severe underlying systemic disease (lupus arteritis, MS, cancer, rheumatoid arthritis)

A-31   Cerebrovascular Accident in the Young Adult (Cont'd)

 b. Noninflammatory
  i. Fibromuscular dysplasia
  ii. Carotid or vertebral artery dissection
  iii. Moyamoya disease
  iv. Homocystinuria
  v. Pseudoxanthoma elasticum

4. Coagulopathy (includes all hypercoagulable states): 10%
 a. Particularly venous infarction in young women with history of pregnancy, peripartum or smoking
 b. Antithrombin III deficiency
 c. Thrombocytosis
 d. Sickle cell disease
 e. Paroxysmal nocturnal hemoglobinuria
 f. Homocystinuria
 g. Chronic systemic disease
 h. Nephrotic syndrome
 i. SLE with lupus
 j. Risk factors of dural sinus thrombosis[*]
  Infection usually local (otitis media, sinusitis, peritonsillar abscess)
  Pregnancy & puerperium
  Birth control pills
  Dehydration & cachexia (includes burns)
  Cardiac disease (including CHF)
  Ulcerative colitis
  Periarteritis nodosa
  Sickle cell trait
  Trauma
  Iatrogenic (S/P radical neck surgery, transvenous pacemaker, craniotomy)
  Malignancy
  Protein C deficiency (may be an artifact of dehydration)
  Diabetes mellitus: Especially with ketoacidosis

A-31   Cerebrovascular Accident in the Young Adult (Cont'd)

5. Mechanical, trauma

   a. Neck manipulation

   b. Dissection

6. Causes of cerebral emboli[†]

   Source Distal to Lungs

   a. Emboli (from cardiac mural thrombus, carotid dissection, open heart surgery, post angiogram)

   b. Infection (infective endocarditis/subacute bacterial endocarditis [SBE])

   c. Thrombi

   d. Tumor (atrial myxoma, chorioepithelioma, marantic endocarditis)

   Source Proximal to Lungs (Requires Right to Left Shunt [Rare])

   a. Amniotic fluid embolism

   b. Fat emboli (following trauma)

   c. Thrombi (from IVC or other thrombophlebitis)

---

* Adapted from Greenberg MS. Handbook of Neurosurgery, p 672. Lakeland, Florida. 1991.

† Adapted from Reeder MM, Bradley WG. Reeder and Felson's Gamuts in Radiology: Comprehensive Lists of Roentgen Differential Diagnosis, p 617. New York, Springer-Verlag, 1993.

A-32   Intracranial Vascular Lesions

1. Vascular malformations
    a. Arteriovenous: Serpiginous, multiloculated flow void
    b. Venous angioma: Parallel line sign of misregistered slow flow
    c. Cavernous hemangioma: Calcification with hyperintense center and hypointense hemosiderin ring (T2)
    d. Telangiectatic or capillary hemangioma: Thin spiderlike foci of flow void or increased signal
2. Aneurysms: Lamellated foci of alternating signal void, bright signal (clot or slow flow) and hypointense signal (hemosiderin and vessel wall)
3. Dolichoectasia: Basivertebral > carotid, flow void without clot, thrombus, or hemorrhage (may produce mass effect on brain stem)
4. Moyamoya collaterals: Punctate foci of signal void (fast flow), frontal, sub-frontal, and centrosylvian distribution
5. Hemangiopericytoma: Dural based, homogeneous enhancement, mixed hyperintense T2 signal (resembles angioblastic meningioma on histology)

A-33   Tipoffs to Subtypes of Vascular Malformation

Arteriovenous Malformation
1. Tortuous hypointense flow void
2. Multiple large caliber draining veins with flow void or flow phenomenon

Capillary Telangiectasia
1. Small clustered linear foci of flow void, less than 1-2 mm in diameter
2. Irregular foci of hypointense hemosiderin
3. Infratentorial brain stem location

Cavernous Angioma
1. Hypointense globular calcification
2. Hemosiderin rim
3. Central hyperintensity

Venous Angioma
1. Draining transcerebral vein, linear in shape
2. Parallel black and white lines representing phase shift effect of oblique flow phenomenon
3. Variable appearance of small hypo- or hyperintense medullary veins emptying into transcerebral vein
4. Poorly defined increased signal at the tip of a transcerebral vein due either to blood pooling or hemorrhage
5. Associated hemorrhage less common than with arteriovenous malformation (but can occur, particularly in infratentorial venous angioma)

A-34   Intravascular Dural Venous Sinus Signal

Hypointense T1 and T2
1. Patent flow void^a (time-of-flight and turbulent dephasing)
2. Intravascular calcification

Iso-/Hypointense T1, Hypointense T2
1. Patency^b (complex first echo flow phenomenon)
2. Acute clot

Hyperintense T1, Hypointense T2
1. Patency^a (first echo slice entry phenomenon)
2. Subacute clot (field dependent T2 relaxation shortening simulates patency on T2)

Hypointense T1, Hyperintense T2
1. Patency^b (second or even echo rephasing)
2. Hyperacute clot^c (proteinaceous water-like signal)

Hyperintense T1, Hyperintense T2
1. Patency^b (first echo slice entry phenomenon and second echo rephasing)
2. Chronic clot

Hypointense T1, Isointense T2
1. Patency^c (complex second echo flow phenomenon)
2. Hyperacute clot^a in transition from hyperacute to acute phase

Hyperintense T1, Isointense T2
1. Patency^c (first echo slice entry and second echo complex flow phenomenon)
2. Early subacute clot in transition from acute to subacute phase

a Very common
b Common
c Uncommon or rare

A-35   Tipoffs to the Diagnosis of Intracranial Aneurysm

1.   Round or dumbbell shape
2.   Lamellated alternating T1 hyperintense signal (flow or subacute clot) with intermediate or hypointense signal (fibrin, hemosiderin, flow void)
3.   Anatomic contiguity with known vascular structure
4.   Foci of flow void within the lesion
5.   Slice entry phenomenon

A-36   Tipoffs in the Diagnosis of Vascular (Carotid, Vertebral) Dissection

1. Absence of flow void in the carotid or vertebral arteries
2. Visualization of both dark and bright signal in the vertebral or carotid arteries in all planes and on all pulsing sequences
3. Presence of multiple lacunar or scattered infarctions in the supratentorial space in a young patient
4. Infratentorial infarction involving the restiform body and medulla (PICA distribution) in a young patient
5. Unilateral headache with anterior or posterior neck pain and incomplete Horner's syndrome (carotid dissection) or bulbar (Wallenberg's)* syndrome (vertebral dissection)
6. History of pre-existing trauma, upper respiratory infection or neck manipulation not uncommon

* Wallenberg's is a syndrome produced by occlusion of the posterior inferior cerebellar artery marked by ipsilateral loss of temperature and pain sensation of the face and contralateral loss of these sensations in the extremities and trunk. Ipsilateral ataxia, dysphagia, dysarthria and nystagmus are present.

A-37   Etiologies of Communicating Hydrocephalus

Common

1. Subarachnoid hemorrhage
2. Normal pressure hydrocephalus

Uncommon

1. Meningitis
2. Posterior fossa extra-axial masses
3. Subdural hematoma
4. Venous pathway occlusion
5. Congenital abnormalities of extraventricular pathways
6. Neoplastic meningeal carcinomatosis
7. Increased CSF protein

A-38 **Findings in Parkinson's Disease**

1. Generalized atrophy
2. Alteration in brain iron stores with exaggerated putaminal hypointensity
3. Loss of the normal signal hypointensity in the dorsal lateral substantia nigra on T2 (40%)
4. Narrowing of the normal hyperintense signal of the zona compacta of substantia nigra on T2 (10%)

A-39 **Parkinson Plus Syndromes**

1. Progressive supranuclear palsy
2. Striatonigral degeneration
3. Shy-Drager syndrome (multisystem atrophy)
4. Olivopontocerebellar atrophy

A-40   Parkinsonism & Pseudoparkinsonism: MR Findings

Common

1. Parkinson's disease: Atrophy, T2 hypointensity (iron-related) in the putamen, increased or exaggerated decreased T2 signal in zona compacta of substantia nigra

Uncommon

1. Hypothyroidism: Diffuse atrophy, exaggerated signal hypointensity (iron-related) in globus pallidus, putamen, substantia nigra, and red nucleus
2. Olivopontocerebellar atrophy: Pontomedullary and inferior cerebellar atrophy

Rare

1. Progressive supranuclear palsy: Tectal atrophy or pointing, increased periaqueductal T2 signal intensity secondary to gliosis, exaggerated or decreased signal (iron-related) in putamen or superior colliculus
2. Striatonigral degeneration: Diffuse atrophy with exaggerated hypointensity (iron-related) in substantia nigra, caudate nucleus and putamen
3. Shy-Drager syndrome: T2 signal hypointensity (iron-related) in putamen, zona compacta of substantia nigra (most severe in multisystem atrophy), variable increased subcortical white matter and basal ganglia T2 signal
4. Hallervorden-Spatz disease:* Diffuse atrophy, exaggerated and early appearance of T2 signal hypointensity (iron-related) in globus pallidus, red nucleus, and substantia nigra zona reticulata

* T2 hypointensity secondary to brain iron should not appear in the globus pallidus or other normal anatomic locales before age 10.

A-41   Subtypes of Multisystem Atrophy: Clinical & MR Findings

1.   Parkinsonian: Amyotrophy syndrome

    a.   Extremely rare

    b.   Affects nigrostriatum

    c.   Anterior horn cell degeneration

2.   Striatonigral degeneration

    a.   Severe caudate atrophy like Huntington's chorea demonstrates decreased
         neostriatal signal due to increased iron, striatonigral degeneration does not

    b.   Patients severely Parkinsonian or refractory to therapy but without tremor or
         ataxia

    c.   Neostriatum degenerates but does not appear to accumulate iron either patho-
         logically or on MR

3.   Shy-Drager

    a.   Putaminal atrophy and hypointense T2 or T2* signal far more common and
         pronounced than in classic Parkinson's disease

    b.   Very similar to olivopontocerebellar atrophy pathologically but Shy-Drager
         exhibits globus pallidus signal alteration

    c.   Decreased pars compacta may be seen as in Parkinson's disease

    d.   Autonomic dysfunction present in only 40% of cases: Two types of Shy-
         Drager, one with and one without autonomic dysfunction

4.   Olivopontocerebellar degeneration affects inferior cerebellar structures and the
     pons in 30-55%

    a.   May overlap with heredofamilial Friedrich's or Joseph's disease

    b.   May be associated with putaminal hypointensity like Shy-Drager

    c.   Clinically severe ataxia, does not respond to Parkinsonian medication

5.   Progressive supranuclear palsy

    a.   Pseudobulbar palsy with variable ophthalmoplegia

    b.   Severely Parkinsonian but without tremor and refractory to conventional
         Parkinsonian therapy

    c.   Tectal attenuation with collicular plate and midbrain atrophy

    d.   Hypointense signal in the putamen, variably in superior colliculus

A-42   Parkinson's & Related Diseases*

1. Parkinson's disease
2. Olivopontocerebellar degeneration
3. Striatonigral degeneration
4. Progressive supranuclear palsy
5. Shy-Drager syndrome
6. Drug-induced
7. Toxic (carbon monoxide, manganese)
8. Ischemia
9. Trauma
10. NPH
11. Neoplasm
12. Riley-Day
13. Guam type
14. Post-encephalitis Parkinsonism (most victims no longer living)

* Adapted from Greenberg MS. Handbook of Neurosurgery, p 73. Lakeland, Florida, Greenberg
Graphics, 1991.

A-43   Dystonic Syndromes

1. Leigh's disease
    a. A defect in pyruvate metabolism resulting in increased lactate levels and acidosis
    b. Manifests clinically with severe dystonia
    c. Pathologic gliosis and vacuolation affect the putamen, midbrain and periaqueductal region, and cortex
    d. Increased signal rather than decreased signal is seen in the putamen, midbrain and occasionally cortical regions
2. Wilson's disease
    a. Increased putaminal signal reported at low field and variably decreased or increased signal at high field
    b. Moderate amounts of copper in the putamen will not produce T2 shortening but large amounts will
3. Hallervorden-Spatz disease: Decreased and increased globus pallidus signal more common than putaminal signal
4. Post-infection dystonia: Atrophy and increased putaminal signal; otherwise non-specific
5. Infarct-induced dystonia: Hemorrhagic or non-hemorrhagic lesions result in mixed increased and decreased T2 signal that is heterogeneous and associated with focal atrophy
6. Metabolic disorders for which glutaric aciduria is a prototype
    a. This potentially treatable disorder is manifested by local acidosis, hypoglycemia and hyperammonemia with resultant gliosis
    b. Increased T2 signal in the putamen and midbrain

A-44   Dementias: Etiologies

Remediable (Depending on Severity)

1.   Intoxication: Medications (Aldomet, digitalis, lithium, etc), polypharmacy (methyldopa, cimetidine, narcotics)

2.   Infections: Bacterial, protozoal (e.g., syphilis), fungal

3.   Metabolic/nutritional: Hypo-/hyperthyroid, hypo-/hyperglycemia, electrolyte abnormalities, vitamin deficiencies

4.   Structural: Hydrocephalus, tumors, subdural hematomas, hypertension

5.   Vascular: Hypertension

Non-remediable

1.   Alzheimer's

2.   Pick's disease

3.   Multiple sclerosis

4.   Huntington's chorea

5.   Parkinson's disease

6.   AIDS dementia complex

7.   Multi-infarct dementia

8.   Slow virus dementias (e.g., Creutzfeldt-Jakob)

9.   Progressive multifocal leukoencephalopathy

* Adapted from Greenberg MS. Handbook of Neurosurgery, p 85. Lakeland, Florida, Greenberg Graphics, 1991.

A-45   Pearls in Relatively Common Dementias: MR Findings

Common

1. Vascular (multi-infarct) dementia: Diffuse atrophy, exaggerated T2 hypointensity (iron-related) in normal anatomic locales, deep white matter and cortical infarction of variable ages in multiple vascular territories involving the supra- and infratentorial spaces

2. Alzheimer's disease: Diffuse atrophy with a parietotemporal predilection, variable deep white matter signal hyperintensity

3. Parkinson's disease: Atrophy, variable decreased or increased signal in the substantia nigra

Uncommon

1. Pick's disease: Atrophy of the frontotemporal region but sparing the posterosuperior temporal gyrus and caudate nucleus

2. Huntington's chorea: Atrophy and T2 hypointensity (iron-related) in the caudate nucleus variably affecting the putamen

3. Vascular (subcortical arteriosclerotic encephalopathy): History of hypertension with diffuse supratentorial atrophy and confluence of multifocal areas of periventricular T2 hyperintensity with scattered multifocal signal hypointensity due to prior hypertensive hemorrhage in the basal ganglia, thalamus, and/or brain stem

4. Normal pressure hydrocephalus (chronic communicating hydrocephalus): Ventricular enlargement with rounded enlarged temporal and frontal horns with periventricular transependymal T2 hyperintensity, exaggerated bizarre hypointense aqueductal and intraventricular flow void on T2, effaced sulci with superiorly bowed corpus callosum in the sagittal projection

5. Viral (HIV): History of AIDS with patchy periventricular and parieto-occipital T2 signal hyperintensity with associated atrophy; associated hyponatremia and exaggerated antidiuretic hormone release is common

6. Wernicke-Korsakoff dementia: Generalized atrophy with superior vermian and mamillary body predilection, increased periaqueductal and medial thalamic OR putaminal T2 signal hyperintensity

A-46   Clinical Pearls in Dementia & Movement Disorders

1. Alzheimer's disease
    a. Usually between 50 and 70
    b. Variable white matter signal alteration with parieto-temporal atrophy, 80-90% have hippocampal atrophy with dilatation of the choroidal fissure
    c. Fibrillary tangles, senile plexus, Hirano bodies, granulovacuolar degeneration
2. Pick's disease
    a. Peak age of onset 60 years, females greater than males, less common than Alzheimer's, occasionally heredofamilial
    b. Frontotemporal distribution sparing the superior temporal gyrus
    c. Neuronal intracytoplasmic argentophilic Pick's bodies seen pathologically
3. Multi-infarct dementia
    a. Dementia
    b. Moderate to marked white matter microangiopathic T2 hyperintensity with variable aged infarctions and multiple vascular territories
4. Huntington's chorea
    a. Onset between 40-60 y.o.
    b. Autosomal dominant
    c. Marked atrophy and/or diminutive size of the caudate nucleus and putamen
5. Sydenham's chorea
    a. Post-rheumatic fever
    b. Symmetric or asymmetric increased T2 signal in the putamen
6. Wernicke-Korsakoff syndrome
    a. Associated with alcoholism and thiamine deficiency
    b. Severe mamillary body atrophy with variable increased signal in the putamina and thalami unilaterally or bilaterally
7. Leigh's disease (subacute necrotizing encephalopathy)
    a. A defect in pyruvate metabolism with increased lactate levels and acidosis
    b. Manifests clinically with severe dystonia
    c. Gliosis and vacuolation affect putamen, midbrain, periaqueductal area, cortex
    d. Increased signal rather than decreased signal is seen in the putamen, midbrain and occasionally cortical regions

A-47   Pearls in the Diagnosis of Brain Iron

1.   Infancy: Iron is absent

2.   Young adulthood (over age 12): Globus pallidus, substantia nigra, zona reticulata, red nucleus, dentate nucleus

3.   Aged brain: Adult distribution includes the putamen, fifth layer of gray matter, all areas previously mentioned

4.   Iron accumulates where structures with GABA-ergic efferents function (globus pallidus, red and dentate nuclei, substantia nigra, putamen, caudate nucleus, and fifth layer of subcortical gray matter)

5.   Signal changes related to iron may vary as Fe^{3+}-hemosiderin-ferritin (the physical state of iron, whether particulate or clumped, will also affect the hypointensity created by iron)

A-48   Causes of Increased Brain Iron

1.   Multiple sclerosis: Thalamus, putamen
2.   Glioma or neoplasm: Transfer receptors around glioma periphery
3.   Radionecrosis: Microangiopathic hemorrhage, brain siderosis
4.   Simple hemorrhage: Chronic hemorrhage associated with macrophage accumulation of iron around the periphery
5.   Parkinson's disease: Putamen, zona compacta, substantia nigra
6.   Parkinson-plus: Putamen, zona compacta, substantia nigra
7.   Hallervorden-Spatz: Globus pallidus, substantia nigra, zona reticulata
8.   Huntington's chorea: Caudate nucleus, putamen
9.   Motor neuron disease: Putamen
10. Alzheimer's disease: Cerebral cortex
11. Diffuse increased brain iron can be seen
     a.   Hallervorden-Spatz
     b.   Hypothyroidism
     c.   Hemochromatosis
     d.   Parkinson-plus syndromes

A-49   CSF Pathways Obstruction Versus Ex Vacuo Hydrocephalus*

1. Dilatation of the anterior third ventricle

2. Inferior bowing and displacement of the hypothalamus with reduction of mamillopontine distance (less than 1 cm)

3. Depression of the posterior fornix with increase in the superior inferior dimensions of the lateral ventricles

4. Uniform smooth thinning and elevation of the corpus callosum

5. Dampened intraventricular flow void due to CSF movement

6. Periventricular high signal on proton density and T2

* Adapted from Gammalte TE, Allen MB, Brooks BS, et al. MR Evaluation of Hydrocephalus. AJNR 8:591-597, 1987.

A-50   Pearls in the Diagnosis of Aqueductal Stenosis

1. Subtypes
    a. Congenital
    b. Tumor
    c. Radiation
    d. Inflammation
2. CSF flow void absent on T2, MR movies may be useful in confirmation
3. Mamillopontine distance is decreased and usually less than 1-2 cm in the sagittal projection
4. The third ventricle is ballooned
5. Enlargement of the pineal, chiasmatic and infundibular recesses in the sagittal projection
6. The corpus callosum is bowed upward in the sagittal projection
7. Within the aqueduct, look for webs, masses and tectal deformity
8. In patients with nontumoral aqueductal stenosis, the tectum may be gliotic and assume the shape of a rounded or ovoid mass simulating glial neoplasm

A-51 Subtypes of Hydrocephalus

Obstructive

1. Noncommunicating

    a. Masses

    b. Aqueductal stenosis

        i. Decreased mamillopontine distance less than 1 cm

        ii. Upward bowing of the corpus callosum

        iii. Bowing of the third ventricular cisterns

        iv. Effacement of the aqueduct of Sylvius

2. Communicating

    a. Acute communicating hydrocephalus (secondary to recent hemorrhage)

    b. Chronic or normal pressure hydrocephalus (NPH), Hakim's disease

        i. Noncompliant ventricles with exaggerated pulsation phenomena

        ii. Triad of ataxia, dementia and incontinence present in 20%

Nonobstructive

1. Ex vacuo

    a. Associated with atrophy which may be focal, diffuse or central

    b. Temporal horns are not dilated, and the frontal horn ratios are not abnormal

2. Overproduction hydrocephalus (associated with choroid plexus tumors)

A-52   Pearls in the Diagnosis of Pseudotumor Cerebri

Key Features

1. Elevated intracranial pressure in the absence of intracranial mass
2. Usually self-limited, recurrence is common
3. Preventable cause of (often permanent) blindness from optic atrophy
4. Risk of blindness is not reliably correlated to duration or number of recurrences

Diagnostic Criteria

1. Increased CSF pressure
2. Normal CSF protein
3. Elevated ICP along (papilledema, headaches, no focal findings)
4. Usually normal CT and MR (occasionally slit ventricles, infantile form large ventricles and fluid spaces over the brain)

Symptoms

1. Headaches
2. Dizziness
3. Nausea
4. Visual changes
5. Diplopia

Findings on MR

1. Increased T2 relaxation in brain parenchyma diffusely
2. Increased T2 signal, optic streaks

* Adapted from Greenberg MS. Handbook of Neurosurgery, p 578. Lakeland, Florida, Greenberg Graphics, 1991.

A-53   Pearls in Normal Pressure Hydrocephalus

Key Features

1. Classic triad: Dementia, gait disturbance, urinary incontinence
2. Communicating hydrocephalus on CT or MR
3. Normal pressure on random LP
4. Symptoms remediable with CSF shunting

Etiologies

1. SAH
2. Trauma
3. Meningitis
4. Posterior fossa surgery
5. Tumors
6. Alzheimer's disease (seen in 15% of Alzheimer patients)
7. Aqueductal stenosis

Findings on MR

1. Enlarged ventricles including temporal horns
2. Abnormal frontal horn ratio
3. Effaced sulci
4. Transependymal migration
5. Augmented aqueductal & intraventricular flow

Findings on Cisternography

1. Ventricular influx ± flow into sylvian cisterns but no convexity flow = "positive scan"
2. Delayed convexity flow is a "mixed" pattern

* Adapted from Greenberg MS. Handbook of Neurosurgery, p 216. Lakeland, Florida, Greenberg Graphics, 1991.

A-54   Hydrocephalus Ex Vacuo Versus Hydrostatic Hydrocephalus

Hydrocephalus Ex Vacuo

Enlargement of the ventricles due to loss of normal cerebral tissue

Usually as a function of normal aging

Accelerated by certain disease processes (e.g., Creutzfeldt-Jakob)

Not true hydrocephalus

Hydrostatic Hydrocephalus

Ballooning of frontal horns ("Mickey Mouse" ventricles)

Suggested

1. When the size of both temporal horns (TH) is ≥ 2 mm in width and the Sylvian and interhemispheric fissures and cerebral sulci are not visible, *or*

2. When both temporal horns are ≥ 2 mm and FH/ID > 0.5 (where FH is the largest width of the frontal horns and ID is the internal diameter from inner table to inner table)

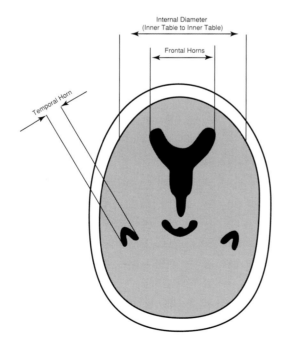

Fig. A-54.1*
  * Greenberg MS. Handbook of Neurosurgery, p 199. Lakeland, Florida, Greenberg Graphics, 1991.

A-55 Intracranial Arteriovenous Anatomy

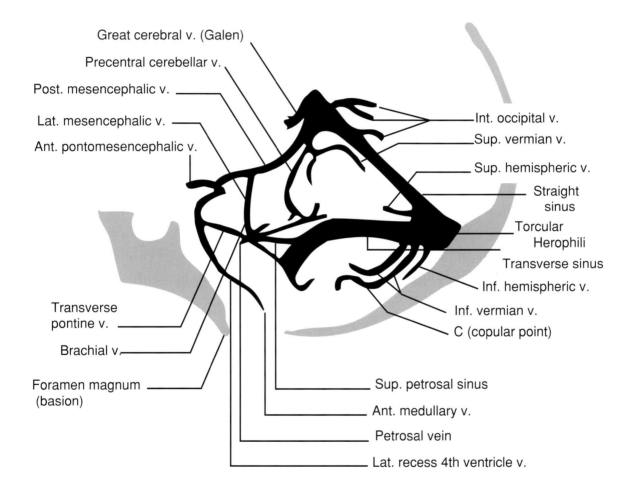

Great cerebral v. (Galen)
Precentral cerebellar v.
Post. mesencephalic v.
Lat. mesencephalic v.
Ant. pontomesencephalic v.
Int. occipital v.
Sup. vermian v.
Sup. hemispheric v.
Straight sinus
Torcular Herophili
Transverse sinus
Inf. hemispheric v.
Inf. vermian v.
C (copular point)
Transverse pontine v.
Brachial v.
Foramen magnum (basion)
Sup. petrosal sinus
Ant. medullary v.
Petrosal vein
Lat. recess 4th ventricle v.

Fig. A-55.1 Posterior Fossa Venous Anatomy*

* Drawing adapted from Greenberg MS. Handbook of Neurosurgery, p 281. Lakeland, Florida, Greenberg Graphics, 1991.

A-55   Intracranial Arteriovenous Anatomy

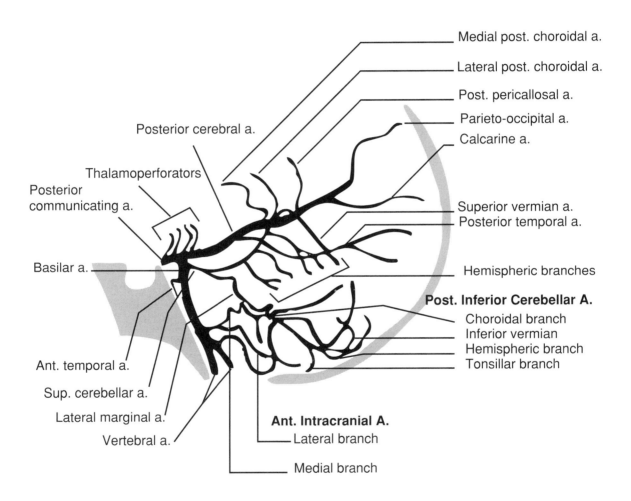

Medial post. choroidal a.

Lateral post. choroidal a.

Post. pericallosal a.

Parieto-occipital a.

Calcarine a.

Posterior cerebral a.

Thalamoperforators

Posterior communicating a.

Superior vermian a.
Posterior temporal a.

Basilar a.

Hemispheric branches

Post. Inferior Cerebellar A.

Choroidal branch
Inferior vermian
Hemispheric branch
Tonsillar branch

Ant. temporal a.

Sup. cerebellar a.

Lateral marginal a.

Vertebral a.

Ant. Intracranial A.
Lateral branch

Medial branch

Fig. A-55.2   Posterior Cerebral Artery Anatomy*

* Drawing adapted from Greenberg MS. Handbook of Neurosurgery, p 280. Lakeland, Florida, Greenberg Graphics, 1991.

A-55 **Intracranial Arteriovenous Anatomy**

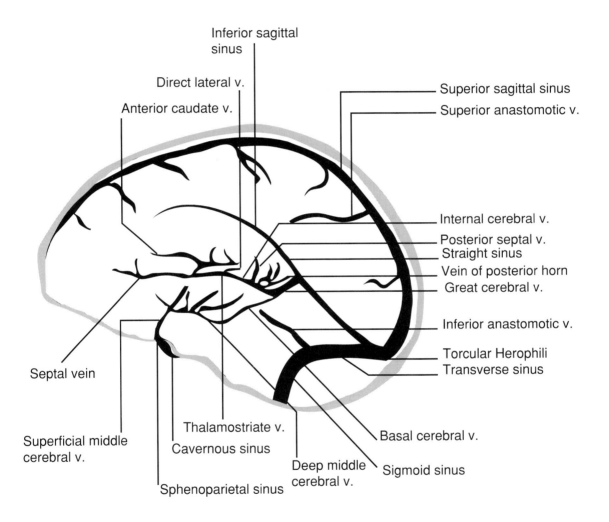

Fig. A-55.3 **Sagittal Venous Anatomy***

* Drawing adapted from Greenberg MS. Handbook of Neurosurgery, p 281. Lakeland, Florida, Greenberg Graphics, 1991.

CATEGORY A: THE BRAIN

Section 3:   The Sella   Page

A-56   Sellar Lesions by Signal

Common

1. Adenoma: Iso- or hypointense T1, hyperintense T2

2. Craniopharyngioma: Hyperintense T1, hyperintense T2 > hypointense T1, hyper-intense T2 > mixed hypo-, iso-, or hyperintense T1 and T2

3. Empty sella: Very hypointense T1, very hyperintense T2, homogeneous, midline stalk

4. Normal parasellar carotid arteries: Very hypointense T1 and T2

Uncommon

1. Aneurysm (Sheehan's or Simmonds' infarction or hemorrhage): Hyperintense T1, hyperintense T2, rare fluid-fluid levels with dependent T2 hypointensity

2. Meningioma: Hypointense T1, iso- or hypointense T2, enhances

3. Metastases: Hypointense T1, iso-, hypo-, or hyperintense T2, may enhance

Rare

1. Abscess: Hypo- or hyperintense T1, hyperintense T2

2. Carotid cavernous fistula: Hypointense T1 and T2

3. Chordoma: Isointense T1, mixed iso- and hyperintense T2

4. Hypothyroidism: Isointense T1 and T2

5. Hypothalamic/chiasmatic glioma: Isointense T1, iso- or mild hyperintense T2

6. Hypogonadism: Isointense T1 and T2

7. Nasopharyngeal carcinoma: Isointense T1, mildly hyperintense T2

8. Arachnoid cyst: Very hypointense T1, very hyperintense T2, homogeneous

9. Pituilith: Very hypointense T1 and T2

10. Choristoma (granular cell tumor, myoblastoma): Iso- or hyperintense T1, iso- or hyperintense T2, inhomogeneous, enhances

11. Lymphoid hypophysitis (pregnancy): Intermediate T1, iso- or hyperintense T2

12. Teratoma: Hyperintense T1, mixed T2

13. Dysgerminoma: Isointense T1, hyperintense T2, inhomogeneous

14. Parasitic infection (cysticercosis): Hypointense T1, hyperintense T2

15. Epidermoid: Hypointense T1, hyperintense T2, inhomogeneous

A-57   Sellar, Suprasellar & Perisellar T1 Hyperintensity

Common

1. Normal posterior neurohypophysis*

2. Fat in the posterior clinoid, anterior clinoid or tuberculum sellae

3. Chemical shift artifact

4. CSF flow phenomenon

Uncommon

1. Regenerating ectopic neurohypophysis

    a. Apoplexy

    b. Trauma

    c. Dwarfism

2. Rathke's cyst

3. Craniopharyngioma

4. Dermoid

5. Hemorrhagic chromophobe adenoma

6. Aneurysm

7. Lipoma

8. Cavernous sinus thrombosis (subacute to chronic)

* Antidiuretic hormone vasopressin or neurophysin complex histologically contains lipid-bearing granules that increase with dehydration or stress and increase the intensity of the normal or ectopic posterior pituitary lobe signal hyperintensity on T1.

A-58   Criteria for Sellar Microadenoma

Direct Criteria

1. T1 hypointensity < 1 cm in size
2. Hypointense on CEMR < 8 minutes, can be isointense 8-40 minutes and hyperintense on CEMR > 40 minutes

Indirect Criteria

1. Stalk deviation
2. Abnormal gland height (greater than)
   a. 6-7 mm male or prepubescent
   b. 7-11 mm gravid female postpuberty
   c. 10-13 mm female, peripartum
3. Floor deviation
4. Gland size asymmetry

A-59   Pearls in the Diagnosis of Pituitary Microadenoma

1.   Hypointense more common on T1, hyperintense on T2
2.   Contrast-enhanced T1 shows adenoma hypointensity in the first 3-8 minutes which eventually is isointense at 20 minutes and hyperintense on delayed imaging at 40 minutes

     Time Course of Normal Pituitary Gland Enhancement

     a.   Within the first 30 seconds: Enhancement occurs in the posterior pituitary via the inferior hypophyseal trunk
     b.   30-60 seconds: Enhancement of the pars intermedia via the superior hypophyseal trunk
     c.   60-120 seconds: Enhancement of the anterior pituitary normally occurs via the portal hypophyseal venous plexus

3.   Stalk: Deviation by itself is not a useful criterion since stalk deviation may be seen in a high percentage of normals (20-30%)
4.   Gland height: Normal man, less than 7 mm; gravid female, 8-11 mm; peripartum female, 10-13 mm
5.   Gland convexity: Focal downward erosion of the floor is more reliable than focal upward contour alterations
6.   Delayed imaging of the pituitary (30-40 minutes) may produce hyperintensity at the site of adenoma due to pooling of contrast in the lesion (an isointense phase may be seen between 10-30 minutes)
7.   May be secreting or non-secreting

     a.   Primary secreting microadenomas usually have prolactin levels of 100 picograms/deciliter
     b.   Normal lab values are usually below 20-30 picograms/dl
     c.   Although uncommon, compression of the pituitary may produce secondary prolactin elevation up to 100 picograms/dl
     d.   Levels above 100-120 picograms/dl are usually due to primary prolactin secreting tumors

A-59   **Pearls in the Diagnosis of Pituitary Microadenoma (Cont'd)**

Pituitary Gland & Components

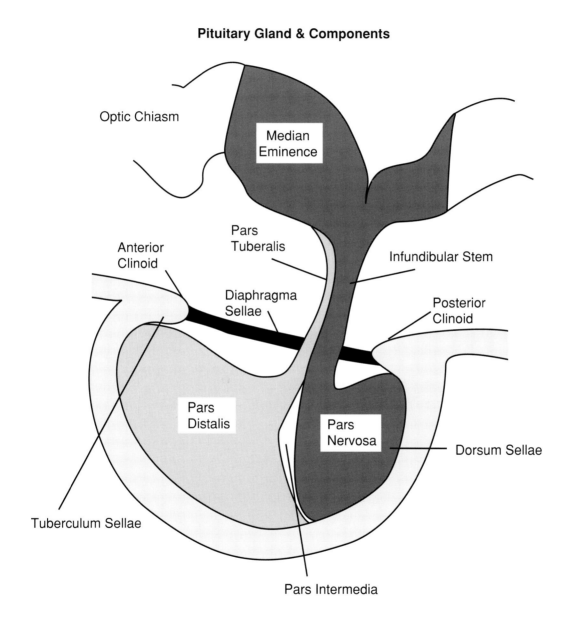

Fig A-59.1*

* Drawing from Elster AD. Modern Imaging of the Pituitary. Radiology 187:2, 1993.

A-60   Pituitary Adenomas: Frequency*

1.   Prolactin-cell adenoma (27%)

2.   Null cell adenoma, including oncocytoma (26%)

3.   Growth hormone-cell adenoma (13%)

4.   Corticotroph adenoma (10%)

5.   Gonadotroph adenoma (9%)

6.   Mixed growth hormone and prolactin-cell adenoma (8%)

7.   "Silent" corticotroph adenoma (5%)

8.   Thyrotroph adenoma (1%)

9.   Plurihormonal adenoma (1%)

* Adapted from Elster AD. Modern Imaging of the Pituitary. Radiology 187:6, 1993.

A-61   Pearls in the Diagnosis of Pituitary Macroadenoma

1. Greater than 1 cm
2. Isointense on T1
3. Iso- or hyperintense on T2 with mild to moderate enhancement
4. Diaphragma sellar notching helps differentiate extrasellar mass growing down from pituitary mass growing up
5. Complications of macroadenoma
   a. Chiasmatic compression
   b. Cavernous sinus invasion
      i. Prolactin levels > 2,000 picograms/dl implies cavernous invasion
      ii. Abuts the lateral dural sinus walls
      iii. Loss of speckled signal in the cavernous sinus distribution
   c. Pituitary hemorrhage or apoplexy
   d. Pituitary adenoma recurrence
   e. Differential diagnosis of macroadenoma
      i. Craniopharyngioma (white-white)
      ii. Meningioma (dark-isointense)
      iii. Aneurysm (lamellated)
      iv. Metastases (isointense-bright)

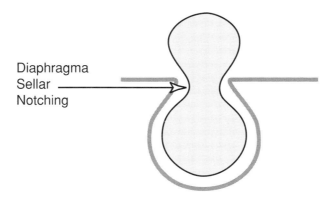

Diaphragma
Sellar
Notching

Fig. A-62.1

A-62   Diabetes Insipidus: Varied Appearances

1. Stalk transection or discontinuity: Trauma
2. Pronounced stalk enhancement with normal appearance on noncontrast MR: Idiopathic DI
3. Thickened stalk (greater than 3 mm) with pronounced enhancement on CEMR: Idiopathic diabetes insipidus
4. Increase in size and signal within the posterior neurohypophysis on T1 and T2: Nephrogenic diabetes insipidus
5. Isointense signal around and posterior to the stalk: Tuber cinereum hamartoma
6. Bulky masslike enhancement of stalk and hypothalamus: Sarcoid, breast or lung carcinoma, histiocytosis X
7. Hypothalamic hyperintense T2 signal and/or enhancement: Hypothalamic astrocytoma or glioma, metastatic disease
8. Ectopic pars nervosa (trauma, dwarfism, developmental)

A-63   Pituitary Gland Height*

1. Under 12 years of age: Less than or equal to 6 mm
2. Adolescent boys 12 to 21 years of age: Less than or equal to 7 mm
3. Adolescent girls 12 to 21 years of age: Less than or equal to 10 mm
4. Pregnant, peripartum/puerperium: Less than or equal to 12 mm

* Convex upper margins may be seen in teenage girls with spherical pituitary shape in the sagittal projection.

A-64   **Intrasellar Pituitary Signal Void or Hypointensity**

Common

1.   Volume averaging of the parasellar carotid artery dura and CSF

Uncommon

1.   Aneurysm of the paracavernous carotid artery

Rare

1.   Vascular malformation of the paracavernous carotid artery
2.   Primitive trigeminal artery aneurysm
3.   Pituilith
4.   Intrasellar calcified meningioma
5.   Pituitary gas associated with abscess formation or prior surgery
6.   Intrasellar calcified craniopharyngioma
7.   Postsurgical intrasellar susceptibility effect (clip, metal, etc.)

A-65   Cystic Pituitary Masses

Empty Sella
1. Homogeneous T1 hypointensity, T2 hyperintensity: Pure water signal
2. Midline pituitary stalk
3. Paucity of solid pituitary tissue
4. No evidence of chiasmatic or suprasellar mass effect
5. Enhancement of normal pituitary tissue only

Arachnoid Cyst
1. Homogeneous T1 hypointensity, T2 hyperintensity: Pure water signal
2. Sellar, suprasellar, retrosellar, and perisellar mass effect are common
3. Effaced and displaced pituitary stalk, multidirectional
4. Enhancement of normal pituitary tissue

Cystic Pituitary Adenoma or Neuroectodermal Tumor
1. Moderate T1 hypointensity, T2 hyperintensity: Proteinaceous water signal (therefore no exact CSF match)
2. Displaced pituitary stalk
3. Hormonal abnormalities frequently present
4. Intra- and suprasellar mass effect and/or extension
5. Foci of nodular enhancement from solid components

Cystic Craniopharyngioma
1. May have foci of T1 hyperintensity
2. May have hypointense T2 calcification
3. Suprasellar +/- intrasellar extension
4. Mixed enhancement

Dermoid
1. Hyperintense T1, hyperintense T2
2. Predominantly suprasellar
3. Nonenhancing

A-65   Cystic Pituitary Masses [Cont'd]

Epidermoid

1.   Hypointense T1, hyperintense T2
2.   Inhomogeneous
3.   Minimal peripheral enhancement
4.   Irregular shape

Cystic Optic Chiasmatic/Hypothalamic Glioma

1.   Neurofibromatosis frequently associated
2.   Origin in, or involvement of, the optic chiasm or hypothalamus
3.   Mild enhancement

A-66 Pearls in the Diagnosis of Rathke's Cyst

1. Signal intensity
   a. Cystic type: Hypointense T1, hyperintense T2 (60%)
   b. Fatty type: Hyperintense T1, hypointense T2 (30%)
   c. Hydrolyzed fat type: Hyperintense T1, hyperintense T2 (10%)
2. Homogeneous signal (70%), inhomogeneous signal* (30%)
3. Hypointense calcification on T2 not present
4. Location
   a. Intrasellar (90%)
   b. Infrasellar (8%)
   c. Suprasellar (2%)
5. Single epithelial layer

* Inhomogeneity represents thickening of the cyst wall, desquamated cells or epidermoid-like material.

A-67 Pearls & Etiology of Empty Sella

1. Primary or secondary
2. Secondary causes
   a. Radiation
   b. Tumor
   c. Surgery
3. MR findings
   a. Water signal within pituitary fossa
   b. Midline pituitary stalk
   c. Chiasmatic prolapse (particularly common after surgery)

A-68   Suprasellar Arachnoid Cyst Versus Aqueductal Stenosis

Arachnoid Cyst	**Aqueductal Stenosis**
Oval or square appearance to the suprasellar cistern	Enlarged diamond-shaped suprasellar cistern
Cisternal eccentricity	Cisternal symmetry
Splaying of the cerebral peduncles	No peduncular splaying
Carotid terminus separation	No carotid terminus separation
Trigeminal or crural cistern widening	No trigeminal or crural cistern widening
Anterior displacement of the optic chiasm	Downward or slight posterior displacement of the optic chiasm
Diamond shaped mid third ventricle	Enlarged but normal shaped mid third ventricle
Asymmetric dilatation of lateral ventricles, asymmetric expansion of foramen of Monro	Symmetric lateral ventricular dilatation
A pseudo third ventricle enlarged out of proportion to remaining ventricle	Third and lateral ventricles evenly enlarged
Dilatation of the third ventricle and effaced suprapineal recess	Large pineal recess
Superolateral displacement of the forniceal columns	Nominal displacement of the forniceal columns
Flow void in the cerebral aqueduct of Sylvius may remain	Flow void in the cerebral aqueduct of Sylvius absent
Variable displacement of mamillary body (more common superoposterior)	Downward displacement of mamillary body with mamillopontine distance < 1-2 cm

A-69   Pearls in the Diagnosis of Hamartoma

1. Peak age: 12-18 years
2. Location: Tuber cinereum, anteroinferior to the mamillary body
3. Signal
    a. Isointense on T1 and T2 (suprasellar)
    b. Isointense T1, mild hyperintense T2 (subcortical location)
4. Shape: Pedunculated or ovoid (lying between the pituitary stalk and mamillary body)
5. Male predominance
6. Clinical: Isosexual precocious puberty, episodes of spontaneous laughter and oculopalpebral clonus (gelastic seizures), partial complex temporal lobe epilepsy (25%) most often seen in lesions greater than 1.5 cm

A-70   Pearls in the Diagnosis of Optic/Hypothalamic Glioma

1. Peak age: 2-10 years
2. Signal: Isointense T1, mildly hyperintense T2
3. Bilateral optic gliomas: Neurofibromatosis
4. Unilateral optic glioma: 25% have neurofibromatosis
5. Bilateral perioptic T2 hyperintense signal: Dural ectasia
6. Cyst formation in glioma: 10% optic chiasm, 30% of cases following radiation
7. Calcification in glioma: 15% of patients with neurofibromatosis
8. Multiplicity in glioma: 25% (most associated with neurofibromatosis)
9. Enhancement in glioma: Variable, most often nominal to mild

A-71   **Pearls in the Diagnosis of Craniopharyngioma**

1. Peak age: Biphasic, 3-5 years and 50-60 years

2. Location

    a. Suprasellar (80%)

    b. Sellar/suprasellar (15%)

    c. Sellar (4%)

    d. Third ventricle (0.5%)

    e. Nasopharynx (0.5%)

3. Signal

    a. Hyperintense T1 & T2: Hydrolyzed cholesterol and/or blood (65%)

    b. Intermediate T1, hyperintense T2: Keratin (20%)

    c. Hypointense T2: Calcification (75%)

    d. Hypointense T1, hyperintense T2: Cyst formation (40%)

    e. Intermediate T1 and T2: Solid tumor (15%)

4. Calcification (75%): Twice as frequent in children as adults (Rathke's cysts do
    not calcify)

5. Origin: Rathke's cells or pouch having multilayered complex epithelium
    (Rathke's cysts have a simple single-layered epithelium)

6. Enhancement: Variable, none to mild

7. Hemorrhage: (10%)

8. Differential diagnosis: Meningioma (homogeneous, marked enhancement);
    aneurysm (flow void or clot); pituitary adenoma (more homogeneous signal, non-
    calcified, usually no hyperintense T1 signal)

A-72   Pearls in the Diagnosis of Ectopic Pinealoma

1. Occurs in the second to third decade of life and is more common in females, unlike pineal (ectopic) germinoma which is far more common in males
2. Primary germinoma has been described in the basal ganglia and thalamus
3. Most sellar germinomas have an associated pineal lesion which likely has seeded the CSF, although true ectopic germinoma likely exists
4. Lesions enhance with contrast MR
5. Occasionally may be associated with hormonal production (HCG)
6. Radiation sensitive
7. Propensity to seed the cerebrospinal fluid

CATEGORY A: THE BRAIN

A-73   Pearls in the Diagnosis of Trigeminal Neuroma

1. 50% involve the gasserian ganglion
2. 50% have an extradural location in the middle fossa
3. 25% are intradural and involve a portion of the ganglion and extend into the cerebellopontine angle
4. 25% involve both the middle and posterior fossae
5. Hyperintense on T2 (meningioma is more often isointense)
6. Enhancement is pronounced (not as pronounced as meningioma and does not usually produce dovetail enhancement like meningioma)
7. Any straddling mass involving the middle and posterior fossae is most likely a trigeminal neuroma

Anatomy

1. Cranial nerve V

    Extends from the brain stem to the anterolateral surface of the pons to Meckel's cave (a dural invagination in the posterior inferior aspect of the cavernous sinus contains CSF, motor and sensory trigeminal rootlets, and the gasserian ganglion) to the orbit, pterygopalatine fossa, muscles of mastication, face and scalp

2. Trigeminal nerve divisions

    a. The mandibular nerve V-3 extends under the posterior inferior cavernous sinus to enter the foramen ovale

    b. Anteriorly, the maxillary nerve V-2 exits from the inferior aspect of the cavernous sinus to enter foramen rotundum, the pterygopalatine fossa and the infraorbital fissure, where it divides into the infraorbital and zygomatic nerves

    c. At the PPF, cranial nerve V-2 communicates with the pterygopalatine ganglion and its branches

    d. The ophthalmic nerve (cranial nerve V-1) extends inferolaterally to the intracavernous internal carotid artery, then to the anterior clinoid process with cranial nerves III, IV and VI, and finally to the superior orbital fissure, where cranial nerve V-1 divides into frontal, lacrimal and nasociliary nerves

A-74   Cerebellar Sarcoma, Adult Medulloblastoma or Primitive Neuroectodermal Tumor of the Adult

1. Pediatric medullobastoma usually arises from the fourth ventricular roof and the inframedullary velum distribution

2. There is usually a thin plane of hypointensity separating the lesion from the fourth ventricular floor (not ordinarily present in ependymoma)

3. Pediatric medulloblastoma occurring before age 2 has a particularly bad prognosis

4. Medulloblastoma tends to be slightly more homogeneous than ependymoma which appears more speckled due to hyperintensity from hemorrhage and calcification

5. Adult or hemispheric medulloblastoma is hyperdense on CT and isointense on T2 MR (may mimic meningioma)

6. There is a biphasic peak of medulloblastoma in both pediatric and young adult groups

7. The adult form of the disease has a more benign course (approximately 50-60% survival rate at 10 years)

8. As many as 30% of medulloblastomas may seed the subarachnoid and subependymal spaces, easily recognized with gadolinium-DTPA

A-75   Pearls in the Diagnosis of Cerebellar Astrocytoma

1. 11% of primary CNS tumors in children
2. Prognosis excellent with surgical resection and a 10-year survival of 94%
3. Accounts for one-third of childhood posterior fossa tumors with no gender predilection
4. Late peak in the first decade and early in the second decade
5. Up to 80% are cystic with hemispheric astrocytomas more often cystic than their vermian counterparts
6. Most common histologic appearance is that of the juvenile type, called fibrillary astrocytoma, closely resembling juvenile pilocytic astrocytoma of the third ventricle
7. A less common form in 15% of cases, particularly in adolescence, is diffuse astrocytoma with fibrillary stellate or piloid cells (prognosis is poor, with possible anaplastic degeneration in these lesions)
8. Loose association with malignant cerebellar astrocytoma and neurofibromatosis
9. Proteinaceous cyst intermediate signal on spin density, hypointense on T1 and hyperintense on T2, with an intermediate signal intensity nodule that may occasionally be cystic and enhances (cystic nodules are seen in 5%)
10. Lesion eccentricity and size > 6 cm favors astrocytoma over hemangioblastoma, young age favors astrocytoma over hemangioblastoma
11. Circumferential hyperintense edema, usually mild
12. May be associated with erythropoietin secretion and polycythemia

A-76   Pearls in the Diagnosis of Hemangioblastoma

1. 7% of infratentorial tumors

2. This is a tumor of adults rather than children, and is extremely rare under the age of 30

3. 20% have Hippel-Lindau disease, and 5% of these are multiple

4. Associated findings in Hippel-Lindau disease include retinal angioma, pheochromocytoma, renal cell carcinoma, and cysts of the pancreas, lung, epididymis, liver, and kidney

5. 60-70% of lesions are cystic, with the internal constituents consisting of a gelatinous and hemorrhagic material

6. MR appearance

    a. Hypointense T1 and hyperintense T2 with intermediate signal-enhancing nodule

    b. The nodule abuts the pial surface, and cystic nodules are rare

    c. Tipoff to the diagnosis is punctate hyperintense foci of flow void due to hypervascularity, as well as the fact that the lesions occur in adults and tend to be smaller than cerebellar astrocytomas

7. Diagnosis includes ependymal- or nonependymal-lined cyst, cerebellar astrocytoma and arachnoid cyst

A-77   Pearls in the Diagnosis of Brain Stem Gliomas

1.   10-15% of CNS tumors in children

2.   Usually astrocytoma or glioblastoma multiforme

3.   Astrocytic, fibrillary and pilocytic types are common

4.   Up to 40% are falsely malignant

5.   Pontine and medullary tumors more aggressive than midbrain lesions

6.   Thalamic extension from midbrain tumors is common, while pontomedullary tumors infiltrate the cerebellum

7.   Small subset of benign pilocytic gliomas have a favorable prognosis

8.   MR produces hyperintense T2 but enhancement is variable

9.   Lesions are usually isodense on CT and may be diagnosed only by changes in morphology

10.   Infiltrative type is more common in the pons, while the cystic type is more common in the tectum

11.   Hemorrhagic necrosis is associated with a poor prognosis

12.   Size criteria
      a.   Midbrain tegmentum: 11-15 mm
      b.   Pons: 24-29 mm
      c.   Pontomedullary junction: 11-17 mm
      d.   Medullary junction: 8-11 mm

A-78   Cystic Lesions of the Brain Stem Diagnosed by Tectal Position on Sagittal MR

1. Quadrigeminal plate cistern arachnoid cyst: Tectum and collicular plate pushed anteriorly
2. Aqueductal stenosis with diverticular enlargement of the third ventricle: Tectum and collicular plate pushed posteriorly
3. Tectal glioma: Cyst within the collicular plate
4. Ependymal- and nonependymal-lined cyst: Located within the parenchyma or substance of the tegmentum and midbrain

A-79   Brain Stem, Cranial Nerve & Related Syndromes

1. Weber's: Cranial nerve III palsy with contralateral hemiparesis
2. Benedikt's: Similar to Weber's plus red nucleus lesion
3. Millard-Gubler: Facial and abducens palsy with contralateral hemiplegia (usually ischemic infarct, occasionally tumor)
4. Foster-Kennedy: Usually from olfactory groove or medial third sphenoid wing tumor, now rare due to CT
5. Bell's palsy (facial nerve palsy syndrome): The most common cause of facial paralysis
6. Parinaud's (sylvian aqueduct syndrome): Convergence, accommodation and supranuclear upward gaze palsy
7. Wallenberg's (PICA syndrome, lateral medullary syndrome)
8. Miller-Fisher: Bilateral VII & VIII neuritis
9. Rhombencephalitis & trigeminal neuritis: Usually due to herpes simplex neuritis
10. Optic perineuritis: Usually due to herpes zoster ophthalmicus
11. Optic neuritis: Usually due to multiple sclerosis

A-80   The Cerebellum & Brain Stem*

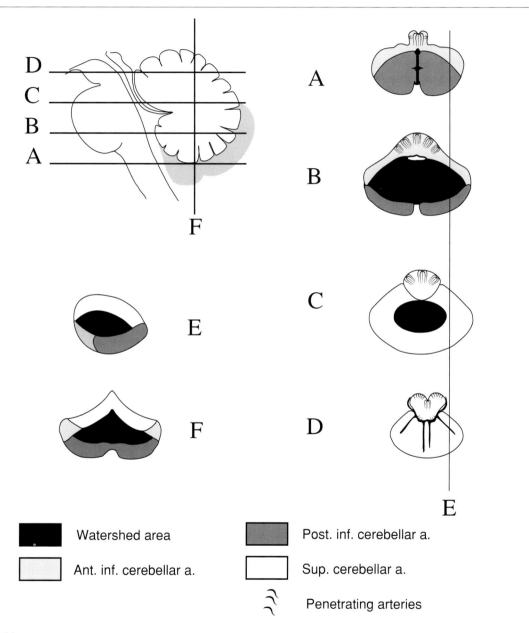

Fig. 80.1*

* Drawing adapted from Savoiardo M, Bracchi M, Passerini, et al. The Vascular Territories in the Cerebellum and Brainstem: CT and MR Study. AJNR 8:203, 1987.

CATEGORY A: THE BRAIN

Section 5: Hemorrhage   Page

A-81   Intracranial Hemorrhage 1.0-1.5T

Hyperacute (2-10 hours)

T1 iso- to hypointense

T2 hyperintense

Acute (10 hrs-3 days)

T1 hypointense (circumferential hypointense edema)

T2 very hypointense (circumferential hyperintense edema)

Early Subacute (3-10 days)

T1 iso- to hypointense center with hyperintense rim (extreme peripheral circumferential
       hypointense edema)

T2 hypointense (circumferential hyperintense edema)

Late Subacute (10-21 days)

T1 hyperintense (circumferential hypointense edema)

T2 iso- to hyperintense (circumferential hyperintense edema ± hemosiderin ring)

Chronic (2 weeks-months)

T1 hyperintense (nominal circumferential hypointense edema)

T2 iso- to hyperintense (black hemosiderin ring surrounded by nominal circumferential
       hyperintense edema)

Remote (months to years)

T1 hypointense (water-like)

T2 hyperintense (water-like) with black hemosiderin ring

A-82   Intracranial Hemorrhage 0.5T

Hyperacute (2-10 hours)

T1 iso- to hypointense

T2 hyperintense

Acute (10 hours-3 days)

T1 hypointense (circumferential hypointense edema)

T2 iso- or hypointense (circumferential hyperintense edema)

Early Subacute (3-8 days)

T1 iso- to hypointense center with a hyperintense rim (extreme peripheral circumferential hypointense edema)

T2 iso- to mildly hypointense (circumferential hyperintense edema)

Late Subacute (8-14 days)

T1 hyperintense (circumferential hypointense edema)

T2 hyperintense (circumferential hyperintense edema)

Chronic (2 weeks-months)

T1 hyperintense (nominal circumferential hypointense edema)

T2 hyperintense (hypointense hemosiderin ring surrounded by nominal circumferential hyperintense edema)

Remote (months to years)

T1 hypointense (water-like)

T2 hyperintense (water-like) with hypointense hemosiderin ring

A-83   Intracranial Hemorrhage < 0.35 T

Hyperacute (2-10 hours)
T1 iso- to hypointense
T2 hyperintense

Acute (10 hrs-3 days)
T1 hypointense (circumferential hypointense edema)
T2 iso- or hyperintense (circumferential hyperintense edema)

Early Subacute (3-10 days)
T1 iso- to hypointense center with a hyperintense rim (extreme peripheral circumferential hypointense edema)
T2 iso- to mildly hyperintense (circumferential hyperintense edema)

Late Subacute (10-21 days)
T1 hyperintense (circumferential hypointense edema)
T2 hyperintense (circumferential hyperintense edema)

Chronic (2 weeks-months)
T1 hyperintense (nominal circumferential hypointense edema)
T2 hyperintense (nominal circumferential hyperintense edema)

Remote (months to years)
T1 hypointense (water-like)
T2 hyperintense (water-like)

A-84   Signs of Intracranial Neoplastic Hemorrhage

1.   Intermediate signal intensity on T1 and T2
2.   Signal alteration which does not correspond to any known pattern of blood evolution over an appropriate period of time
3.   Delayed temporal resolution of hemorrhage
4.   Bizarre or complex signal intensities
5.   Irregular, absent or complex hemosiderin rings
6.   Persistent or exaggerated edema
7.   Lesion multiplicity
8.   Absence of hypointense calcification
9.   Disproportionate mass effect for lesion size
10. Nodular enhancement

A-85   Etiologies of Intracranial Hemorrhage*

1.   Hemorrhage from chronic hypertension
2.   Hemorrhage from aneurysms
3.   Bleeding from vascular malformations
     a.   Arteriovenous malformation
     b.   Cavernous angioma
     c.   Capillary telangiectasia
     d.   Venous angioma
4.   Abnormally fragile arteries
     a.   Amyloid angiopathy
     b.   Arteritis
     c.   Ehlers-Danlos syndrome and other heredofamilial connective tissue disease
5.   Bleeding diathesis
     a.   Warfarin, heparin, tissue plasminogen activating factor
     b.   Thrombocytopenia
     c.   Hemophilia
     d.   Leukemia
     e.   Fibrinolysis
6.   Drug abuse
7.   Venous and sinus thrombosis
8.   Infectious endocarditis, septic emboli
9.   Head trauma (into contusion site, tear of lenticulostriate arteries)
10. Bleeding into preexisting lesions such as:
     a.   Primary and metastatic tumors
     b.   Granulomas
11. Hemorrhagic stroke, hemorrhage into infarcts

A-85   Etiologies of Intracranial Hemorrhage [Cont'd]

12.   Miscellaneous rare causes

   a.   Migraine

   b.   Medical conditions with acute hypertension such as eclampsia, pheochromo-cytoma, glomerulonephritis

   c.   Vasopressor drugs

   d.   After carotid atherectomy

   e.   Upon exertion

   f.   Severe dental pain, painful urologic examination

   g.   Exposure to cold weather

   h.   Fat embolism to the brain

   i.   Supratentorial hemorrhage after posterior fossa surgery

   j.   After occlusion of arteriovenous fistula

   k.   Carcinoid syndrome

* Adapted from Heinrich PM, O'Reilly GV, Edelman RR, et al. Brain: Spontaneous Hemorrhage. In MRI: Clinical Magnetic Resonance Imaging, p.496. Edelman RR, Hesselink JR, eds. Philadelphia, WB Saunders, 1990.

A-86   Spontaneous Brain Hemorrhage*

100 Unselected Patients: Distribution by Site

Type	No. Cases
Putaminal	34
Lobar	24
Thalamic	20
Cerebellar	7
Pontine	6
Caudate	5
Putaminothalamic	4

* Heinrich PM, O'Reilly GV, Edelman RR, et al. Brain: Spontaneous Hemorrhage. In MRI: Clinical Magnetic Resonance Imaging, p 496. Edelman RR, Hesselink JR, eds. Philadelphia, WB Saunders, 1990.

A-87   Pediatric Spontaneous Intracerebral Hemorrhages*

Causes & Frequency in 72 Patients

Clinical Diagnosis	No.	%
Ruptured arteriovenous malformation	21	29.1
Arterial hypertension	11	15.3
Ruptured saccular aneurysm	7	9.7
Sympathomimetic drug abuse	5	6.9
Tumor	3	4.2
Acute alcohol intoxication	2	2.8
Pre-eclampsia/eclampsia	2	2.8
Superior sagittal sinus thrombosis	1	1.4
Systemic lupus erythematosus	1	1.4
Moyamoya	1	1.4
Cryoglobulinemia	1	1.4
Undetermined	17	23.6
Total	*72*	*100.0*

* Heinrich PM, O'Reilly GV, Edelman RR, et al. Brain: Spontaneous Hemorrhage. MRI: Clinical Magnetic Resonance Imaging, p 495. Edelman RR, Hesselink JR, eds. Philadelphia, WB Saunders, 1990.

A-88 Frequency of Hemorrhage in Intracranial Neoplasms*

1. Pineal choriocarcinoma or teratocarcinoma (90%)

2. Primary intracranial neuroblastoma (85%)

3. Oligodendroglioma (80%)

4. Melanoma (70%)

5. Ependymoma (55%)

6. Glioblastoma multiforme or high-grade astrocytic neoplasm (35%)

7. Metastasis (especially renal cell, thyroid, bronchogenic, melanoma and choriocarcinoma)

* The frequency of intracranial neoplastic hemorrhage increases dramatically after cranial irradiation.

A-89   Maturation of Intracranial Hemorrhage

1. Hyperacute phase (H)
    a. Consists of intact red cells in serum appearing as a proteinaceous solution of water, hypointense on T1 and hyperintense on T2
    b. This hyperacute appearance can last from 2-10 hours
    c. Note that the red cells contain oxygenated hemoglobin, which produces little in the way of T1 or T2 relaxation shortening effects

2. Acute phase hematoma (A)
    a. Contains intact red cells that have deoxygenated with deoxyhemoglobin and methemoglobin within the intact red cell
    b. Leads to a preferential T2 shortening effect known as PT2-PRE (more pronounced on fast scan utilizing gradient echo or field echo, T2 weighted spin echo images, and is a field-dependent phenomenon)
    c. The acute phase appearance may begin from 6-12 hours and may continue for up to 72 hours
    d. Acute hematoma at high field is black on T2 and gray on T1 (at lower fields, the black signal on T2 is less pronounced)
    e. The lower the field, the less black the signal on T2

3. Early subacute phase of hematoma (ES)
    a. Can begin as early as three days and maintain its appearance for 7-10 days
    b. In the early subacute phase peripheral red cells have begun to lyse, while central red cells may remain intact
    c. The free methemoglobin in the periphery of the clot exhibits a proton-electron dipole-dipole interaction that results in T1 shortening and a peripheral hyperintense rim
    d. The center of the clot may remain hypointense on T2 due to intracellular deoxyhemoglobin and methemoglobin, resulting in the field-dependent T2 effect (less pronounced the lower the field)
    e. Only minimal hypointense T1 and hyperintense T2 edema will be seen surrounding the clot

A-89   Maturation of Intracranial Hemorrhage (Cont'd)

4.   Late subacute phase (S)

   a.   Can begin as early as 7 days, usually lasts 14 days but can last for 21 days

   b.   Red cell lysis is complete: The clot is now homogeneously white on T1

   c.   In the early subacute phase there is a white rim and a gray center on T1

   d.   On T2, the degree of black signal has waned due to red cell lysis and the absence of intracellular deoxy- and methemoglobin

      i.   The clots may appear from gray to white

      ii.   May be isointense to the brain

      iii. Occasionally, isointensity on T2 can appear in the early subacute phase

      iv. Edema is pronounced, hypointense on T1 and hyperintense on T2 surrounding the clot

5.   Chronic phase hematoma (C)

   a.   Can begin as early as 2-3 weeks and last for 4-6 months

   b.   Typically white on T1 and T2 due to complete red cell lysis, proton-electron dipole-dipole interaction of free methemoglobin on T1 and water signal on T2

   c.   A paramagnetic effect of T2 shortening is seen due to hemosiderin-laden macrophages around the periphery of the clot

   d.   Edema begins to subside

   e.   Hematomas may enhance as a rim on T1 C+ MR as early as the subacute phase and in the chronic phase

6.   Remote hematoma (R)

   a.   Begins as early as 4-6 months and persists for years

   b.   A proteinaceous water-like signal similar to the hyperacute phase of hematoma

   c.   Edema has waned

   d.   There is negative mass effect

   e.   The hematoma now appears as a simple or proteinaceous cyst, rounded or slitlike

   f.   The identifying feature is the presence of a hemosiderin rim

   g.   The remote hematoma may collapse completely, and only hemosiderin remains

A-89   Maturation of Intracranial Hemorrhage (Cont'd)

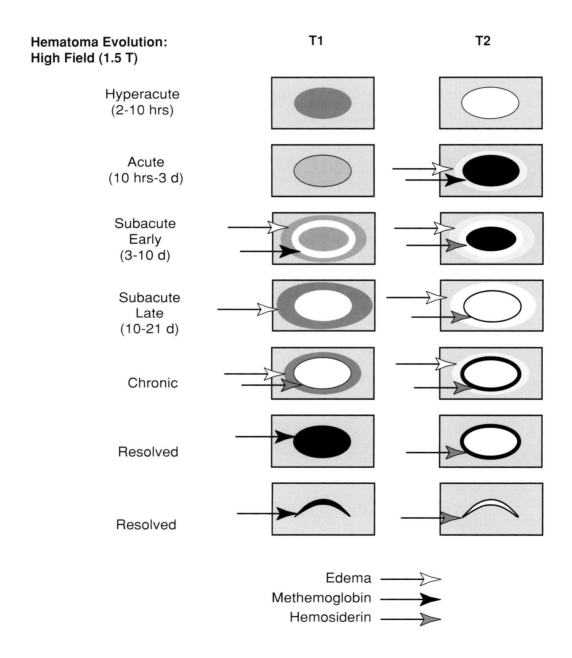

Fig. A-89.1

A-89   **Maturation of Intracranial Hemorrhage (Cont'd)**

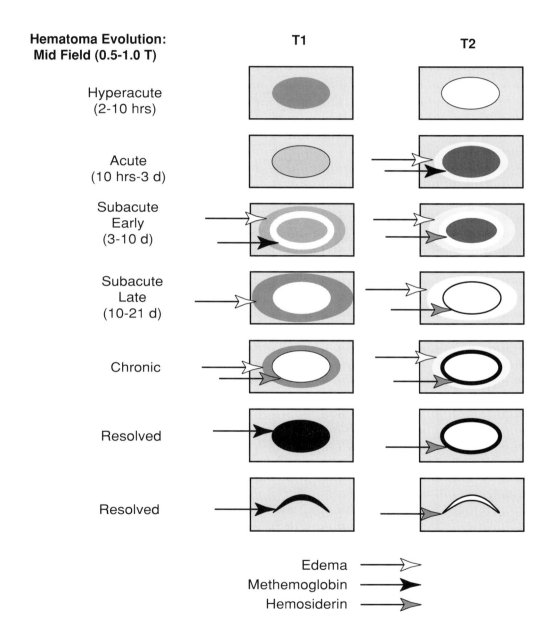

Fig. A-89.2

A-89   Maturation of Intracranial Hemorrhage (Cont'd)

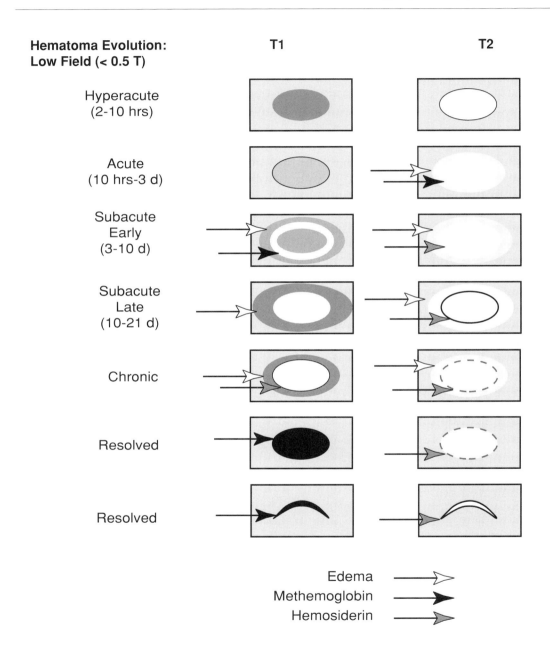

Hematoma Evolution: Low Field (< 0.5 T)

	T1	T2
Hyperacute (2-10 hrs)		
Acute (10 hrs-3 d)		
Subacute Early (3-10 d)		
Subacute Late (10-21 d)		
Chronic		
Resolved		
Resolved		

Edema →
Methemoglobin →
Hemosiderin →

Fig. A-89.3

A-90   Pearls, Tricks & Rules of Hemorrhage

1.   On T1, the clot signal goes from gray to white

2.   On T2, the clot goes from black to white at high field and from gray or white to white on mid- and low field, respectively

3.   Exposure to air may accelerate maturation of clot signal

4.   At lower fields, there is less preferential T2 shortening effect, and clots are less black on T2

5.   Diffusion into surrounding tissues and variable rates of red cell lysis produce more heterogeneous and unpredictable effect in the body

6.   Sequences without a 180° pulse, such as gradient echo and field echo, bring out the susceptibility effect of T2 hypointensity due to preferential T2 effect earlier in the age of the clot

7.   Edema peaks in the subacute phase

8.   Hemosiderin rim peaks in the chronic phase

9.   Proteinaceous water-like signal can be seen in either the hyperacute or the remote phase

10.   Ringlike contrast enhancement occurs in the late subacute and chronic stages

11.   Blackest T2 signal is seen in the acute phase

12.   Fast scan gradient echo will bring out the susceptibility effects of T2 shortening in the clot and in hemosiderin effects earlier

13.   Isointense phases of clot on T2 occur in transition from hyperacute to acute and from the subacute to the chronic

CATEGORY A: THE BRAIN

Section 6: Inflammation, Myelin Disorders   Page

A-91 **Pearls in the Diagnosis of Herpes Encephalitis & Herpetic Neuralgia**

1. MR is the examination of choice since CT is poor at visualizing temporal lobes

2. Temporal lobe hyperintensity on T2 is seen in the Ammon's horn distribution and involves the uncus and parahippocampus, centrosylvian extension is not uncommon

3. Bilateral involvement is seen in 40% of cases

4. Coronal T2 images are far more sensitive than CT in making the diagnosis, and occasionally the earliest sign will be subtle contrast enhancement in the parahippocampus

5. Trigeminal neuritis and ophthalmic zoster equals rhombencephalitis: Commonly manifested as T2 pontine hyperintensity and fifth nerve enhancement on T1

6. Ramsay Hunt syndrome: T1 enhancement of the 7th and 8th nerves, cochlea and the vestibules

A-92   Patterns of Myelination*

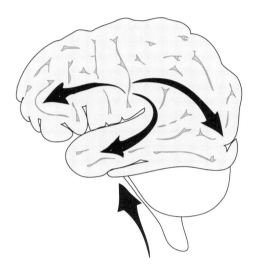

Myelination progresses in a cau-docranial direction from the brain stem, through the posterior limb of the internal capsule and to the hemispheric white matter, proceeding from the central sulcus toward the poles.

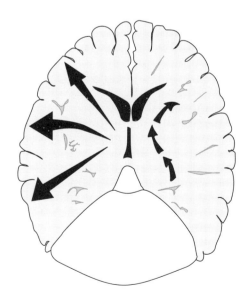

Myelination advances from deep to superficial and from posterior to anterior

* From Ballesteros MC, Hansen PE, Soila K. MR Imaging of the Developing Human Brain. Radiographics 13:612, 1993.

A-93   Progression of Myelination on MR*

Areas	Fetal	Postnatal
Medulla		
Cerebellum		
Pons Mesencephalon		
Posterior Limb Internal Capsule		
Basal Nuclei		
Centrum Semiovale		
Optic Radiations		
Splenium Corpus Callosum		
Anterior Limb Internal Capsule		
Genu Corpus Callosum		
Peripheral Occipital White Matter		
Peripheral Parietal White Matter		
Peripheral Frontal White Matter		
Peripheral Temporal White Matter		

* From Ballesteros MC, Hansen PE, Soila K. MR Imaging of the Developing Human Brain. Radiographics 13:613, 1993.

A-94   Myelination: General Rules of Thumb

1. Myelination continues from prenatal phase into the second decade of life (the most rapid myelination is within the first two years)
2. Process proceeds caudocranial, deep to superficial and posterior to anterior (it follows the order of phylogenic evolution)
3. MR appearance of myelination lags slightly behind histology due to the need for a threshold of myelin necessary before detection on MR
4. Unmyelinated white matter is hyperintense on T2 and hypointense on T1 in contrast to the adult myelinated brain

A-95   Terminology: Deep White Matter Signal Intensity

1.   Unidentified bright objects (UBOs): A wastebasket term that includes hyperintense foci of deep white matter microangiopathic signal alteration

2.   Ependymitis granularis: Triangular perifrontal hyperintensities common in normal individuals secondary to focal ependymal breakdown, local decreased myelin content, and preferential centripetal drainage of interstitial fluid

3.   Periventricular lesions (PVL): Used to describe any confluent or nonconfluent periventricular hyperintensity be it from demyelination, vascular disease, or transependymal migration from hydrocephalus

4.   Transependymal migration (TM): A subset of PVL refers to fluid which, by virtue of increased CSF pressure, preferentially migrates centripetally into the interstitium producing frontal and occipital smooth signal hyperintensity

5.   Leukoaraiosis (LA): Periventricular white matter lesions (PVL's) that are causally related to cerebral hypoperfusion and microangiopathy

6.   Subcortical arteriosclerotic encephalopathy or Binswanger's disease: A clinical and radiographic subset of LA, UBOs or PVLs that are confluent, severe, coalescent (this entity is rare)

7.   État criblé: Foci of hyperintensity on T2 that are hypointense on T1 since chronic hypertension results in focal periarteriolar atrophy; the perivascular spaces enlarge and create a speckled appearance to the inferior aspect of the frontoparietal brain (especially around the anterior commissure)

A-96   Tipoffs to the Diagnosis of Multiple Sclerosis

Major Tipoffs

1.   Ovoid lesions whose major axis or long axis is perpendicular to the anteroposterior dimension of the brain

2.   Right angle demyelination extending perpendicular to the ventricular system along the *Dawson's finger** white matter

3.   Clustered parasagittal supraventricular location, "septocallosal"

4.   Lesions in the middle cerebellar peduncles, either unilateral or bilateral

Minor Tipoffs

1.   Central atrophy

2.   Increased brain iron

3.   Lesions in the brain stem or cervical cord (15%) - posterolateral & asymmetric

4.   All lesions possessing no, nominal or mild mass effect

5.   Enhancement without mass effect in the posterolateral cervical cord

6.   Ring enhancement in the brain

* Dawson's finger refers to periventricular white matter.

A-97   Pearls in the Diagnosis of Multiple Sclerosis

1. Normal MRI without contrast in the brain or spine imaging in <5%

2. There is no such thing as asymptomatic MS when plaques are present, but the patient has no clinical symptoms of MS and develops MS one or two years later

3. When MS is seen on MR, the patient has or has had symptoms consistent with the diagnosis

4. Diagnosis is made on MR when complementary tests are supportive

    a. Eye signs or internuclear ophthalmoplegia, a disorder of eye movement characterized by impaired adduction on the side of an MS plaque with dissociated nystagmus of the adducting eye (the same eye movement disorder in an older age group is usually due to cerebral vascular disease)

        • The medial longitudinal fasciculus (MLF) consists of four vestibular nuclei on the floor of the fourth ventricle and at the pontomedullary junction
        • Fibers from nuclei form the MLF, which extends cephalad and caudad adjacent to the midline and the midbrain and connects the abducens, trochlear, and oculomotor nuclei
        • Ocular motion is coordinated with head motion and these structures have a role in vertical gaze via the interstitial nucleus of Cajal in the posterior commissure
        • In internuclear ophthalmoplegia (INO), disconjugate gaze is demonstrated

    b. History of optic neuritis

    c. Waxing or waning of clinical sensory syndrome

    d. Bowel or bladder dysfunction

    e. Positive oligoclonal bands, auditory or visual evoked response tests

    f. Sensorineural hearing loss

5. Multiple sclerosis in children

    a. A female predominance

    b. More severe course

    c. More infratentorial plaques

    d. Less atrophy and less conspicuous increase in brain iron

A-98   Pearls in the Diagnosis of Amyotrophic Lateral Sclerosis (ALS)

Key Features

1.   Mixed upper and lower motor neuron disease
2.   No cognitive, sensory or autonomic dysfunction
3.   Usually atrophy and fasciculations in upper extremities, spasticity in lower extremities
4.   Caused by degeneration of neurons in cervical spine or medulla
5.   Annual incidence 0.4-1.76/100,000

Clinical

1.   Voluntary muscles, sparing eye and urinary sphincter muscles
2.   Initially with weakness and atrophy of hands, spasticity and hyper-reflexia of lower extremities (hyporeflexia is possible)
3.   Dysarthria and dysphagia, tongue atrophy and fasciculations may occur
4.   Age onset usually after 50
5.   Autosomal dominant in 5%

MR Findings

1.   The presence of lower-motor neuron findings in the tongue in the presence of a normal MRI is highly suggestive of ALS
2.   Hyperintense T2 foci in the corticospinal tract ± T1 hypointensity
3.   Anterolateral cord atrophy

Differential Diagnosis

1.   Progressive bulbar palsy
2.   Juvenile amyotrophy (monomelic amyotrophy, benign focal amyotrophy): Atrophy in hand or forearm in boys, self-limited course

A-99   Clues to Diagnosing Demyelination or Myelinoclasis

1.   Multiple sclerosis: Waxing and waning symptoms, positive oligoclonal bands, visual or auditory evoked response, optic neuritis, visual deficit, bowel or bladder dysfunction
     MR findings: Right angle demyelination, rounded plaques, periventricular location, bilateral involvement of the middle cerebellar peduncles, increased brain iron

2.   Progressive multifocal leukoencephalopathy (PML): History of immunosuppression
     MR findings: Confluent, asymmetric and peripheral to central progression of T2 hyperintensity with scalloping of outer margins

3.   Acute disseminated encephalomyelitis (ADE): Recent history of childhood viral infection or vaccination (measles, mumps, etc.)
     MR findings: Rounded hyperintense T2 signal, progressive and unrelenting with hypointensity on T1 within two weeks

4.   Acute hemorrhagic leukoencephalitis: Same as acute disseminated encephalomyelitis but with foci of hyperintense T1 hemorrhage

5.   Subacute white matter encephalitis: History of HIV or CMV infection
     MR findings: Bilateral diffuse patchy to confluent hyperintensity, supra- and infratentorial spaces with poorly defined margins

6.   Radiation encephalopathy: History of radiation ≥ 5800 rads six to eight months previously
     MR findings: Confluent T2 signal hyperintensity with forceps major predilection; sparing of the splenium of corpus callosum and peripheral margin scalloping; relative posterior fossa, basal ganglia and internal capsule sparing; hypointense T2 hemosiderin deposits due to microangiopathy

A-99   Clues to Diagnosing Demyelination or Myelinoclasis [Cont'd]

7.   Marchiafava-Bignami disease: History of alcohol abuse or drinking from iron- or lead-contaminated stills
     MR findings: Atrophy or T1 hypointensity and T2 hyperintensity in the corpus callosum with or without atrophy

8.   Central pontine myelinolysis: History of alcoholism, hypothermia, and rapid correction of hyponatremia
     MR findings: Confluent central T2 hyperintensity in the pons with peripheral rim-sparing (trident or bird-shaped)

9.   Anoxia: History of hypoxemia
     MR findings: Symmetric T2 hyperintensity with a predilection for the parieto-occipital white matter, globus pallidus, and periaqueductal brain

A-100   Pearls in Dysmyelinating Disease

Macrocephaly
1. Canavan's disease
2. Alexander's disease

Signal Alteration Masslike or Round in the Thalamus
1. Krabbe's disease
2. Sandhoff's disease

Parieto-occipital Predilection
1. Classic adrenoleukodystrophy

Enzymatic or Chromosomal Defects
1. Pelizaeus-Merzbacher disease: CNS myelin-specific proteolipid protein (DNA probe detectable)
2. Canavan's disease: Aspartoacylase deficiency, increased urine and plasma N-acetylaspartic acid
3. Metachromatic leukodystrophy: Arylsulfatase-A deficiency (during screening)
4. Tay-Sachs disease: Hexosaminadase
5. Canavan's disease

Sex-linked Inheritance*
1. Adrenoleukodystrophy
2. Pelizaeus-Merzbacher diseae

* Most dysmyelinating disorders are inherited as autosomal recessive.

A-101   Characteristics of Brain Abscess

1. Homogeneous signal
2. Hypointense T1, hyperintense T2 (50%) or hypointense T1, mildly hypointense T2 (50%)*
3. Peripheral pseudocapsule signal: Mildly hyperintense T1 and mildly hypo- or isointense T2
4. Pseudocapsule shape: Extremely thin, smooth and thinner on the nonpial surface
5. Peripheral or ring enhancement with rim caliber or thickness consistently thin
6. Satellite lesions (25%)
7. Leptomeningeal or ventricular wall contrast enhancement (10-15%)

A-102   Criteria for Herpes Encephalitis

Direct Signs
1. Bilateral (50%) or unilateral (30%) white matter edema with involvement of the uncal protuberance
2. Hyperintense T2 or T2 relaxation prolongation involving the amygdala, gyrus ambiens and limbus
3. Enhancement of the parahippocampal gyral gray matter on T1 either unilaterally or bilaterally

Indirect Signs
1. White matter edema in the centrosylvian region
2. Signal alteration does not correlate with a known vascular territory

* T2 hypointensity related to stable oxygen-free radicals producing paramagnetic susceptibility effect.

A-103   Escobar Classification of Neurocysticercosis

	Clinical	MR Description
Stage I	Vesicular	Intermediate signal intensity mural nodule and small proteinaceous cyst with thin capsule
Stage II	Colloidal vesicular	Intermediate signal intensity nodule w/ heavily proteinaceous fluid cyst and thick hypointense capsule, moderate perilesional hyperintense T2 edema
Stage III	Granular nodular	Intermediate signal intensity mass with foci of hypointense calcification on T2 or T2*[a] imaging, thick hypointense capsule, mild hyperintense T2 edema
Stage IV	Calcified	Punctate hypointense foci on T2 and T2* imaging

NOTE: Escobar classification is a pathologic classification based on the macroscopic cyst appearance.

a While T2* is a T2-appearing sequence, it does not utilize a 180° refocusing RF pulse, does not give true T2 contrast, and is governed by susceptibility effects.

A-104   Spectrum of Radiation Effect

1.   Radiation white matter effects: Scalloped white matter hyperintense T2 signal with sharp margins, forceps major predilection with sparing of the splenium of the corpus callosum
2.   Mixed foci of bland and hemorrhagic infarction or foci of punctate T2 hypointensity (iron) secondary to remote microangiopathic infarction *(parenchymal siderosis)*
3.   Coagulation necrosis: Masslike intermediate T2 signal surrounded by hyperintense edema with enhancement and poorly defined margins
4.   Marrow change: Hyperintense T1 (predominant yellow marrow)

A-105   Pearls in the Diagnosis of Behçet's Disease

1.   Age: Peak 30 years, range 15-45 years
2.   Prevalence among Mediterranean, Near Eastern and Asian populations (especially Japanese)
3.   MR findings
     a.   Bilateral symmetric T2 hypointensity in cerebral peduncles or thalami (80%)
     b.   Leptomeningeal contrast enhancement (less than 5%)
4.   HLA-linked disease
5.   Triad
     a.   Plantar and palmar erythema
     b.   Keratitis/corneal erosion
     c.   Central nervous system vasculitis and aseptic meningitis (25%)

A-106   AIDS: Neurologic Involvement

Viral Infections

1. Subacute encephalitis: Parenchymal peripheral hyperintensity
2. Atypical aseptic meningitis: Leptomeningeal enhancement
3. Herpes simplex encephalitis: Temporal lobe hyperintensity, gyriform enhancement
4. Progressive multifocal leukoencephalopathy: Confluent white matter hyperintensity, no mass effect
5. Viral myelitis: Poorly defined T2 hyperintensity, poorly defined enhancement
6. Varicella zoster encephalitis: Parenchymal peripheral T2 hyperintensity

Non-viral Infections (Usually Ring-enhancing Nodules)

1. Toxoplasma gondii
2. Cryptococcus neoformans
3. Candida albicans
4. Coccidiomycosis
5. Treponema pallidum
6. Atypical mycobacteria
7. Mycobacterium tuberculosis
8. Aspergillus fumigatus
9. E. coli bacteria

Neoplasms

1. Primary CNS lymphoma: Mass effect, deep, periventricular, enhancing
2. Systemic lymphoma with CNS involvement: Leptomeningeal enhancement
3. Kaposi's sarcoma (including brain mets): Rounded nodules

Strokes

1. Infarct
2. Intracerebral hemorrhage

* Adapted from Greenberg MS. Handbook of Neurosurgery, p 249. Lakeland, Florida, Greenberg Graphics, 1991.

A-107   Inflammatory Disease in HIV

1. Primary HIV Infection
    a. Multifocal patchy white matter disease, usually asymmetric
    b. Enhancement is variable, may be nonexistent
    c. Lesions may resemble multiple sclerosis

2. Lymphoma
    a. Lesions are confluent rather than patchy
    b. Enhancement usually pronounced and homogeneous
    c. May be round or ovoid
    d. Propensity for deep white matter, particularly periventricular corpus callosum
    e. Mass effect more conspicuous than HIV infection

3. Toxoplasmosis and fungal disease
    a. Lesion seen as nodules or ringlike
    b. Enhancement usually ringlike
    c. Lesion multiplicity with involvement of supra- and infratentorial spaces

4. Tuberculosis and other mycobacterial infection
    a. Multiple nodules, usually smaller than toxoplasmomas
    b. Homogeneous nodular or ring enhancement
    c. More common early in the HIV disease process (atypical mycobacteria more frequent later in the disease process)

5. Progressive multifocal leukoencephalopathy
    a. Confluent periventricular white matter disease, often with peripheral involvement (i.e., peripheral to central evolution)
    b. No mass effect, usually asymmetric

CATEGORY A: THE BRAIN

A-108   The Absence of the Septum Pellucidum*

Developmental

Holoprosencephaly

Septo-optic dysplasia

Dysgenesis of the corpus callosum

Apert syndrome

Brain hypoplasia

Cortical dysmorphogenesis (gray matter heterotopia)

Schizencephaly (including Gruner syndrome)

Lissencephaly

Congenital hydrocephalus

Chiari malformation Type II

Acquired

Significant long-standing hydrocephalus

Leptomeningitis

Trauma

Porencephaly

* Sarwar M. The Septum Pellucidum: Normal and Abnormal. AJNR 10-1001, 1989.

A-109   Disorders of Migration & Associated Findings

Lissencephaly

1. Smooth brain with no gyri
2. Microcephaly
3. Hourglass appearance of cerebral hemispheres
4. Absent opercula, claustra and extreme capsules
5. Atrophy of the corpus callosum
6. Heterotopic nodules of gray matter
7. Colpocephaly (developmental enlargement of the atria of lateral ventricles)

Pachygyria

1. Thickened flattened gyri
2. Shallow sulci

Polymicrogyria

1. Numerous small gyri that occasionally may appear fused into larger gyri and simulate pachygyria

Heterotopic Gray Matter

1. Islands of neural tissue or gray matter, nodular in appearance and located within the white matter from the subependymal to the subcortical region

Schizencephaly

1. Full thickness clefts lined by gray matter so that the ependyma of the ventricular system connects to the cortical pia, a *pial-ependymal zipper*
2. Pachygyria lining the cleft
3. Ventricular diverticulum
4. Absence of the septum pellucidum
5. Atrophy of the corpus callosum
6. Atrophy of the pyramidal tracts

A-110   Leptomeningeal Disease in Children

Common

1. Meningitis
2. Leukemia
3. Medulloblastoma
4. Retinoblastoma
5. Lymphoma
6. Ependymoma
7. Neuroblastoma

Uncommon

1. Gliomas of the brain stem or corpus callosum
2. Oligodendrogliomas

A-111   Anterior Fontanelle Mass

1. Meningocele/encephalocele: Very hypointense T1, hyperintense T2
2. Subgaleal dermoids: Hyperintense T1, hyperintense T2
3. Lipoma: Hyperintense T1, hypointense T2
4. Sebaceous cyst: Hypointense T1, hyperintense T2
5. Hemangioma/lymphangioma: Mixed T1 and T2 signal
6. Melanotic progonoma: Hyperintense T1, hypointense T2
7. Sinus pericranii: Isointense T1, hyperintense T2

A-112   Findings Associated with Agenesis or Hypoplasia of the Corpus Callosum

1. Interhemispheric lipoma (40%)
2. Interhemispheric cysts (6%)
3. Sphenoidal encephalocele
4. Absence of the hippocampal formation and anterior commissure (3%)
5. Probst bundles (white matter lining the medial border of the lateral ventricles)
6. Agyria, pachygyria, polymicrogyria or gray matter heterotopia
7. High riding third ventricle
8. Single fused or azygous anterior cerebral artery
9. Colpocephaly
10. Splayed frontal horns of lateral ventricles
11. Optic atrophy
12. Coloboma
13. Schizencephaly
14. Loss of horizontal orientation of the cingulate gyrus
15. Arrhinencephaly
16. Porencephaly

A-113   Findings in Phakomatosis

Hippel-Lindau Disease

1. Hemangioblastoma: Proteinaceous cysts, hypointense on T1, hyperintense on T2 with intermediate signal intensity nodules that enhance in the cerebellum (50%), brain stem (8%) or spinal cord (4%); hypointense flow void on T1 and T2 due to lesion hypervascularity

2. Retinal neoplasm: Enhancement on T1 (30-50%), angiomas (hemangioblastoma), retina, brain, lungs, spleen, kidney, liver

3. Renal cell carcinoma: 35% of all patients, T2 signal hyperintensity

4. Pheochromocytoma: 15%, hyperintense on T2

5. Cerebral hemangioblastoma: Rare, occurring in less than 0.3%

6. Solid hemangioblastoma: Intermediate T1, mild T2 hyperintensity (20%)

7. Cysts of the pancreas, lungs, liver, kidney, spleen, adrenal, epididymis: Hypointense T1, hyperintense T2

8. Carcinoma of the pancreas: 2%

9. Other neoplasms: Ependymoma, islet cell tumor of pancreas, medullary carcinoma of the thyroid, epididymal cystadenoma

10. Polycythemia: 9-20%

Neurofibromatosis

1. Craniospinal neurofibromas (VIII > V > VII > IX > X): Hyperintense T2 with hypointense T2 centers, moderately pronounced enhancement

2. Meningiomas: Iso- to hypointense T2, pronounced homogeneous enhancement

3. Gliomas: Intra-axial signal hyperintensity or isointensity on T2

4. Craniospinal or orbital dural ectasia: Water signal cavities hypointense on T1, hyperintense on T2

5. Hamartoma or low-grade glioma/dysplasia: Mild T2 signal hyperintensity with nominal enhancement (predilection for optic pathway)

6. Lacunar and nonlacunar infarction (UBOs and cortical infarcts)

7. Thoracic kyphoscoliosis: Normal vertebral T1 hypointensity with or without plexiform neurofibroma masses, epidural and paraspinous

8. Arachnoid cyst: Hypointense T1, hyperintense T2, homogeneous

A-113   Findings in Phakomatosis (Cont'd)

Neurofibromatosis (cont'd)

9. Moyamoya disease: Speckled T2 hypointensity of vascular collaterals intermixed with hyperintense lacunar infarction

10. Herniation of the temporal lobe or subarachnoid spaces into the posterior orbit

11. Skin lesions: Café-au-lait, cutaneous nodules, Lisch nodules (iris pigmentation)

Sturge-Weber Syndrome

1. Venous angioma of the leptomeninges with ipsilateral cutaneous nevi: Cortical T2 signal hyperintensity with variable peripheral enhancement

2. Hemiatrophy

3. Choroid plexus angiomatosis: T2 hyperintensity with asymmetric choroid plexus enhancement

4. Mesial temporal sclerosis or gliosis: Subtle T2 hyperintensity

5. Accelerated myelination in the ipsilateral involved hemisphere

Tuberous Sclerosis (Bourneville's Disease)

1. Subependymal calcification: Punctate T2 signal hypointensity

2. Subcortical-cortical hamartoma: Slight hypointensity T1, slight hyperintensity T2

3. Altered myelinization: Hyperintense T2

4. Micro- and macroinfarctive disease: Hyperintense T2 lacunar infarction (round) or cortical infarction (wedge or gyriform shape)

5. Neoplasm

    a. Giant cell astrocytoma: Mixed hypointense T2 (calcium), intermediate signal T1 (solid tumor), homogeneous T1 hypointensity or T2 hyperintensity (cyst)

    b. Ependymoma: Mixed T1 and T2 signal from hemorrhage and cyst formation

6. Meningioma: Iso- to hypointense T2

7. Sebaceous cysts: Marked hyperintensity, well-circumscribed in subcutaneous or subgaleal fat

8. Skin lesions: Subungual fibromas, Shagreen patches, adenoma sebaceum

9. Other: Angiomyolipoma of the kidneys, rhabdomyoma of the heart

A-114   MR Findings & Pearls in Sturge-Weber Syndrome

Clinical

1. Facial nevus flammeus
2. Seizures
3. Mental retardation
4. Dementia
5. Hemianopsia
6. Glaucoma
7. Hemiparesis
8. Hemiatrophy
9. Male predominance of 1.5:1

Plain Film Findings

1. Sinus hypertrophy
2. Bone hypertrophy
3. Calcification

MR Findings

1. Gyriform enhancement and mixed T2 hyper- and hypointensity secondary to pial angiomatosis
2. Cerebral hemiatrophy with or without mesial temporal sclerosis may be seen in a minority of patients
3. T1 retinal choroidal signal hyperintensity or subretinal hemorrhage or effusion
4. Vascular anomalies
   a. Pial or leptomeningeal angiomatosis
   b. Absence or decreased cortical veins
   c. Prominence of the deep venous system with exaggerated flow void
   d. Choroid plexus enlargement, enhancement, and increased T2 due to angiomatous malformation

A-114   MR Findings & Pearls in Sturge-Weber Syndrome (Cont'd)

Other Findings

1. Gyriform calcification on CT
2. Diffuse hemicephalic temporo-parieto-occipital hypometabolism on positron emission tomography
3. Retinal calcification on CT (rare)
4. Diffuse persistent staining on angiography due to slow cerebral drainage

A-115   Cerebral Hemiatrophy

1. Idiopathic
2. Chronic seizures
3. Dyke-Davidoff-Masson syndrome
4. Slow-growing cerebral neoplasms with Wallerian degeneration

A-116   Pearls in the Diagnosis of Arachnoid Cyst

1. Location: Middle fossa, retrocerebellar, parietal, suprasellar, quadrigeminal plate
2. Homogeneous water-like signal, hypointense on T1 and very hyperintense on T2 (Remember that pulsation in the cyst may create the false impression of a nodule inside)
3. There should be no evidence of intra-axial edema
4. The margins of the lesion are smooth, sharp and straight, particularly in the middle fossa cysts along the posterior margin
5. Suprasellar cysts are oval or square in shape, splay the cerebral peduncles and carotid termini, and push the mamillary body upward and posterior
6. Differential diagnosis
    a. Epidermoid: Hypointense T1, mixed hyperintense T2, does not match CSF fluid
    b. Ependymal- or nonependymal-lined cyst: Intra-axial
    c. Craniopharyngioma: Mixed T1 and T2 signal, variable hyperintense fat
    d. Dermoid tumor: Hyperintense T1 & T2
    e. Cystic glioma: Hypointense T1, hyperintense T2, intra-axial with surrounding edema

A-117   Arachnoid Cysts: Presentations

Middle Fossa Cysts

1. Seizures
2. Headaches
3. Hemiparesis

Suprasellar Cysts with Hydrocephalus

1. Intracranial hypertension
2. Craniomegaly
3. Developmental delay
4. Visual loss
5. Precocious puberty
6. Bobble-head doll syndrome

Diffuse Supra- or Infratentorial Cysts with Hydrocephalus

1. Intracranial hypertension
2. Craniomegaly
3. Developmental delay

* Adapted from Greenberg MS. Handbook of Neurosurgery, p 133. Greenberg Graphics, Lakeland, Florida. 1991.

A-118   Sylvian Fissure Cysts on CT*

Type I   Small, biconvex, located in the anterior temporal tip, no mass
              effect, communicates with subarachnoid space on water-soluble
              CT cisternogram (WS-CTC)

Type II   Involves proximal and intermediate segments of Sylvian fissure
              (complete open insula given rectangular shape), partial communi-
              cation on WS-CTC

Type III   Involves entire Sylvian fissure, marked midline shift, bony expan-
              sion of middle fossa, elevation of lesser wing of sphenoid, outward
              expansion of squamous temporal bone, minimal communication
              on WS-CTC; surgical treatment usually does not result in total re-
              expansion of brain (may approach Type II lesion)

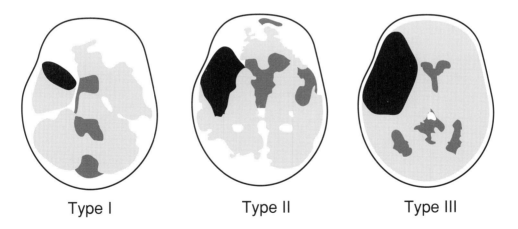

Type I   Type II   Type III

Fig. A-118.1

* Adapted from Greenberg MS. Handbook of Neurosurgery, p 134. Lakeland, Florida, Greenberg
Graphics, 1991.

A-119   Chiari Type I-II Malformations on MR*

Finding	Type I	Type II
Caudal displacement of medulla	Unusual	Yes
Caudal displacement of inferior vermis	No	Yes
Spina bifida (myelomeningocele)	May be present	Rarely absent
Hydrocephalus	May be absent	Rarely absent
Medullary kink	Absent	Present 55%
Course of upper cervical nerves	Usually normal	Usually cephalad
Age of presentation	Young adult	Infancy
Presentation	Cervical pain	Progressive hydro-cephalus, respiratory distress

* Adapted from Greenberg MS. Handbook of Neurosurgery, p 134. Lakeland, Florida, Greenberg Graphics, 1991.

A-120   Arnold-Chiari (Chiari II) Malformation on CT & MR*

Primary Findings

1. "Z" bend deformity of medulla †
2. Cerebellar peg
3. Tectal fusion
4. Enlarged massa intermedia
5. Elongation or cervicalization of medulla
6. Low attachment of tentorium
7. Agenesis or dysgenesis of corpus callosum †

Associated Findings

1. Hydrocephalus
2. Syringomyelia
3. Trapped fourth ventricle
4. Cerebellomedullary compression

* Adapted from Greenberg MS. Handbook of Neurosurgery, p 144. Lakeland, Florida, Greenberg Graphics, 1991.
† Best appreciated on MR

A-121   Pearls in the Diagnosis of Chiari Malformation

1. Chiari I: Ectopia with or without cyst formation
2. Chiari II (Arnold-Chiari): Caudal displacement of the fourth ventricle, peg-shaped and fused tonsils, craniocervical junction anomalies such as Klippel-Feil, ± meningocele
3. Chiari III-IV: Cerebellar hypoplasia or occipital encephalocele

A-122   Childhood Diseases of the Basal Ganglia

Acute

    Hypoxia

    Hypoglycemia

    Carbon monoxide poisoning

    Hemolytic-uremic syndrome

    Osmotic myelinolysis

    Encephalitis

Chronic

Inborn Errors of Metabolism

    Leigh's disease

    MELAS

    Glutaric acidemia Type II

    Methylmalonic acidemia

    Maple syrup urine disease

    Wilson's disease

Degenerative diseases

    Juvenile Huntington's chorea

    Sequelae of acute insults

    Basal ganglia calcification

Dysmyelinating diseases

    Canavan's disease

    Metachromatic leukodystrophy

Other

Neurofibromatosis Type I

Hallevorden-Spatz disease

* Adapted from Ho VB, Fitz CR, Chuang SH, et al. Bilateral Basal Ganglia Lesions: Pediatric Differential Considerations. RadioGraphics 13:273, 1993.

CATEGORY A: THE BRAIN

Section 8: Supratentorial Neoplasia   Page

A-123   Pearls in the Diagnosis of Partial Complex Temporal Lobe Epilepsy

1. Lesions are usually located in the temporal lobe
2. Coronal imaging is key
3. 50% to 75% have anatomic lesions
4. As many as 50% may have parahippocampal sclerosis (mesial temporal sclerosis/gliosis)
5. 10% cured with resection
6. 65% improve following surgery
7. 95-100% have an abnormal positron emission tomography (PET) scan showing temporal lobe hypometabolism
8. Most common MR in patients with first-time seizures is normal (second most common is parahippocampal atrophy and third most common is mesial temporal gliosis)

A-124   Paraneoplastic Syndromes Affecting the Nervous System*

Cerebrum or Cerebellum

1. Encephalitis
2. Limbic encephalitis
3. Pan-cerebellar degeneration[†‡]
4. Opsoclonus-myoclonus[†]

Spinal Cord

1. Poliomyelitis
2. Subacute necrotizing myelitis
3. Ganglionitis[†]

Peripheral Nervous System

1. Chronic sensory-motor
2. Pure sensory
3. Pure motor (rare, nearly always due to lymphoma, primarily Hodgkin's)
4. Guillain-Barré
5. Eaton-Lambert myasthenic syndrome[†]
6. Myasthenia gravis
7. Polymyositis[†]
8. Type II-b muscle fiber atrophy

* Adapted from Greenberg MS. Handbook of Neurosurgery, p 100. Lakeland, Florida, Greenberg Graphics, 1991.

† In patients without a previous history, work-up for occult malignancy has a high yield.

‡ The most common primary neoplasms in pan-cerebellar degeneration are shown in the table below.

Women	Men
Ovarian cancer	Lung cancer
Breast cancer	Hodgkin's lymphoma
Uterine cancer	
Hodgkin's lymphoma	

A-125   Leptomeningeal Enhancement & Thickening*

Focal

1. Leptomeningeal carcinomatosis (e.g., breast, lung, melanoma): Lumpy
2. Lymphoma: Lumpy or smooth
3. Meningitis: Smooth
4. Postoperative scarring: Smooth
5. Subjacent acute infarction (pial collaterals): Smooth

Diffuse

1. Leptomeningeal carcinomatosis (breast, lung, melanoma): Lumpy
2. Meningitis (bacterial [common]; fungal and viral [rare]): Smooth
3. Post radiation: Smooth
4. Post shunt: Smooth
5. Post subarachnoid hemorrhage: Smooth
6. Post surgery: Smooth
7. Post trauma: Smooth
8. Sarcoidosis: Lumpy or smooth

* Adapted from Reeder MM, Bradley WG. Reeder and Felson's Gamuts in Radiology: Comprehensive Lists of Roentgen Differential Diagnosis, p 629. New York, Springer-Verlag, 1993.

A-126   The Dura on MR

Nonenhancing Hypointensity

1.   Calcified meningioma

2.   Dense calcification

3.   Melanoma metastasis

4.   Ossification due to prominent inner table

5.   Post traumatic siderosis

Enhancing Lesion*

1.   Benign meningeal fibrosis (following shunt, subarachnoid hemorrhage or surgery)

2.   Dural metastasis (e.g., neuroblastoma)

3.   Local tumor spread (e.g., from glioblastoma)

4.   Meningioma

5.   Normal (especially at high field with high dose gadolinium)

* Adapted from Reeder MM, Bradley WG. Reeder and Felson's Gamuts in Radiology: Comprehensive Lists of Roentgen Differential Diagnosis, p 629. New York, Springer-Verlag, 1993.

A-127 Imaging Dural Masses*

Abscess/Empyema

CT: Low attenuation extra-axial mass, variable rim enhancement, sinusitis usual

MR: Slightly hyperintense to CSF on T1, bright on T2, marked rim enhancement

Angiography: Avascular mass, possible early draining veins

Comments: Fevers, headaches, meningismus, history of sinusitis or surgery

Postoperative Fibrosis

CT: Craniotomy defects, dural abnormalities usually not seen

MR: Thickened, enhancing dura subjacent to a craniotomy site

Angiography: No angiographic findings

Comments: History of previous surgery

Hemangiopericytoma

CT: Lobulated, intense homogeneous enhancement, bone erosion, may have narrow dural attachment

MR: Intratumoral signal voids

Angiography: Multiple irregular feeding vessels

Comments: Includes most tumors previously identified as angioblastic meningioma

Capillary Hemangioma

CT: Slightly hyperdense mass with intense enhancement

MR: Hyperintense on T2, intense enhancement, draining veins

Angiography: Enlarged meningeal feeders, intense staining, lobular architecture

Comments: Infants or very young children

Hematoma

CT: Mass of increased or diminished attenuation, convex or concave inner border, enhancing wall or membranes in chronic stages

MR: Signal intensity function of age, subacute-chronic bright on T1 (almost specific)

Angiography: Avascular mass

Comments: History of trauma or acute onset of severe headache

A-127   Imaging Dural Masses (Cont'd)

Meningioma

CT: Round, convex or flat dural mass, intense contrast enhancement, bone changes common (hyperostosis, erosion)

MR: Iso- or hypointense to gray on T1, highly variable signal intensity on T2, intense enhancement, "dural tail" sign usually present, cerebral edema often present

Angiography: Supplied by meningeal vessels with occasional pial recruitment, radial pattern of arterial feeders, dense staining persists late into venous phase

Comments: The most common meningeal neoplasm, usually middle aged females

Metastasis

CT: Enhancing dural mass, adjacent bone destruction common

MR: Slightly brighter than CSF on T1, intense enhancement

Angiography: Usually hypovascular

Comments: Miliary seeding more common than isolated mass

Pachymeningitis

CT: Thickened, enhancing tentorium or other dural regions

MR: Hypointense dural thickening with marked enhancement

Angiography: Narrowing of dural sinuses or carotid siphon

Comments: Headaches, cranial nerve deficits, elevated sed rate

Vascular Malformation

CT: Enhancing round or tubular structures, adjacent hematoma or subarachnoid hemorrhage, calcifications often present

MR: Signal voids, areas of hemorrhage

Angiography: Arteriovenous shunting, enlarged feeding vessels and draining veins

Comments: Acute onset of severe headache, may present with seizures

* Modified from Willing. Capillary Hemangioma, AJNR 14:534, 1993.

A-128   Signs of Meningioma

1.   Iso- or hypointensity on T2 images

2.   Inward white matter buckling

3.   Speckled T2 signal hyperintensity (microcyst formation)

4.   Focal T2 hypointensity (macrocalcifications)

5.   Prominent circumferential flow void (hypervascularity)

6.   Cisternal widening

7.   Calvarial hypointense T1 and T2 (sclerosis) or hyperintense T2 (edema or hyperemia)

8.   Pseudocapsule formation due to desmoplasia or fibrosis, displaced dura, CSF, and vessels

9.   Variable edema (edema can be pronounced)

10.   En plaque variant, ridge

    a.   Wraps around structures especially basilar skull vessels

    b.   Aggressive

    c.   Propensity for sphenoidal ridge

    d.   Fibrovascular histology more common

A-129   Intraventricular Tumors by Location*

Third Ventricle

Colloid cyst

Craniopharyngioma

Astrocytoma

Teratoma

Choroid plexus papilloma

Cysticercosis

Dermoid

AVM

Fourth Ventricle

Medulloblastoma

Ependymoma

Epidermoid

Cysticercosis

Astrocytoma

Subependymoma

Choroid plexus papilloma (adults)

Lateral Ventricle: Atrium

Meningioma

Astrocytoma

Choroid plexus papilloma

Choroid plexus carcinoma

Arachnoid cyst

Ependymal cyst

A-129   Intraventricular Tumors by Location (Cont'd)

Lateral Ventricle: Body

Ependymoma

Choroid plexus papilloma

Choroid plexus carcinoma

Ependymal cyst

AVM

Lateral Ventricle: Frontal Horn

Astrocytoma

Meningioma

Subependymoma

Dermoid

* Adapted from Greenberg MS. Handbook of Neurosurgery, p 178. Lakeland, Florida, Greenberg Graphics, 1991.

A-130   Pearls in the Diagnosis of Metastatic Disease

Hemorrhagic Metastases*

1. Choriocarcinoma: 90-95%
2. Melanoma: 85%
3. Hypernephroma: 65%
4. Thyroid carcinoma: 55%
5. Lung carcinoma: 15%
6. Breast carcinoma: 10%
7. Alimentary tract carcinoma: 5-10%
8. Other: Less than 5%

Subtypes With a Lower Propensity Toward Brain Metastases

1. Squamous cell carcinoma
2. Sarcoma

Primary Brain Tumors Which May Metastasize Peripherally

1. Medulloblastoma
2. Cerebellar sarcoma
3. Glioblastoma multiforme

Subependymal or Intraventricular Tumor Spread

1. Melanoma
2. Lymphoma
3. Breast carcinoma
4. Lung carcinoma

Leptomeningeal or Dural Carcinomatosis

1. Breast carcinoma
2. Lung carcinoma (adenocarcinoma)
3. Melanoma
4. Lymphoma

A-130   Pearls in the Diagnosis of Metastatic Disease [Cont'd]

Brain Metastases Without Edema
1.   Squamous cell carcinoma

Cystic Metastases
1.   Lung carcinoma (oat cell)
2.   Radiated metastases†

Isointense Metastases
1.   Metastatic colon carcinoma (70%)
2.   Prostate carcinoma (60%)
3.   Osteogenic sarcoma
4.   Melanoma (30%)

Pure Cortical Metastases
1.   Melanoma
2.   Choriocarcinoma
3.   Lung carcinoma

Intraventricular Choroidal Metastases
1.   Lung carcinoma
2.   Colon carcinoma
3.   Breast carcinoma
4.   Melanoma

* Hemorrhagic metastases are listed in the order of the frequency of their propensity to hemorrhage. For instance, choriocarcinoma is the metastasis which most often hemorrhages; however, hemorrhagic metastases from lung or breast carcinoma occur more often since the prevalence of metastatic disease from these entities is higher. The incidence of hemorrhage in metastatic disease increases dramatically after irradiation regardless of cell type. Other predisposing factors to hemorrhagic metastases include large lesions, rapid growth, coagulopathy, hyperintension, and chemotherapy.

† Radiated metastases, particularly in the brain stem, may undergo degeneration.

A-131   Complex Partial Seizures

Common

1. Normal MRI (50%)
2. Mesial temporal sclerosis (gliosis) (6%), hyperintense N(h) and T2
3. Temporal lobe dilation, unilateral (6%)
4. Cerebellar atrophy (4%)
5. Cerebral atrophy (3%)

Uncommon

1. Neoplasms with temporal lobe predilection
    a. Ganglioglioma
    b. Oligodendroglioma
    c. Glioma
    d. Benign and juvenile fibrillary astrocytoma
2. Thrombosed arteriovenous malformation (hypointense hemosiderin on T2)
3. Cavernous malformation

Rare

1. Cerebral hemiatrophy
2. Sturge-Weber: Gyriform peripheral signal enhancement
3. Tuberous sclerosis: Subependymal T2 hypointensity, subcortical T2 hyperintensity
4. Lacunar infarction
5. Other vascular malformations

A-132   Classification of Glioma Grade

Major Criteria of High-grade Tumor

1. Mass effect
2. Necrosis (hypointense T1, hyperintense T2)

Minor Criteria of High-grade Tumor

1. Hemorrhage (hyperintense T1)
2. Poorly defined border
3. Crosses the midline
4. Extensive edema
5. Extensive irregular enhancement*

A-133   Pearls in the Diagnosis of Oligodendroglioma

1. Peak age: 30-50 years
2. Calcification: 80%
3. Cyst formation: 10%
4. Edema: 50%
5. Location: Frontotemporal centrum
6. Hemorrhage: 80-90%
7. Margins: Poorly defined, therefore, all areas of T2 relaxation prolongation should be radiated
8. Enhancement: Moderate and inhomogeneous
9. Differential diagnosis
    a. Meningioma (pseudocapsule, extra-axial)
    b. Ganglioglioma (males, temporal lobe and anterior third ventricle predilection)
    c. Calcified glioma (less infiltrative, more mass effect, less calcification)
    d. Arteriovenous malformation (hypointense flow void signal, T2 dependent hemosiderin)

* Absence of enhancement does occur with high-grade tumors.

A-134   Pearls in the Diagnosis of Subependymoma

1.   Location: 75% infratentorial, 25% supratentorial (lateral ventricle or septum pel-
      lucidum)
2.   Often asymptomatic and smaller than ependymoma
3.   Not associated with edema, invasion or hydrocephalus
4.   Intermediate T1 signal, hyperintense T2 signal
5.   Polypoid oval or rounded shape

A-135   Pearls in the Diagnosis of Choroid Plexus Papilloma

1. Peak age: 2-10 years

2. Gender: Slight male predominance

3. Location

   a. Adults: Fourth ventricle most common

   b. Pediatric: Left lateral ventricular trigone and third ventricle most common

4. Signal: Intermediate T1, hyperintense T2

5. Malignant choroid plexus tumor (signs): Glomus displacement, parenchymal brain edema, glomus invasion, mixed necrosis or hemorrhage

6. Hydrocephalus or unilateral hydrocephalus (45%) due to

   a. Cerebrospinal fluid overproduction

   b. Intermittent hemorrhage

7. Enhancement: Moderate to marked homogeneous

8. Calcification: 5%

9. Differential diagnosis

   a. Meningioma (lower T2 signal, hypointense pseudocapsule)

   b. Choroid plexus xanthogranuloma (cystlike signal, no hydrocephalus, no enhancement)

   c. Ependymoma or subependymoma (no hydrocephalus)

   d. Arteriovenous malformation, cavernous angioma or hemangioma (hypointense flow void, hypointense T2 dependent hemosiderin, inhomogeneous enhancement)

   e. Cavernous hemangioma: Intermediate T1, hyperintense T2, central enhancement, hemosiderin rim

A-136   Pearls in the Diagnosis of Ganglioglioma

1. Age: 15-30 years
2. Gender: Slight male predominance
3. Location: Temporal lobe or anterosuperior third ventricle
4. Signal: Nonspecific hypointense T1 and hyperintense T2
5. Enhancement: Variable and nominal to moderate
6. Cyst formation: 10%
7. Hemorrhage: Rare
8. Calcification: 10-20%
9. Insidious seizure history and lesion in the correct location are tipoffs to diagnosis
10. Differential diagnosis
    a. Oligodendroglioma: More edema
    b. Vascular malformation: Less mass effect, no edema, flow void, hemosiderin
    c. Colloid cyst: Smaller size, hyperintense T1

A-137   Spectrum of Intracranial Ganglionic Tumors

1. Gangliocytoma: A hamartoma with neuronal but no glial elements and no cystic or calcified mass, cerebellum or temporal location
2. Ganglioglioma: Mildly undifferentiated neuronal cells, nominal T1 and T2 relaxation prolongation, no edema
3. Ganglioneuroblastoma: Undifferentiated neuronal cells
4. Anaplastic ganglioglioma: Undifferentiated neural and glial cells
5. Neuroblastoma: Markedly undifferentiated neural cell, forms cysts, calcified, hemorrhagic, pediatric age group

A-138   Summary of Nonastrocytic Glial Neoplasms

1. Oligodendroglioma
   a. 89% calcified
   b. Hypointense T2 signal is variable due to calcification
   c. Hemorrhagic tendency
   d. 50% associated with moderate to marked edema
   e. Cerebrospinal fluid seeding may occur
   f. Propensity for the frontotemporal centrum
   g. Small areas should be radiated that exhibit edema since tumor can be present in any of these hyperintense foci

2. Giant cell astrocytoma
   a. History of tuberous sclerosis with peripheral hypointense T1 and hyperintense T2 tubers (the tubers may be subtle hyperintense edema)
   b. Subependymal hypointense T2* calcification
   c. Lesion or mass in the foramen of Monro which may be infiltrative or cystic and has calcification and solid components

3. Ganglioma
   a. Anterior third ventricle or temporal lobe propensity
   b. 30% of patients are less than 30 years old
   c. 20% may calcify
   d. Long-standing history of chronic seizures
   e. T1 and T2 relaxation prolongation
   f. Lesion may dedifferentiate into neuroblastoma or glial neoplasm
   g. Lower grades of ganglioglioma represent hamartomas and are sometimes referred to as gangliocytoma (when very mature, ganglion and glial cells that do not appear neoplastic are present)

A-138   Summary of Nonastrocytic Glial Neoplasms (Cont'd)

4. Choroid plexus tumors
    a. Males greater than females
    b. Supratentorial tumor in children
    c. Predilection for the left ventricular trigone and third ventricle in children, fourth ventricle in adults
    d. Hydrocephalus due to recurrent hemorrhage or CSF overproduction
    e. Invasion of surrounding tissue = malignancy
    f. Displaced choroid plexus glomera = malignancy

5. Ependymoma
    a. 5-10% of intracranial tumors, and 5% of all gliomas
    b. 60% infratentorial and 40% supratentorial
    c. Mean age of incidence is 5-7 years, with a second peak at 34 years (the actual childhood peak is in the first two years of life)
    d. Male predominance of 1.7:1 is present for ependymoblastoma (considered a subset of PNET tumor)
    e. Signal intensity is mixed, inhomogeneous, hypointense on T1 with foci of hyperintense hemorrhage and inhomogeneous hyperintensity on T2 (lesions generally enhance)
    f. Location includes floor and roof of the fourth ventricle, but usually filling out the entire ventricle with exophytic extension to valleculae, foramina of Luschka and CP angle
    g. Supratentorial ependymoma is more often malignant than its posterior fossa counterpart (50% may be malignant)
    h. Epithelial, papillary and cellular histologic types all have a similar prognosis
    i. Cystic ependymoma with calcification is seen in 44%
    j. Supratentorial meningioma has a greater tendency toward cyst formation

A-139   Pearls in the Diagnosis of Primary & Secondary Brain Lymphoma

1. Location
    a. Deep white and gray matter (70%)
    b. Leptomeningeal signal: Intermediate T1 and isointense to hyperintense T2 (30%)
2. Enhancement: Marked
3. Margin: Sharply marginated intra-axial lesions which may be large, and round or oval in shape
4. Edema: Mild to moderate
5. Cyst formation: Extremely rare
6. Hemorrhage: Extremely rare
7. Calcification: Rare
8. Multiplicity: Extremely common
9. Tipoff: Clinical history of immunosuppression or AIDS

A-140   Criteria & Signs of Colloid Cyst

Criteria

1. Most anterosuperior third ventricle location
2. Size < 1.5 centimeters
3. No or nominal contrast enhancement

Indirect Signs

1. Intermittent hydrocephalus
2. Paramagnetic

A-141   Appearance of Colloid Cysts by Signal Intensity

1. Paramagnetic type, most common (60%): Hyperintense T1, hypointense T2, peripheral hyperintense T2 rim*
2. Cystic type, uncommon (20%): Hypointense T1, hyperintense T2
3. Isointense type, rare (10%): Isointense T1 and isointense or minimally hyperintense T2
4. Mixed type, rare (less than 10%): Hyperintense T1, isointense T2

* Fluid levels with T2 hypointensity layering dependently are seen in 30-40% of cases.

A-142   Pearls in MR Diagnosis of Colloid Cysts

1. Signal intensity similar to hemorrhagic cysts or cystic craniopharyngioma
2. Paramagnetic type, most frequent
3. Most anterosuperior third ventricle location
4. Intermittent hydrocephalus
5. Minimal enhancement on CEMR
6. Internal constituents include calcium, magnesium, copper, iron, manganese, and sodium
7. Rare in the pediatric population
8. May simulate melanoma metastases

A-143   Intracranial Neuroectodermal Neoplasms

1. Medulloblastoma
2. Neuroblastoma
3. Pineoblastoma
4. Ependymoblastoma
5. Medulloepithelioma
6. Spongioblastoma
7. Ganglioneuroblastoma

A-144   Pearls in the Diagnosis of Arachnoid Cyst

1. Location: Extra-axial
    a. Middle cranial fossa, peritemporal
    b. Cerebral convexity
    c. Posterior fossa, retrocerebellar
    d. Suprasellar
    e. Quadrigeminal plate cistern
2. Signal: Matches ventricular nonpulsatile CSF
3. Enhancement: None
4. Margin: Sharp with moderate to marked mass effect
5. Edema: None
6. Cyst formation: Always
7. Hemorrhage: Extremely rare
8. Calcification: Extremely rare
9. Multiplicity: Rare
10. Tipoffs: Straight posterior margin of middle fossa cyst with hypoplasia or mass effect on temporal lobe and bulging temporal calvarium
11. Differential diagnosis
    a. Ependymal and nonependymal-lined cysts: Intra-axial
    b. Dermoid: Hyperintense T1 & T2
    c. Teratoma: Calcification, not simple water signal, mixed T1 hyperintensity
    d. Craniopharyngioma: Calcification, hyperintense T1, not simple water, mixed T2 signal
    e. Cystic glioma: Intra-axial, mild edema
    f. Parasitic cyst: Not simple water, calcified, often intra-axial, enhances

A-145   Suprasellar Arachnoid Cyst Versus Third Ventricular Enlargement

1. MR criteria
    a. Water signal, homogeneous low on T1 and high on T2
    b. Stalk displacement common
    c. Mass effect
2. Key differential diagnoses include aqueductal stenosis with ballooned third ventricle or cystic pituitary adenoma (signal of cystic adenoma does not exactly match CSF)
3. Tipoffs to the diagnosis of arachnoid cyst
    a. Oval or square suprasellar cistern
    b. Cistern eccentricity
    c. Splayed peduncles
    d. Splayed carotid termini
    e. Splayed trigeminal and crural cistern
    f. Anterior displacement of the chiasm and posterior displacement of mamillary body
    g. Diamond-shaped third ventricle
    h. Pseudo third ventricle which is too big and represents the cyst rather than the ventricle

A-146   Intracranial Cysts on MR*

1.   Arachnoid cyst: Extra-axial, no edema, non-enhancing

2.   Cystic neoplasm (low tumor density): Edema, enhances

3.   Chronic subdural hematoma or hygroma: Extra-axial

4.   Suprasellar cyst from dilated third ventricle

5.   Interhemispheric cyst from porencephaly

6.   Posterior fossa cyst form of Dandy-Walker malformation

7.   Enlarged cisterna magna

8.   Post-infarct cystic encephalomalacia

9.   Cysts associated with isodense tumors

   a. Ganglioma: May calcify

   b. Cerebellar hemangioblastoma

   c. Cystic astrocytoma: Enhancing nodule

10.   Cysticercosis: Calcification

* Adapted from Greenberg MS. Handbook of Neurosurgery, p 172. Lakeland, Florida, Greenberg Graphics, 1991.

A-147   Pineal Masses by Signal, Sex, Other

Males

Common

1.   Germinoma: Hypointense T1, mildly hyperintense T2, enhances, elevated HCG, may seed CSF

Uncommon

1.   Teratoma: Mixed signal with fat (hyperintense T1, hypointense T2), may calcify (T2 hypointense), and contain cysts (hypointense T1, hyperintense T2)
2.   Teratocarcinoma: Hypointense T1, hyperintense T2, elevated alpha-fetoprotein

Females

Common

1.   Pineocytoma: Iso- or hypointense T1, iso- or hyperintense T2, calcifies, enhances

Uncommon

1.   Pineoblastoma: Hypointense T1, hyperintense T2, enhances but does not calcify, large size, invasive
2.   Falcotentorial meningioma: Iso- or hypointense T1; iso-, hypo-, or hyperintense T2; inhomogeneous; calcifies, enhances

A-147   Pineal Masses by Signal, Sex, Other [cont'd]

Males or Females

Very Common

1.   Pineal cyst: Homogeneous cyst signal (hypointense T1, hyperintense T2), does not enhance or calcify, usually < 2 cm

Uncommon

1.   Metastases (breast, lung, choriocarcinoma, melanoma): Isointense T1, hyperintense T2, enhances

Rare

1.   Pineal glioma: Mildly hypointense T1, mild to moderately hyperintense T2, rare calcification, variable enhancement

2.   Choriocarcinoma: Hemorrhagic signal common (hyperintense T1, hypo- or hyperintense T2), enhances, marked HCG elevation, may seed CSF

3.   Embryonal cell carcinoma: Hypointense T1, hyperintense T2, enhances, mild HCG elevation

4.   Trilateral retinoblastoma: Hyperintense T1, hypointense T2, history of prior ocular retinoblastoma

A-148   Summary of Germ Cell Neoplasm & Inclusion Phenomena

1. Dermoid
    a. Often midline
    b. White-white differential diagnosis, hyperintense T1 & T2
    c. May rupture
    d. Associated with sinus tract formation posteriorly
    e. Not associated with pineal gland location: These are teratomas!

2. Teratoma
    a. Most commonly in the peripineal region, rare around the sella
    b. Contains ectoderm, mesoderm and endoderm
    c. Frequently calcifies (hypointense T2)
    d. Intermediate signal intensity nidus
    e. May exhibit fat/fluid level
    f. Differential diagnosis
        i.   Choriocarcinoma
        ii. Teratocarcinoma
        iii. Trilateral retinoblastoma

3. Epidermoid
    a. Location: Intradiploic, middle fossa, petrous, CP angle, suprasellar, fourth ventricle, spinal subarachnoid space is rarest
    b. Lesions lateralize, have thinner walls, are serpiginous, not associated with sinus tract and rarely rupture, which distinguishes them from dermoid tumor
    c. Lesions have a Swiss cheese appearance with inhomogeneous internal architecture and long T1 and T2 relaxation (like proteinaceous water)
    d. Fat signal in less than 5%, unlike dermoid (fat signal is uniformly present)
    e. Enhancement is nominal to nonexistent
    f. Diagnosis: Dermoid tumor, cholesterol granuloma, arachnoid cyst, glioma

4. Lipoma
    a. Usually asymptomatic
    b. May involve suprasellar region, corpus callosum, quadrigeminal plate or CP angle
    c. Matches the subgaleal fat in signal intensity on all pulsing sequences

A-149   Epidermoids, Dermoids and Teratomas

Epidermoid	**Dermoid**	**Teratoma**
Lateralized or eccentric	Midline	Midline
Calvarial, middle fossa, petrous bone, CPA, 4th ventricle predilection	Subfrontal or infratemporal predilection	Pineal or peripineal predilection
Water signal	Hydrolyzed cholesterol signal	Mixed fat, water, solid signal
Hypointense T1	Hyperintense T1	Mixed hyperintense T1
Hyperintense T2	Hyperintense T2	Mixed hyperintense T2
Tumor rupture rare	Tumor rupture not rare	Tumor rupture rare
Thin walls	Thick walls	Moderately thick walls
Squamous epithelial lining with keratin, variable lipid cholesterin	Squamous epithelial lining, skin appendages, hydrolyzed cholesterol	Ectodermal, mesodermal, endodermal elements with foci of fat
No contrast enhancement	No contrast enhancement	Nominal enhancement
Irregular margins	Round margins	Round or variable margins
No edema	No edema	No edema
Calcify: 5%	Calcify: 10-20%	Calcify: 80%
No hormonal secretion	No hormonal secretion	Elevated AFP

A-150   Pearls in the Diagnosis of Epidermoidomas

1. Location: Extra-axial

   a. Intradiploic calvarium

   b. Middle fossa/temporal lobe

   c. Petrous bone or cerebellopontine angle

   d. Suprasellar

   e. Fourth ventricle

   f. Intraspinal subarachnoid space

2. Signal

   a. Proteinaceous water-like (97%)

   b. Foci of fatlike hyperintense T1 signal (4%)

3. Enhancement: None to nominal, margins only

4. Margins: Irregular, sharp

5. Edema: None

6. Cyst formation: Solid epidermoids occur in 2% of cases radiographically

7. Hemorrhage: Extremely rare

8. Calcification: 3-7%

9. Differential diagnosis

   a. Arachnoid cyst: Pure water signal, more mass effect

   b. Dermoid: Hyperintense T1 and T2

   c. Abscess: Intra-axial, associated edema

   d. Teratoma: Fat signal, cyst signal, calcification, pineal location

   e. Lipoma: Matches signal of subcutaneous fat

   f. Cystic astrocytoma: Intra-axial location

A-151   Radiation Necrosis & Recurrent Neoplasm

Radiation Necrosis   **Recurrent Neoplasm**

Hypointense T1, iso- to hyperintense   Variable T1 and T2
    T2, variable central hypointensity

Enhancement is corrugated, wavy   Masslike & nodular
    & irregular (wrinkled configuration)

Edema has a predilection for the forceps   Edema has no respect for the forceps
    major and spares the splenium of the   major or corpus callosum
    corpus callosum extending to the
    gray matter junction

Ametabolism or severe hypometabolism   Metabolism on PET usually equals or
    relative to white matter on PET   exceeds that of white matter

Appears as early as one month, usually   May recur early or late
    appears by one year

CATEGORY A: THE BRAIN

Section 9: Infratentorial Neoplasia   Page

A-152 Intracranial Signal Intensity Posterior Fossa (Water or Water-like Cysts)

Intra-axial

1. Cerebellar astrocytoma: Hemispheric, pediatric (< 10 years), eccentricity, size > 5-6 cm, intermediate signal nodule, nodule enhances on CEMR, no flow void in vascular feeders, mild edema, proteinaceous water-like signal

2. Hemangioblastoma: Hemispheric, adults (> 30 years), mild eccentricity, size < 5-6 cm, intermediate signal nodule, nodule enhances on CEMR, flow void in vascular feeders, mild edema, proteinaceous water-like signal, 10% multiple

3. Ependymal- or nonependymal-lined cyst: Mild eccentricity, size < 5-6 cm, no vascular feeders, no edema, water signal, homogeneous

Extra-axial

1. Epidermoid: Fourth ventricle or cerebellopontine angle, proteinaceous water-like signal, *Swiss cheese* inhomogeneity, no or nominal enhancement, mass effect mild, no edema

2. Arachnoid cyst: Retrocerebellar, cerebellopontine angle or quadrigeminal plate, water signal, homogeneous, no enhancement, moderate mass effect, no edema

3. Trapped fourth ventricle: Attached to the fourth ventricle, water signal, homogeneous, no enhancement, marked mass effect, no edema

A-153   Cerebellopontine Angle Masses by Signal

Common

1.   Neuroma, VIII, V or VII nerve: Iso- or hypointense T1, iso- or hyperintense T2

2.   Meningioma: Iso- or hypointense T1, iso- or hypointense T2 (inhomogeneous)

Uncommon

1.   Epidermoid: Hypointense T1, hyperintense T2 (inhomogeneous)

2.   Arachnoid cyst: Very hypointense T1, very hyperintense T2 (homogeneous)

3.   Lipoma: Hyperintense T1, hypointense T2

4.   Aneurysm or ectasia: Hyper- or hypointense T1, hyper- or hypointense T2 (lamellated signal)

5.   Exophytic brain stem or cerebellar glioma: Isointense T1, hyperintense T2

6.   Chordoma: Hypointense T1, hyperintense T2

7.   Glomus tumor: Iso- or hypointense T1, hyperintense T2 (speckled signal)

8.   Exophytic ependymoma: Hypointense T1, hyperintense T2 (inhomogeneous)

9.   Petrosal vein: Hyperintense T1 & T2

10.   Hemangioma: Iso- or hyperintense T1 & T2

A-154   Pearls in the Diagnosis of Neuromas, Acoustic & Trigeminal

Acoustic Neuroma

1. Age: Peak 40-60 years

2. Accounts for 85% of all neoplasms in the cerebellopontine angle

3. Predilection for superior vestibular branch of VIII nerve complex (60%)

4. Heredity

    a. Neurofibromatosis, detectable on chromosome 6

    b. Familial bilateral acoustic neuromas not associated with neurofibromatosis

5. Less than 5%

6. Enhancement: Relatively homogeneous, moderate to marked

7. Intermediate T1, intermediate to hyperintense T2

8. Cyst formation: 5%

9. Shape: Round or ovoid

10. Differential diagnosis

    a. Meningioma: Flat dural margin, intermediate T2 signal, more pronounced homogeneous enhancement

    b. Epidermoidoma: Only late hearing loss, proteinaceous cyst signal, nominal enhancement

    c. Vertebrobasilar dolichoectasia: Flow void signal, brain stem & vascular kinking

    d. Exophytic glioma (intra-axial origin)

    e. Glomus tumor with upward extension (speckled flow void signal, involves jugular bulb)

    f. Arachnoid cyst: Pure water signal

A-154   Pearls in the Diagnosis of Neuromas, Acoustic & Trigeminal [cont'd]

Trigeminal Neuroma

1. Peak age: 30-40 years
2. Second most common intracranial neuroma
3. 50% arise from the gasserian ganglion
4. 50% arise from extradural middle fossa masses
5. 25% arise from the trigeminal root ganglion and appear from the intradural CP angle
6. 25% involve both the middle and posterior fossa angle, called the *straddling neuroma*
7. Female predilection
8. Differential diagnosis is primarily meningioma which has the following features
   a. More pronounced enhancement
   b. A dural margin and *dovetail* enhancement
   c. Less pronounced facial hyperesthesia, corneal anesthesia or hyperesthesia
9. Tipoff: Any solid enhancing mass straddling the middle and posterior fossa with ticlike symptoms

A-155   Cerebellar Astrocytoma & Hemangioblastoma

Astrocytoma
1. Peak age: 3-8 years
2. Proteinaceous cyst signal: Hypointense T1, hyperintense T2
3. Associated intermediate signal nodule on T1 and T2 with moderate enhancement
4. Size greater than 6 cm with cerebellar eccentricity
5. Daughter nodules or cysts may occur
6. Wall of the cyst may enhance (40%)
7. Hypovascular: No punctate foci of flow void
8. Calcification may occur (20%)
9. Hydrocephalus moderately common (40%)
10. Rare association with Turcot syndrome
11. Multiplicity rare
12. May be associated with erythropoietin secretion and polycythemia (5%)

Hemangioblastoma
1. Peak age: 30-50 years (rare less than 30 years unless associated with Hippel-Lindau disease)
2. Proteinaceous cyst signal: Hypointense T1, hyperintense T2
3. Associated intermediate signal nodule with marked enhancement
4. Size less than 6 cm with paravermian location
5. Daughter nodules or cysts rare
6. Wall of the cyst may occasionally enhance (10%)
7. Multiple pinpoint foci of flow void due to hypervascularity
8. Calcification rare
9. Hydrocephalus uncommon (less than 10%)
10. Not uncommonly associated with Hippel-Lindau disease
11. Multiplicity common with Hippel-Lindau disease
12. Primary tumor hormone secretion does not occur but may be associated with hypertension or polycythemia secondary to pheochromocytoma or renal cell carcinoma in Hippel-Lindau disease (5%)

A-156   Pearls in the Diagnosis of Hemangioblastoma

1. 7% of infratentorial tumors

2. This is a tumor of adults rather than children, and is extremely rare under the age of 30

3. 20% have Hippel-Lindau disease, and 5% of these are multiple

4. Associated findings in Hippel-Lindau disease include retinal angioma, pheochromocytoma, renal cell carcinoma, and cysts of the pancreas, lung, epididymis, liver, and kidney

5. 60-70% of lesions are cystic, with the internal constituents consisting of a gelatinous and hemorrhagic material

6. MR appearance
   a. Hypointense T1 and hyperintense T2 with intermediate signal-enhancing nodule
   b. The nodule abuts the pial surface, and cystic nodules are rare
   c. Tipoff to the diagnosis is punctate hyperintense foci of flow void due to hypervascularity, as well as the fact that the lesions occur in adults and tend to be smaller than cerebellar astrocytomas

7. Diagnosis includes ependymal- or nonependymal-lined cyst, cerebellar astrocytoma, and arachnoid cyst

A-157   Pearls in the Diagnosis of Medulloblastoma & Ependymoma

Medulloblastoma

1.   Peak age: 3-5 years

2.   Origin: Roof of the fourth ventricle, inferior medullary velum

3.   Exophytic growth unusual

4.   Signal: Intermediate or mildly hyperintense T2

5.   Hemorrhage: Uncommon; therefore, foci of T1 hypointensity are uncommon

6.   Enhancement: Moderate and homogeneous

7.   Cysts: Rare to uncommon (punctate hypointense T2 microcyst uncommon)

8.   Plane of demarcation from the floor of the fourth ventricle

9.   Parenchymal/hemispheric medulloblastoma (cerebellar sarcoma): Uncommon

10. Subarachnoid tumor spread/drop metastases: 20%

11. Hyperintense pseudocapsule on N(h): 45%

12. Calcification: 10%

13. May metastasize outside the craniospinal axis (sclerotic metastases to bone)

Ependymoma

1.   Peak age: 4-5 years

2.   Origin: Intraventricular fourth ventricle

3.   Exophytic growth common involving valleculae, CP angle & cisterna magna

4.   Signal: Hyperintense inhomogeneous T2 intensity

5.   Hemorrhage: Common foci of T1 hyperintensity, hemorrhagic predilection in myxopapillary form

6.   Enhancement: Marked and inhomogeneous

7.   Cyst formation: Common punctate foci of T2 hyperintense microcyst formation

8.   Poor plane of demarcation from the floor of the fourth ventricle

9.   Parenchymal ependymoma: Rare but ependymoblastoma has a supratentorial predilection, may form a cast of the ventricle and invade the brain parenchyma

10. Subarachnoid tumor spread/drop metastases: 35%

11. No pseudocapsule seen

12. Calcification: 50%

13. No metastases outside the craniospinal axis

A-158   Range of Normal Anteroposterior Brain Stem Diameters

1.   Midbrain tegmentum: 11-15 mm
2.   Pons: 24-29 mm
3.   Pontomedullary junction: 14-17 mm
4.   Cervicomedullary junction: 8-11 mm

A-159   Pearls in the Diagnosis of Brain Stem Gliomas

1.   Peak age: 6-8 years
2.   Signal: Hyperintense on T2 (95%), exophytic tumor produces brighter signal
3.   Growth patterns
      a. Cystic tectum (20%)
      b. Infiltrative, pons (70%)
4.   Dedifferentiation of glioblastoma multiforme 5-7% of pediatric cases
5.   Location
      a. Pontomedullary (80%)
      b. Midbrain (60%)
      c. Cerebellum (40%)
      d. Cervical cord (35%)
      e. Posterior thalamus (30%)
6.   Enhancement: Variable and may not be present
7.   Calcification: Less than 4%
8.   Differential diagnosis
      a. Vascular malformation (flow void or hemorrhage signal, non-expansile)
      b. Metastases (adults with history of primary neoplasm, contrast enhancement)

A-160   Pearls in the Diagnosis of Glomus Tumor

1.   Age: 30-50 years
2.   Signal
     a.   Intermediate T1, hyperintense T2
     b.   Punctate speckled salt and pepper areas pinpoint flow void due to hypervascularity
3.   Location
     a.   Jugular foramen (50-60%) = glomus jugulare
     b.   Tympanic branch or Jacobson's nerve, glomus tympanicum (20-30%)
     c.   Auricular branch or Arnold's nerve, glomus vagale (10%)
     d.   Periganglia cells of the carotid bifurcation = glomus caroticum (less than 10%)
4.   Female predilection
5.   Multiplicity (10%) particularly with multiple endocrine adenomatosis (3%)
6.   Eight percent harbor other neoplasms
7.   Most common primary middle ear neoplasm
8.   Second most common temporal bone neoplasm
9.   Enhancement: pronounced, early, mottled
10.   Associated thrombosis or flow phenomenon in the jugular vein
11.   Shape: Triangular shape in the coronal projection
12.   Differential diagnosis
     a.   Neuroma: No punctate flow void, more rounded shape
     b.   Meningioma: Flat dural margin, homogeneous enhancement, wraparound vessels with infiltrative growth pattern
     c.   Normal slow flow in jugular vein

A-161   Pearls in the Diagnosis of Chordoma

1. Age: 30-40 years
2. Location
    a. Sacrum 50%
    b. Clivus 30%
    c. Cervical (C2) 20%
3. Intermediate T1 signal, mottled hyperintense T2 signal
4. Calcification 30-50%
5. Enhancement: None to mild
6. Shape: Cauliflower-like shape in the C2 and clival regions
7. Tipoffs: Cauliflower-shaped or exophytic mass involving intervertebral disc (sacrum) or straddling the clivus or C2 anteriorly and posteriorly in the sagittal projection

CATEGORY B: THE SPINE

Page

B-1 **Abnormal Disc Protrusions: Dictation Suggestions & Descriptions**

1. Tear in the annular fibrosis
   a. May be hyperintense on T2 or gradient echo, may enhance with contrast
   b. In the axial projection, a small beaklike interruption in the posterior disc margin, usually hyperintense
   c. Protrusions that are not contained are associated with annular tears
2. Disc bulge
   a. Diffuse contour alteration of disc space in the axial view, but no focal protrusion is noted
   b. Seen in the axial projection protruding diffusely
   c. Determine if there is neural compromise or significant canal stenosis (encroaching on the thecal sac)
   d. Seriousness of protrusion: If the spinal canal is small, protrusion encroaches on nerve roots in the thecal sac (clumping) or cord and there is correlation with patient's symptoms, protrusion is deemed significant
   e. If a diffuse protrusion is covered by bone, it is a spondylitic protrusion or bony bar, not a disc bulge
3. Focal soft disc abnormalities (protrusions)
   a. Subligamentous protrusion is the equivalent of "subligamentous herniation"
   b. When dictating, you may choose to describe this as "a disc herniation of the subligamentous protrusion type"
   c. In the axial plane, the protrusion is relatively central, not inordinately large and has a broad base
   d. On single sagittal slice, the diffuse disc protrusion and focal disc protrusion are nearly indistinguishable
   e. On serial sagittal slices, the remainder of the slices will be normal in patients with the focal disc protrusion but will persist on multiple sections for the diffuse protrusion or bulge

B-1   Abnormal Disc Protrusions: Dictation Suggestions & Descriptions (Cont'd)

4.   Focal soft disc abnormality (disc extrusions)

   a.   Broad pedicle disc extrusion (herniation of the transligamentous extrusion type) is differentiated from subligamentous protrusion by the pinching in of the disc material by the PLL which may leave the disc with a broad sagittal pedicle, narrow pedicle or no pedicle at all

   b.   No hypointense line covering the disc since the PLL is interrupted

   c.   In the axial projection, this transligamentous extrusion is often eccentric and is larger in size than the more central subligamentous protrusion

5.   Disc extrusion (narrow pedicle)

   a.   Produces a waist, the disc has a mushroom appearance

   b.   Intermediate signal on T1, may be hyperintense on T2, STIR or field echo

   c.   In the axial plane, it often appears larger and is eccentric in location

   d.   Sagittal projection best to determine pedicular thickness

6.   Disc sequestration or free fragment

   a.   No pedicle (free fragment)

   b.   Frequently hyperintense on gradient echo and T2 spin echo (perhaps related to edema), sometimes hyperintense on T1 due to hemorrhage

   c.   In the axial projection, the lesion is completely detached from the parent disc space

7.   Disc sequestration and migration

   a.   A transligamentous disc herniation without communication may migrate cranially or caudally (best seen on sagittal images)

   b.   In the axial projection, a section at the level of the pedicle shows a mass in the center of the spinal canal demonstrating that this material has migrated away from its disc space

   c.   Sequestrations may be very hyperintense on gradient echo sequences

Note: High grade herniations are not as bright on T2 fast spin echo sequences as they are on field echo or gradient echo.

**B-1   Abnormal Disc Protrusions: Dictation Suggestions &
                    Descriptions (Cont'd)**

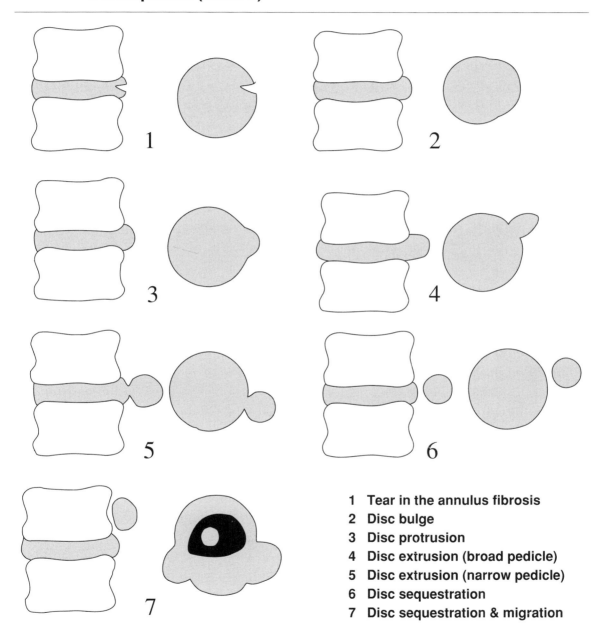

1   Tear in the annulus fibrosis
2   Disc bulge
3   Disc protrusion
4   Disc extrusion (broad pedicle)
5   Disc extrusion (narrow pedicle)
6   Disc sequestration
7   Disc sequestration & migration

Fig. B-1.1

B-2   Nomenclature for Describing Disc Disease on MR

1.   Protrusion or herniation: An anatomic term that describes the position of one structure relative to another and can imply the presence of a contour abnormality related to disc or bone

     a.   Spondylotic protrusion: Spur or calcific bony bar extending off posterior vertebral body or disc margin

     b.   Subligamentous protrusion: A focal contour alteration of the retrodiscal space that is intermediate in signal on T1, slightly hyperintense on T2 or fast scan gradient echo imaging, hugs the posterior vertebral body margin in the axial projection and has a broad stalk or area of communication to the parent disc space

     c.   Diffuse protrusion (another name for diffuse annular bulge)

2.   Annular bulge: A diffuse protrusion or contour alteration of the parent disc space with a smooth rounded appearance which may extend posteriorly or anteriorly

3.   Annular rent: Rip or tear in the annulus fibrosis that appears as an area of slight hyperintensity on T2 or gradient echo fast scan imaging and may enhance in linear fashion with administration of contrast material

4.   Hard disc: A wastebasket term that usually refers to disc disease of the cervical spine which appears calcified (hypointense on T2 or gradient echo fast scan, covered by bone in the sagittal projection on fast scan imaging) and includes true focal spur (or broad bony bar) or calcified disc fragment that adheres to the posterior disc margin, since the two may be indistinguishable

5.   Bony bar: Another term for spondylotic protrusion, usually broad-based and extending across the anterior spinal canal

B-2   Nomenclature for Describing Disc Disease on MR (Cont'd)

6.   Disc broad extrusion: A focal contour alteration of the retrodiscal space that is polypoid in shape and appears to be pinched by the posterior longitudinal ligament through which it extends

   a.   Simple extrusion: Extrusion or transligamentous disc herniation that has a broad stalk or attachment to the parent disc space

   b.   Narrow pedicle extrusion: Transligamentous herniation with a narrow stalk of attachment to the parent disc space

   c.   Sequestration or free fragment: An isolated extrusion that no longer communicates with the parent disc space, i.e., there is no stalk

   d.   Migrated free fragment or migrated sequestration: Extrusion without communication to the parent disc space that has extended cranially, caudally, or posteriorly from the retrodiscal space*

* Most sequestered discs, whether they are migrated or not, exhibit hyperintensity on gradient echo fast scan imaging, T2 and occasionally on T1. At times, a sequestrated disc fragment may migrate under the posterior longitudinal ligament.

B-3   Grading System of Focal Soft Disc Disease*

Grade   **Description**

I   Contour alteration of the disc space with a broad pedicle = sub-
            ligamentous protrusion or broad pedicle transligamentous extru-
            sion

II   Contour alteration of the disc space with a narrow pedicle = nar-
            row pedicle extrusion

III   Intermediate signal mass without communication or pedicle to the
            parent disc space = disc sequestration or free fragment

IV   Intermediate signal mass that does not communicate with the par-
            ent disc space and extends above or below = migrated sequestra-
            tion or free fragment

* Soft disc disease refers to disc protrusions that are not calcified or covered by bone above or below. It
  may be focal as in protrusion or extrusion, or diffuse as in annular bulge.

B-4   Signs of Pseudodiscs

1.   Spondylolisthesis: Disc does not herniate posterior to vertebral body below in the sagittal plane

2.   Conjoined nerve root: Bifurcates from parent root, hyperintense T2 signal due to CSF sheath

3.   Pantopaque: Bright T1, dark T2 signal or invisible on MR (check plain film!)

4.   Spur: Hypointense T2 or fast scan, covers disc in the sagittal plane

5.   Spontaneous epidural hemorrhage: Hyperintense T1, mixed intensity T2, posterior location

6.   Synovial cyst: Slightly hyper- or hypointense T1, hyperintense T2, centered about the posterior facet joint

7.   Epidural abscess: Flat shape, hyperintense T2 disc, edema in anterior and posterior longitudinal ligaments, rim enhancement

8.   Ossification of posterior longitudinal ligament: Linear hypointensity

9.   Epidural veins: Linear, tubular or longitudinal shape in the sagittal plane, nominal mass effect, flow-related signal increase or decrease

10.   Epidural scar: Enhances, not contiguous with parent disc, surgical history

11.   Diastematomyelia: Hypointense spur, two hemisacs or cords

B-5   **Pseudodiscs on MR: Signal Comparison**

	T1	**T2**
Bony spurs, diastematomyelia	hypointense	hypointense
Spondylolisthesis	hypointense	hypointense
PLL calcification	hypointense	slightly hyperintense
Conjoined nerve root *	hypointense	slightly hyperintense
Neuroma	iso- or hypointense	hyperintense
Root cyst	hypointense	hyperintense
Sequestered vacuum phenomenon	signal void	signal void
Pantopaque	hyperintense	hypointense
Abscess	hypointense	hyperintense
Epidural veins	iso- or hyperintense	hyperintense

* One nerve root can have a larger nerve root sleeve producing more pronounced hyperintensity on T2 or gradient echo so this nerve root becomes brighter than the surrounding nerve roots and can be mistaken for a neuroma. Conversely, the conjoined nerve root sleeve can become devoid of water creating confusion with a more hypo- or isointense signal than the surrounding nerve roots.

B-6   **Pearls in the Diagnosis of Synovial Cyst**

1.   Diagnosed by posterior location

2.   Iso- or hyperintense T1 with enhancing rim

3.   Hyperintense, well-marginated T2 with hypointense peripheral rim

4.   Facet arthropathy frequently present and/or fluid

5.   May occasionally protrude posteriorly (may produce a pitfall simulating a soft tissue mass), unilateral or bilateral

6.   Mass aligned directly with the facet joint which demonstrates mild hyperintensity, and the base of the mass appears to sit against the facet interface

7.   Bright signal on T1 (25%) related to proteinaceous and sometimes blood-tinged material that fills these cysts

8.   At surgery, when facet and laminar take-down occurs, the cyst may be accidentally ruptured and will not be seen during surgery

9.   Multiple areas of nerve root clumping due to associated arachnoiditis can be present

B-7   Lumbar Facet Joint Capsules: Types

Ventral Joint

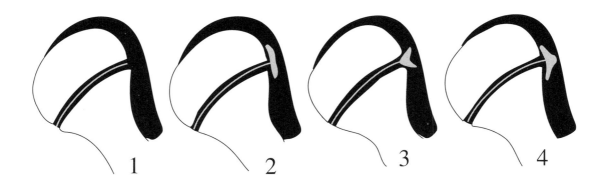

Dorsal Joint

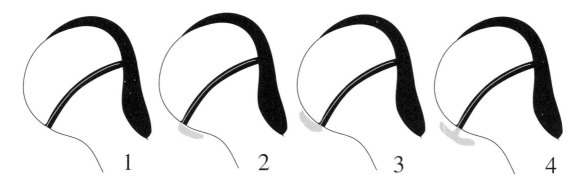

* Xu GL, Haughton VM, Carrera GF. Lumbar Facet Joint Capsule: Appearance at MR Imaging and CT. Radiology 177:415, 1990.

B-8   Pearls in the Diagnosis of Spondylolisthesis

Subtypes of Spondylolisthesis

2. Iatrogenic (surgery, especially facetectomy)

3. Traumatic (thoracocervical)

4. Degenerative (no associated pars defect, but rather severe apophyseal disease)

5. Isthmic (pars): Spondylolisthesis associated with spondylolysis

    a. The portion of the articular process that links the articular pillar with the facet joint is known as the pars interarticularis

    b. Most important in the lower lumbar spine where the inferior pars interarticularis is separated in patients with spondylolysis (usually at L5-S1)

    c. This allows anterior displacement of L5 on S1 (spondylolisthesis) with consequent distortion of disc and thecal sac

    d. Sagittal or sagittal oblique images best suited for foraminal evaluation

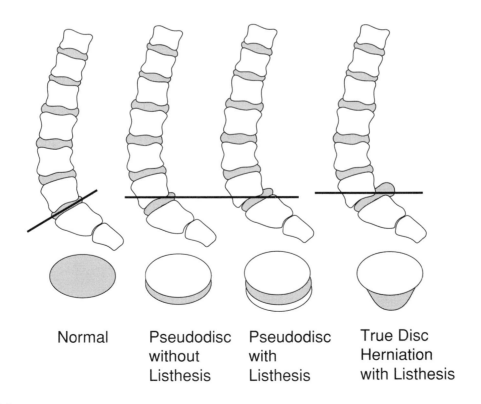

Normal   Pseudodisc   Pseudodisc   True Disc
                  without   with   Herniation
                  Listhesis   Listhesis   with Listhesis

Fig. B-8.1

B-9   Hard Disc on MR

1. Protrusion: Descriptive term (how one structure protrudes relative to another)
2. Focal spondylitic protrusion = spur (if hard in nature)
3. Diffuse spondylitic protrusion = bar (if hard in nature)
4. Hard disc = spur, bar or calcified disc extension (a former disc herniation that has subsequently calcified)
5. On CT, the calcified disc herniation may be impossible to differentiate from a spur or bar but this can be done on sagittal MR

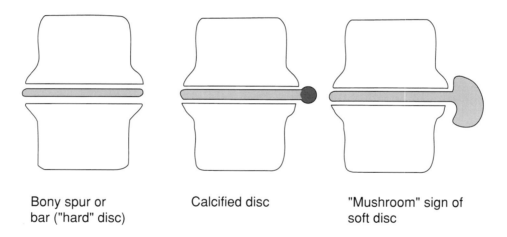

Bony spur or   Calcified disc   "Mushroom" sign of
bar ("hard" disc)   soft disc

Fig. B-9.1

B-10   Soft Disc Disease on MR

1. Diffuse disc protrusions which are concentric are called "bulges"
2. Associated with these bulges may be small tears in the annulus fibrosis called rents
3. Protrusions that occur without annular rents are sometimes referred to as "contained"
4. More focal protrusions
    a. Subligamentous: Central, flat, broad base (sometimes called "contained," but this is not a preferred term)
    b. Transligamentous: Called "extrusion" (extruded through the posterior longitudinal)
5. Herniation: An "old" term still useful because it is understood by clinicians (so we may say herniation of the subligamentous protrusion type or transligamentous extrusion type)

B-11   Postoperative Granulation Tissue Versus Disc Reprolapse*

Disc Reprolapse	Scar
Polypoid shape	Globular shape
Usually communicates with parent disc unless sequestered	Separated from disc by hypointense band when imaging after 16-18 weeks postop
Free fragment or sequestered disc may be hyperintense on T2 with mass effect but disc usually less intense than scar on T2	Tumefactive granulation tissue or scar is usually hyperintense on T2 but may have positive or negative mass effect
Inhomogeneous peripheral rim, delayed with central nonenhancement	Profound homogeneous enhancement within 6-8 minutes
Increase in conspicuity with increased T2 weighting	Decrease in conspicuity with increased T2 weighting
Positive mass effect	Positive or negative (retraction) mass effect

* Until 12-16 weeks after surgery, the native disc space may appear edematous and protrude posteriorly either diffusely or focally. This usually subsides between 16-18 weeks after surgery. A hypointense cleft or line due to repair of the PLL and adjacent complex will separate granulation tissue from the parent disc space after 12-16 weeks postoperative. Before this time, no hypointense cleft may be present to differentiate disc reprolapse versus granulation tissue.

B-12 **Postoperative Neural Enhancement & MR Contrast Agents in the Spine***

Epidural Enhancement

1. Immediate
2. Persists from months to years
3. Peaks at 5-15 minutes after injection
4. Enhancement wanes between 40-60 minutes after injection

Dural Enhancement

1. Immediate
2. Persists from months to years
3. Peaks 5-10 minutes after injection
4. Wanes 40-60 minutes after injection

Pial Enhancement

1. Immediate
2. Persists up to 6-8 months (enhancement wanes and eventually disappears in normal asymptomatic patients by one year)
3. Peaks 5-10 minutes after injection
4. Wanes 40-60 minutes after injection

Nerve Root Enhancement

1. Immediate after surgery
2. Persists 6-8 months (persistent root enhancement after 6 months is abnormal and is seen in patients with radiculopathic symptoms)
3. Peaks 5-10 minutes after injection (but is visible immediately after injection)
4. Wanes 40-60 minutes after injection

Any enhancement of the pia or nerve roots is abnormal after 6 months

* Adapted from Ginkins JR, Osborn AG, Garrett D, et al. Spinal Nerve Enhancement with Gd-DTPA MR: Correlation with Postoperative Lumbar Spine. AJNR 14:383-394, 1993.

B-13   Root Enhancement on MR

1. Postoperative (should decrease by six months in normal patients)
2. Arachnoiditis
3. Drop metastasis
4. Lymphoma
5. Guillain-Barré
6. Sarcoidosis
7. Mycobacterial infection
8. Fungal disease (coccidiomycosis, cryptococcosis, etc.)
9. Parasitic (angylostrongyloides, etc.)

B-14   **Disc & Vertebral Signal in Degenerative Disc Disease (DDD)**

Disc Degeneration

Type I   Isointense T1, hyperintense T2, normal disc volume

Type II   Isointense T1, iso- to hypointense T2, normal disc volume, nuclear cleft

Type III   Isointense T1, hypointense T2, decreased volume, nuclear cleft

Vertebral Body Signal: Linear Endplate Patterns of DDD

1.   Hypointense T1, hyperintense T2 = edema phase

2.   Hyperintense T1, mildly hyperintense T2 = fat phase

3.   Hypointense T1, hypointense T2 = sclerotic phase (on plain film)

Central Pattern of Vertebral Body Marrow Change

1.   Hyperintense bright T1 signal at the center of each vertebral body

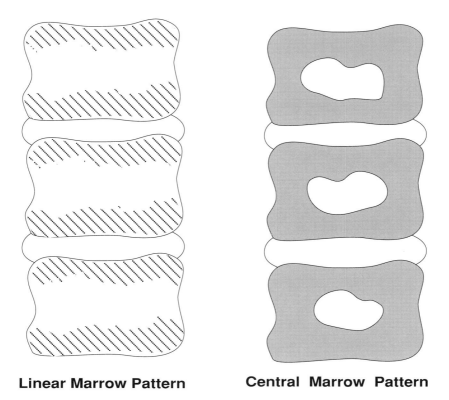

Linear Marrow Pattern   **Central Marrow Pattern**

Fig. B-14.1

B-15   Linear Retrovertebral Extra-axial Hypointensity

Common

1.   CSF pulsation flow void
2.   Thickening or ossification of the posterior longitudinal ligament
3.   Epidural fat (hypointense on T2 only)

Uncommon

1.   Thickened dura
2.   Longitudinal spur
3.   Calcified meningioma
4.   Arteriovenous malformation
5.   Hemosiderin (remote hemorrhage)
6.   Flow void in epidural vein

B-16   Criteria for Arachnoiditis

Direct Signs

1.   Centrally clumped nerve roots: Pseudocord sign

2.   Roots adherent to dural tube periphery: Empty cord sign

3.   Thickened or enlarged nerve roots: Giant root sign

Indirect Signs

1.   Bizarre flow phenomena

2.   Mixed signal with intrathecal Pantopaque (hyperintense T1)

3.   Tumefactive enhancing masses

4.   Multiple intrathecal and extradural masses ("dripping candle wax" sign)

Axial View of the Thecal Sac in Arachnoiditis

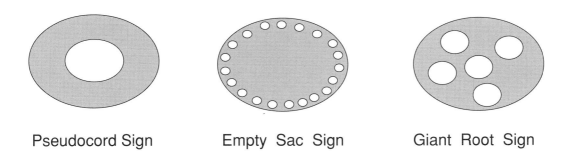

Pseudocord Sign   Empty Sac Sign   Giant Root Sign

Fig B-16.1

B-17   **Criteria for Discovertebral Osteomyelitis**

1. Hypointense T1 disc edema involving > 50% of vertebral body volume
2. Edema has a linear pattern of vertebral involvement
3. Decreased or increased disc volume with hyperintense disc signal
4. Thickening and signal alteration in the anterior longitudinal ligament (ALL)
5. Thickening of the posterior longitudinal ligament with or without epidural soft tissue mass

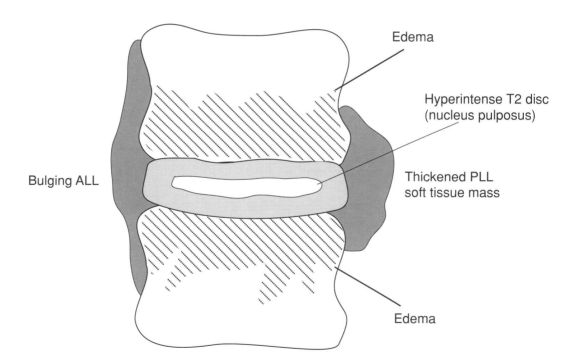

Fig. B-17.1

B-18   Pitfalls in MRI of the Spine

Pseudosyringes

1.   Averaging of central gray matter
2.   Gibb's truncation or edge-ringing phenomenon
3.   Volume averaging of the parasagittal vertebral artery

Flow Phenomena

1.   Simulating thoracic spinal arteriovenous malformation (CSF flow void)
2.   Simulating hemorrhage or mass (CSF slice entry effect)
3.   Simulating posterior spinal mass (CSF loculated by denticulate ligaments)
4.   Simulating low lying cord or conus (slice entry phenomenon in the lumbar spine)

Bright Spots in Vertebral Bodies

1.   Axial focal fat deposition
2.   Type II vertebral endplate (fat signal)
3.   Hahn's notch (slice entry or in-plane flow phenomenon [basivertebral vein])
4.   Hemangioma
5.   Lipoma

Extraskeletal Bright Signal

1.   Pantopaque
2.   Epidural lipomatosis
3.   Filum lipomatosis

Pseudotumors: See Gamut B-20
Pseudodiscs: See Gamut B-4

B-19   Diffuse Vertebral Marrow Signal Patterns

White Marrow (T1)

1.   Radiated marrow

2.   Aplastic anemia

3.   Other causes of marrow aplasia

Gray Marrow (T1)

1.   Normal aged fibrous marrow

2.   Peripheral hemolysis with increased red marrow overproduction

3.   Primary marrow overproduction (polycythemia vera)

4.   Myelophthistic marrow replacement (Gaucher's, leukemia, myeloma)

5.   Diffuse nonsclerotic metastases

6.   Myeloid metaplasia

Black Marrow (T1)

1.   Sclerotic metastases (breast, prostate, etc.)

2.   Osteopetrosis

3.   Myeloid metaplasia (myelofibrosis)

4.   Sarcoidosis

B-20   Cervical Pseudotumors

Common

1.   Arthropathy secondary to degenerative disc disease, rheumatoid arthritis or craniocervical junction anomaly

Uncommon

1.   Bony spur of diastematomyelia
2.   Spontaneous epidural hematoma
3.   Epidural lipomatosis
4.   Gouty tophi
5.   Villonodular synovitis
6.   Tumoral form of calcium pyrophosphate deposition disease
7.   Os odontoideum
8.   Giant intradural disc fragment
9.   Synovial cyst
10. Elastofibroma

B-21   Cervical Arthropathic Pseudotumor MR Criteria

1.   Mass encircling C2 dens spares the clival medullary bone
2.   Iso- or hypointense T1 and T2 signal intensity
3.   Negligible enhancement
4.   Follows the synovial distribution around the dens, and C1-2 joint interface
5.   No intradural involvement
6.   Mass may involve atlantodental interval (ADI)

B-22   Neoplastic & Non-neoplastic Wedge Compression Fractures

Neoplastic Wedge Compression
1. Multiple rounded, oblique or angled hypointense vertebral body foci on T1 in medullary bone
2. Lesion multiplicity with other levels of vertebral involvement
3. Skip areas with intervening normal vertebral bodies
4. Epidural lesion exhibiting intermediate T1 and T2 signal (soft tissue) and enhancement

Non-neoplastic Wedge Compression
1. Linear hypointense T1 and hyperintense T2 signal abutting the endplate (the edema fracture line)
2. Epidural mass, if present, is hyperintense on T1 (medullary bone) or hypointense on T1 and T2 (cortical bone) and nominal in extent
3. Usually single or clustered multilevel involvement without skip areas

B-23   Criteria for Non-neoplastic Compression Fractures

1. Linear hypo- or hyperintense T1 signal at the endplate
2. Linear hyperintense T2 signal at the endplate
3. Normal pedicle signal
4. No soft tissue mass
5. Anterior and posterior vertebral body margins are concave inward, not outward
6. *Middle column sign:* Sparing of signal alteration in the posterior one-third of vertebral body and pedicle (middle column)

B-24   Common Spinal Masses by Signal

Intramedullary

1. Ependymoma: Mixed T1, inhomogenous hyperintense T2

2. Astrocytoma: Iso- or hypointense T1, iso- to hyperintense T2

3. Hemangioblastoma: Hypointense T1, hyperintense T2 (cyst formation, serpiginous or punctate flow void from vascular feeders)

4. Metastases: Isointense T1, iso- to hyperintense T2 (gray nodule with edema)

Intradural

1. Meningioma: Isointense T1, iso-, hypo-, or hyperintense T2

2. Neurinoma: Isointense T1, hyperintense T2

3. Neurofibroma: Isointense T1, mixed hyperintensity T2

4. Lipoma: Hyperintense T1, hypointense T2 (central fibrous hypointensity)

5. Metastases: Isointense T1, iso- to hyperintense T2

Extradural

1. Metastases: Hypointense T1, mild hyperintensity T2

2. Teratoma: Mixed hypo- and hyperintensity T1, mixed hyperintensity T2

3. Epidermoid: Hypointense T1, hyperintense T2

4. Lymphoma: Isointense T1, iso- to hyperintense T2

5. Lipomatosis or lipoma: Hyperintense T1, hypointense T2

Other

1. Arachnoid cyst: Marked T1 hypointensity, markedly homogeneous T2 hyperintensity

2. Chordoma: Heterogeneous T1 isointensity, mixed T2 hyperintensity

3. Arthropathic pseudotumor: Iso- or hypointense T1, iso- to hypointense T2

B-25   Special Diagnostic Features of Spinal Neoplasms

Intramedullary

1. Ependymoma: Hemorrhage (esp. myxopapillary form), conus predilection, cyst formation
2. Astrocytoma: Cervicothoracic, expansile, occasional cyst formation
3. Hemangioblastoma: Cyst formation, flow void from vascular feeders
4. Metastases: Lung, breast, melanoma, primary neoplasms, edema, mass effect

Intradural

1. Meningioma: Flat dural margin, marked enhancement, cervicothoracic
2. Neurinoma: Lumbar, round shape, anterolateral
3. Neurofibroma: Central hypointense fibrous area, neurofibromatosis history
4. Lipoma: Matches fat signal
5. Metastases: History of germinoma, glioblastoma, lymphoma, medulloblastoma, ependymoma, etc.; round shape; multiplicity

Extradural

1. Metastases: Bone lesions, hypointense on T1
2. Teratoma: Fat and cyst signal, calcifies, sinus tract
3. Epidermoid: History of trauma or myelography, proteinaceous water signal, irregular shape
4. Lymphoma: Insinuates and infiltrates foramina, homogeneous, bulky, relative bone sparing
5. Lipomatosis or lipoma: Matches fat signal, associated dysraphism with lipoma

Other

1. Arachnoid cyst: Water signal intensity, expansile, intra- or extradural
2. Chordoma: Cauliflower shape, sacrum and C2 predilection
3. Pseudotumor: Low signal, follows synovium at C-2 interface, history of arthropathy

B-26   Spinal Meningioma & Neural Tumor on MR

Meningioma	Neural Tumor
Sessile with a flat dural margin	Round without a flat dural margin
Broad based and flat	Narrow dural base and round
Enhances profoundly and early with contrast	Enhances profoundly with contrast
More common posterolateral	More common anterolateral
May grow en plaque, an aggressive variant	May grow invasively, a plexiform aggressive variant
Thoracic location more common than cervical	Lumbar or conus region location more common than thoracic or cervical
T2 signal may be iso-, hyper- or hypointense Metastasis extremely rare except fibro-vascular atypical variety	Usually hyperintense Metastasis rare except undifferentiated sarcomatous variety
Less frequent association with neurofibromatosis	More frequent association with neurofibromatosis
Good prognosis for removal unless heavily calcified	Good prognosis for removal

B-27   Pearls in the Diagnosis of Spinal Astrocytoma

1. Thoracic location more common than cervical
    a. Astrocytoma is still the most common primary intramedullary malignant neoplasm of the cervical cord
    b. Ependymoma has a propensity for the lower thoracic and lumbar cord or conus
2. Poorly defined
3. Enhancement is variable but usually occurs less than six minutes after contrast administration
4. Hypointense T1 signal and hyperintense T2 signal
5. T2 signal hyperintensity is variable and mild to moderate
6. Lesion is cigar-shaped
7. On T1, patients who have myelitis may have a normal MR other than mild cord enlargement (and T2 is usually posterior lateral without mass effect in myelitis)
8. Patients with astrocytoma usually demonstrate discrete cord signal alteration
9. Myelitis tends to be less focal, more diffuse and more ill-defined than glioma (it may enhance, especially posterolaterally)
10. Gliosis may be extremely difficult to differentiate from glioma (usually there is a long-standing history of neurologic deficit)
11. Gliosis produces nominal to mild enhancement at best and usually associated with syrinx formation, scar formation or focal atrophy

B-28   Pearls in the Diagnosis of Ependymoma

1. Tendency to involve the filum
2. Hemorrhagic in a significant percentage of the cases, especially the myxopapillary form of the filum
3. Tendency to form cysts
   a. Marginal cysts located at the tumor edge and easily amenable to syringotomy decompression
   b. Central cysts which are located within the lesion and must be excised if they are to be treated
4. Ependymomas tend to have hypointense T1 and hyperintense T2 signal and either show cyst formation or signal inhomogeneity
5. Filum location is a strong tip-off to the diagnosis (these lesions tend to seed the CSF and may be a result of drop metastases)
6. Enhancement is moderate to marked

B-29   Pearls in the Diagnosis of Hemangioblastoma

1. Sixty percent are intramedullary; 40% are extramedullary but intradural

2. Thirty percent have Hippel-Lindau disease

3. Thoracic location in 50% and cervical location in 40%

4. Lesions are single in 80% and multiple in 20%

5. Cyst formation in 40%

6. MR findings

    a. Intermediate signal intensity nodule which enhances

    b. Speckled foci of flow void signal in and about the nodule

    c. Areas of marginal cyst formation above and below the lesion

    d. Round or ovoid shape

B-30   Pearls in the Diagnosis of Spinal Lymphoma

1. Bulky
2. Relative bone sparing
3. Insinuates itself in foramina and small spaces
4. Enhancement is not as consistent as in the brain
5. Propensity for posterior epidural spinal space
6. Homogeneous
7. May have adenopathy anteriorly

B-31   Common Presacral Masses on MR

1. Teratoma
    a. Hyperintense fat signal layers nondependently and appears hypointense on T2 (water signal layers down and is hypointense on T1 and hyperintense on T2)
    b. Calcification is common
    c. Slow layering is common and the layering direction may not coincide with supine position
2. Meningocele: Homogeneous T1 and T2 water signal with saclike communication with the subarachnoid space
3. Hematoma: Dark signal or hypointensity lies dependent on T2 when hematoma is acute at high field
4. Metastases or recurrent colonic neoplasm: Solid signal not corresponding to water and invading the adjacent bone, hypointense T1, mixed T2
5. Fibrosis: Hypointense on T1 and T2

B-32   Spine Neoplasia & Selected Masses by Contrast Enhancement

Intramedullary

1. Ependymoma: Well-marginated, marked homogeneous enhancement
2. Astrocytoma: Patchy, heterogeneous enhancement and more often eccentric compared to ependymoma
3. Hemangioblastoma: Enhancement of a rounded nodule with nonenhancing surrounding cyst
4. Cavernous hemangioma: No or nominal enhancement initially, delayed central enhancement
5. Arteriovenous malformation: Heterogeneous enhancement admixed with flow void

Extramedullary Intradural

1. Meningioma: Immediate, uniform, persistent enhancement
2. Neurinoma: Homogeneous enhancement
3. Drop metastases: Multifocal, rounded, nodular, enhancement

Extradural Lesions

1. Metastases: Variable heterogeneous enhancement
2. Arachnoiditis: Nominal to mild heterogeneous multifocal enhancement
3. Disc extrusion: Minimal or moderate rimlike enhancement
4. Meningocele: No enhancement
5. Lymphoma: Homogeneous enhancement
6. Abscess: Rim enhancement
7. Synovial cyst: Rim enhancement
8. Disc extrusion: Rim enhancement
9. Arthropathic pseudotumor: Mild diffuse enhancement

B-33   Signs of High Grade Block

Direct Signs

1. No hyperintense T2 CSF signal at the level of an extradural mass on T2 or T2 fast scan imaging
2. Extraordinarily sharp interface between cord and CSF without utilization of refocusing pulses due to dampened or reduced CSF pulsations

Indirect Signs

1. Large, dominant extradural mass corresponding to neuropathic level
2. Circumferential encasement of cord or conus with hypointense dural tube providing a plane of separation in the axial plane between cord and neoplasm

B-34   Intraspinal Sequelae of Trauma

Acute

1. Fracture with canal compromise
2. Cord contusion: Hyperintense T2, poorly defined, swollen cord
3. Cord transection
4. Hematomyelia: Acutely hypointense T2 intramedullary cord signal
5. Subdural or epidural hematoma: Mixed T1 and T2 signal hyperintensity

Chronic

1. Stenosis
2. Microcystic myelomalacia: Punctate T1 hypointensity, T2 hyperintensity
3. Atrophy
4. Macrocystic myelomalacia: Hypointense T1, hyper-/hypointense (flow void) T2
5. Cord fissure
6. Pseudotumor: Hypointense T1 and T2, surrounds dens
7. Pseudomeningocele: Marked hypointensity T1, hyperintensity T2, homogeneous
8. Epidermoid: Mixed T1 hypointensity and T2 hyperintensity, inhomogeneous

B-35   Spectrum of Cord Injury

Acute

1.   Cord transection: Complete cord discontinuity

2.   Cord maceration: Compressed, irregularly shaped ragged cord

3.   Cord contusion: Iso- or nominal T1 hypointensity and T2 hyperintensity, moderately well defined, enlarged cord

4.   Acute hematomyelia: Mild T1 hypointensity and T2 hypointensity

Chronic: Cystic Myelopathy

1.   Microcystic myelomalacia: Punctate hypointense T1 and hyperintense T2, less than 5.0 mm in size

2.   Macrocystic myelomalacia or syringohydromyelia: Homogeneous hypointense T1 and hyperintense T2 (cyst) with variable central T2 hypointensity due to flow; cord may or may not be enlarged

Chronic: Noncystic Myelopathy

1.   Gliosis or myelitis: Normal to increased cord size with mild, poorly defined T2 hyperintensity and normal T1 signal

2.   Chronic hematomyelia: Hyperintense T1 and T2 with peripheral hypointense T2 hemosiderin rim

3.   Cord fissure: Folded cord appearance with apparent intra-axial cyst that freely communicates with subarachnoid space, hyperintense T2

4.   Simple cord atrophy: Decreased cord size with normal intermediate cord signal

5.   Noncystic myelomalacia: Isointense T1, hyperintense T2, usually with small cord

B-36   **Sequelae of Extra-axial Acute Spine Trauma**

1.   Epidural masses due to disc fragments
2.   Epidural masses due to hematoma
3.   Subdural hematoma
4.   Pseudomeningocele
5.   Herniation of the cord producing pseudocysts and cord kinking or entrapment

B-37   Delayed Sequelae of Intra-axial Cord Transection

1.   Dorsal tethering: Dorsal cord position

2.   Cord atrophy, hemiatrophy

3.   Micro or macro (syrinx) cyst formation: Hypointense T1, hyperintense T2

4.   Cord fissure or maceration: Irregular cord shape

5.   Cord hernia: Bizarre cord kinking with simulation of arachnoid cyst dorsally

6.   Myelomalacia: Increased T2 cord signal inconspicuous on T1 with decreased cord size

B-38   Prognosis & Staging of Cord Injury Based on Signal

Good Prognosis

1.   Normal signal on T1 and T2

Good Prognosis (Mild Neurologic Impairment)

1.   Normal signal T1, hyperintensity T2

Mixed or Intermediate Prognosis

1.   Markedly hypointense T1 signal, markedly hyperintense T2 signal (longitudinal syrinx formation)

Poor Prognosis

1.   Hypointense T1 signal, hypointense T2 signal (acute hemorrhage 1.5T)
2.   Hyperintense T1, hyperintense T2

Class	Description
I	Normal T1 and T2
II	Normal T1, hyperintense T2
III	Mild hypointense T1, hyperintensity T2
IV	Marked T1 hypointensity, marked T2 hyperintensity (cyst formation)
V	Extensive cord atrophy
VI	Cord transection or maceration

B-39   Pearls: Acute & Hyperacute Cord Injury

1.   Hyperacute extra-axial blood, hyperintense on T2, isointense on T1

2.   Acute hematomyelia hypointense on T2, isointense on T1

3.   Dark signal in the acute phase of an injury (6-48 hours) is related to intracellular deoxyhemoglobin and methemoglobin

4.   Hyperacute lesion related to proteinaceous water-like signal, bright on T2 (and not usually hypointense on T2 until 4-6 hours following injury)

5.   Hyperacute bleed can manifest intermediate isointense T2 signal between 2 and 12 hours after bleed

B-40   Spinal Cord Atrophy

Hemiatrophy

1. Brown-Sequard syndrome: The AMF (anterior median fissure) sharply delineates the midline
2. Juvenile amyotrophy of the distal upper extremity: Rare
3. Chronic multiple sclerosis: Accentuation of surface sulci and widened AMF
4. Amyotrophic lateral sclerosis (ALS): Anterolateral flattening with a normal AMF

Anterior Atrophy

1. Anterior spinal artery syndrome: Bilateral decreased anteroposterior diameter and ventral surface flattening (bean-shaped), widened AMF
2. Cervical spondylosis: Spurs producing central flattening and cord infolding with cord beaking produced by acquired prominence of the lateral tracts
3. Amyotrophic lateral sclerosis: Anterolateral flattening due to anterior horn cell and corticospinal tract atrophy
4. Poliomyelitis: Anterior flattening with long segment stringlike cord

Posterior and Diffuse Atrophy

1. Chronic multiple sclerosis: Both diffuse atrophy and focal degeneration due to chronic plaque formation, accentuation of surface sulci and widening of AMF
2. Post-traumatic atrophy
3. Subacute combined degeneration

B-41   Normal Conus Medullaris Level by Age

1.   0–2-year-old: T12 to L2-3 (average L1-2)
2.   2–12-year-old: L2-T12 (average L1-2)
3.   Adult: L1

A conus level of termination at L2-3 or above is normal at any age

A conus level of termination at L3-4 or below is always abnormal

A conus terminating at L3 may be normal or abnormal

B-42   Findings Associated with Closed Spinal Dysraphism

1. Normal
2. Cerebellar tonsillar ectopia
3. Hydromyelia
4. Meningocele
5. Meningomyelocele
6. Lipomeningomyelocele
7. Diastematomyelia
8. Spinal and sacral bone deficiency
9. Lipoma
10. Neural placodes
11. Occipital encephalocele
12. Lacunar skull
13. Coccygeal cyst
14. Thickened filum or filum band
15. Atretic meningocele
16. Dermoid
17. Filum band
18. Dermal sinus
19. Hemangioma

B-43   Fat-Containing Lesions of the Spine

1. Lipoma: May be associated with dysraphism or isolated in the intradural cervicothoracic region (60%) or isolated in the extradural cervicothoracic region (40%)
   a. Hyperintense T1, hypointense T2
   b. Associated anomalies
      i. Filum band
      ii. Filum lipomatosis
      iii. Coccygeal cyst
      iv. Cord tethering
      v. Dysraphism
      vi. Dermoid
      vii. Sacral dimple
      viii. Meningocele
      ix. Myelomeningocele
      x. Meningocystocele

2. Epidural lipomatosis: May be asymptomatic or may produce myelopathy, can be idiopathic or associated with steroid administration or Cushing's disease

3. Filum lipomatosis: A thin band of hyperintensity along the filum terminale, rarely associated with dysraphism or symptoms

4. Dermoid: Ovoid hyperintensity on T1 and T2 with or without associated signs of dysraphism and with or without hypointense calcification

5. Teratoma: Mixed T1 and T2 signal, usually calcified, fluid-fluid levels common, sacrococcygeal location, dysraphism may not be present

B-44   Findings in Occult Spinal Dysraphism

1. Normal: (50%)

2. Isolated fatty filum terminale: Linear thin T1 hyperintensity (5%)

3. Tethered cord with thickened filum terminale: Intermediate T1 linear signal (2%)

4. Tethered cord with lipomeningocele or intradural lipoma (40%)

5. Thickened cauda equina: Enlarged intermediate signal intensity nerve roots (2%)

B-45   Pearls in the Diagnosis of Diastematomyelia

1. When this condition occurs in the cervical region, it is associated with profound neurologic deficit

2. A dysraphic abnormality consisting of a midline longitudinal cleft often associated with a bony or fibrous spur or septum

3. This cleft through the spinal cord (or conus medullaris or filum terminale) divides the cord into two hemicords

4. The clefting of the spinal cord produces two hemicords each with a central canal, one dorsal horn and one ventral horn

5. If the cord is divided with two dorsal horns and two ventral horns, it is referred to as the theoretical entity of diplomyelia (more theoretical than real)

6. The cleft often contains fibrous or osteocartilaginous material

7. The spur or septum is not always present with diastematomyelia and is not essential to the pathologic definition

8. Females:males = 8:1

9. Neurologic symptoms (present in 90% of cases) are nonspecific and may be related to other causes of cord abnormality such as tethering or associated forms of dysraphism

10. Commonly, there are cutaneous manifestations including hypertrichosis (the most common)

11. 85% of patients have associated anomalies including anomalies of the vertebral bodies, hemivertebra, butterfly vertebra, narrow disc spaces, reduced vertebral height

12. Scoliosis and kyphosis are present in almost half the patients and are directly related to associated segmental abnormalities

B-46   Pearls in the Diagnosis of Klippel-Feil Deformity

1.   Typical appearance is fusion of one or several cervical vertebra

2.   There may be marked kyphosis and hypertrophy of the posterior hypointense ligamentous structures which appear to encroach on the posterior cervical canal

3.   Typical clinical triad includes restricted range of neck motion, short neck, low hair line and low set ears (present in 50% of patients)

4.   Cervical abnormality can be seen with plain films, but MR is useful in determining the presence of associated anomalies such as Arnold-Chiari malformation, syringomyelia, hydromyelia, tethered cord, agenesis of the corpus callosum (renal abnormalities may also coexist)

5.   Cervical spine evaluations should include: Thyroid, epiglottis, pre-epiglottic space, level of the foramen magnum, position of the posterior arch and anterior button of C1, nasopharynx, tip of the clivus

B-47   Pearls in the Diagnosis of Vascular Malformations in the Spine

1. Enhancement from contrast-enhanced MR produces bright signal, flow void produces dark signal; therefore, these two signals are fighting each other
2. The key is to look for the presence of flow void on noncontrast MR
3. Large channels which are multiloculated can mimic syrinx
4. Cavernous vascular malformation associated with large channels which are dilated and may enhance with contrast or may simply present as an old calcified hemorrhage with hypointense hemosiderin
5. Not uncommon with occult dural or pial vascular malformation is Foix-Alajouanine syndrome where chronic vascular steal leads to gliosis manifested as elongated T2 hyperintensity without mass effect and clinical progressive myelopathy

CATEGORY C: THE HEAD & NECK

CATEGORY C: HEAD & NECK

C-1   **Pearls in the Diagnosis of Parathyroid Adenoma**

1. Anatomy
   a. Four glands
   b. Superior glands are dorsal and constant along the posterior thyroid above the junction of the thyroid and the recurrent laryngeal nerve
   c. Inferior glands are ventral, inferior to the junction of the inferior thyroidal artery and recurrent laryngeal nerve
   d. The inferior glands are variable in position
2. Parathyroid adenoma evaluation requires true T2 in two planes (sagittal and axial)
3. Parathyroid adenomas like pheochromocytoma produce some of the brightest signal for solid benign neoplasms on T2
4. T1 hyperintensity suggests diagnosis other than parathyroid adenoma (i.e., exophytic thyroid colloidal cyst)
5. Assure axial and sagittal views that include the tracheoesophageal groove & upper mediastinum

C-2 Normal & Abnormal Thyroid Glands

Diagnosis	Homogeneity*	Signal Intensity	
		Short TR/TE	Long TR/TE
Normal thyroid	H	⊕	⊕>⊕⊕
Focal lesions			
Follicular adenoma	I	⊕[†]	⊕⊕⊕
Hemorrhagic Cyst	H	⊕⊕	⊕⊕⊕[‡]
Cystic colloid nodule	H	⊕⊕[§]	⊕⊕⊕
Functioning nodule	H	⊕	⊕⊕
Carcinoma	I	⊕	⊕⊕⊕[‖]
Thyroglossal duct cyst	I	⊕⊕	⊕⊕⊕
Multinodular thyroid gland	I	⊕ (⊕ to ⊕⊕⊕ nodules)	⊕ to ⊕⊕ w/ mult. ⊕⊕⊕ nodules
Diffuse disorder	I		
Hashimoto thyroiditis	I	⊕–⊕⊕	⊕⊕⊕[#]
Graves disease	H	⊕⊕	⊕⊕⊕

Key

H	Homogeneous
I	Inhomogeneous
⊕	Signal similar to surrounding muscle
⊕⊕	Signal isointense to adjacent fat
⊕⊕⊕	Signal hyperintense to adjacent fat

* Gafter WB, Spritzer CE, Eisenberg B, et al. Thyroid Imaging with High-Field-Strength Surface-Coil MR. Radiology 164:484, 1987.
† Two-thirds had ⊕⊕⊕ foci due to chronic hemorrhage.
‡ Low intensity peripheral ring secondary to hemosiderin after 3 weeks.
§ Low intensity colloid cyst on short TR/TE described (3).
‖ 2/3 showed associated lymphadenopathy of similar intensity to thyroid tumor.
Linear low intensity bands (fibrosis in two-thirds).

C-3   **Pearls of Parotid Pleomorphic Adenomas (Benign Mixed Tumors)**

1. Most common salivary gland neoplasm (70-80% of benign major gland tumors)
2. 84% occur in the parotid gland
3. 90% arise in the superficial lobe lateral to the plane of the facial nerve
4. Slow-growing and painless
5. Female predominance particularly over 50 years of age
6. Round shape
7. Solitary
8. Well demarcated with homogeneous hyperintense T2 signal
9. Larger tumors are lobulated
10. Multicentricity less than 0.5%
11. Malignant degeneration
    a. Malignant mixed tumor
    b. Carcinoma ex pleomorphic adenoma
    c. Metastasizing benign mixed
12. Tipoffs to malignant degeneration
    a. Long-standing history (average 10-15 years)
    b. Pain and facial nerve paralysis
    c. Age 60 years or older
    d. Irregular bulky margins with intermediate T2 signal

C-4   Parotid Neoplasms on MR

Common

1. Benign mixed tumor (pleomorphic adenoma): Hypointense T1, hyperintense T2[a, b]

2. Mucoepidermoid low-grade carcinoma: Hypointense T1, iso- or hyperintense T2[d]

Uncommon

1. Warthin's tumor: Hypointense T1, hyperintense T2[a, c]
2. Acinar cell carcinoma: Isointense T1, iso- or mild hyperintense T2[d]
3. Squamous cell (duct) carcinoma: Isointense T1, iso- or mild hyperintense T2[d]
4. Adenocarcinoma: Isointense T1, iso- or mild hyperintense T2[d]

Rare

1. Adenocystic: Isointense T1, iso- or mild hyperintense T2[d]
2. Mucoepidermoid high-grade carcinoma: Isointense T1, iso- or mild hyperintense T2[d]

a   Sharp margin with pseudocapsule, superficial lobe > deep lobe
b   Female predilection 2:1
c   10% bilateral, 10% malignant degeneration to carcinoma ex pleomorphic adenoma
d   Poorly defined margin, no pseudocapsule

C-5   Multiple Parotid Space Masses on MR

1. Benign lymphoepithelial cysts of AIDS: Hypointense T1, hyperintense T2
2. Metastatic tumor
    a. Skin malignancy
        i.   Squamous cell carcinoma: Intermediate T1, intermediate to mildly hyper-intense T2, inhomogeneous
        ii. Melanoma: Variable hyperintense T1, variable hypo- or hyperintense T2
    b. Non-Hodgkin's lymphoma: Intermediate T1, mildly hyperintense T2, homo-geneous
3. Warthin's tumor: Intermediate T1, very hyperintense T2, homogeneous

C-6   **Parotid Space Masses on MR**

Common

1. Benign tumors
    a. Pleomorphic adenoma or benign mixed tumor: Intermediate or hypointense T1, very hyperintense T2, homogeneous
    b. Warthin's tumor or papillary cystadenoma lymphomatosum: Intermediate or hypointense T1, very hyperintense T2, homogeneous

2. Malignant tumor (metastatic)
    a. Skin squamous cell carcinoma: Intermediate T1, intermediate to mildly hyperintense T2, inhomogeneous
    b. Melanoma: Variable T1 hyperintensity, variable T2 hypo- or hyperintensity, variable homogeneity
    c. Non-Hodgkin's lymphoma: Intermediate T1, mildly hyperintense T2, homogeneous

3. Malignant tumor (primary)
    a. Mucoepidermoid carcinoma: Intermediate T1, mixed intermediate T2 hyperintensity
    b. Adenocystic carcinoma: Intermediate T1, hyperintense T2

C-6   Parotid Space Masses on MR (Cont'd)

Uncommon

1. Benign
   a. Lipoma: Hyperintense T1, hypointense T2, homogeneous
   b. Facial neuroma: Intermediate T1, hyperintense T2, occasional central hypointensity
   c. Oncocytoma: Intermediate T1, mildly hyperintense T2

2. Congenital
   a. First branchial cleft cyst: Variable but usually hypointense T1, very hyperintense T2
   b. Hemangioma, pediatric: Intermediate T1, hyperintense proton density, very hyperintense T2, well marginated
   c. Lymphangioma, pediatric: Hypointense T1, hypo- to isointense proton density, hyperintense T2, less well marginated

3. Malignant (metastatic)
   a. Abscess/cellulitis: Hyperintense T2, well or poorly defined
   b. Benign lymphoepithelial cysts of AIDS: Hypointense T1, very hyperintense T2
   c. Reactive lymphadenopathy: Intermediate T1, intermediate to mildly hyperintense T2

4. Malignant tumor (primary)
   a. Non-Hodgkin's lymphoma: Intermediate T1, intermediate to mildly hyperintense T2, homogeneous
   b. Malignant mixed tumor or carcinoma ex pleomorphic adenoma: Variable hyperintense T2
   c. Acinous cell carcinoma: Variable hyperintense T2
   d. Adenocarcinoma: Variable hyperintense T2

C-7   Parapharyngeal Space Masses on MR

Common

1. Pseudotumor of asymmetric pterygoid venous plexus: Hyperintense T2, hyperintense gradient echo, intermediate T1, enhances

2. Inflammatory disease or abscess: Intermediate T1, hyperintense T2, enhances, perilesional edema

   Abscess may spread from:

   a. Pharyngeal mucosal space: Tonsils, tonsillitis, adenoiditis

   b. Parotid space: Calculus disease

   c. Masticator space: Odontogenic inflammation

3. Benign neoplasm

   a. Pleomorphic adenoma or benign mixed tumor: Hypointense T1, very hyperintense T2, well marginated

4. Malignant neoplasm

   a. Intermediate T1, intermediate to mildly hyperintense T2

   b. Direct spread of malignant neoplasm from adjacent fascial spaces particularly pharyngeal mucosal space, intermediate T1, intermediate to mildly hyperintense T2

      i. Squamous cell carcinoma

      ii. Non-Hodgkin's lymphoma

      iii. Minor salivary gland malignancy

C-7   Parapharyngeal Space Masses on MR (Cont'd)

Uncommon

1.   Congenital

Atypical second branchial cleft cyst: Very hypointense T1, very hyperintense T2, nonenhancing

2.   Benign tumor

a.   Lipoma: Hyperintense T1, hypointense T2

b.   Neural tumors (neuroma, neurofibroma, schwannoma): Intermediate T1, hyperintense T2

3.   Malignant tumor

a.   High grade mucoepidermoid carcinoma and malignant mixed: Mixed intermediate T1 and T2

b.   Direct spread of malignant tumor from adjacent deep fascial space, especially

i.   Masticator space sarcoma

ii. Parotid space mucoepidermoid carcinoma and adenocystic carcinoma

C-8   Pharyngeal Mucosal Space Lesions on MR

1. Benign mixed tumor or pleomorphic adenoma: Hypointense T1, very hyperintense T2

2. Inflammatory
    a. Adenoidal or faucial tonsil hypertrophy: Intermediate T1, intermediate to mild hyperintense T2
    b. Adenoidal or faucial tonsillitis: Hyperintense T2
    c. Adenoidal or faucial tonsil abscess: Intermediate or hypointense T1, hyperintense T2 with or without central hypointensity
    d. Post inflammatory dystrophic calcification: Hypointense T2 or gradient echo
    e. Post inflammatory retention cyst: Variable T1, variable T2 but usually hyperintense

3. Malignant tumor
    a. Squamous cell carcinoma: Intermediate T1, intermediate to mildly hyperintense T2, heterogeneous
    b. Non-Hodgkin's lymphoma: Intermediate T1, intermediate to mildly hyperintense T2, homogeneous
    c. Minor salivary gland malignancy: Intermediate T1, mixed T2 but adenocarcinoma hyperintense

4. Thornwaldt's cyst: Intermediate to hypointense T1, hyperintense T2

5. Pseudotumor
    a. Asymmetric fossa of Rosenmüller: Isointense with contralateral fossa
    b. Mucosal inflammation from radiation-induced or infectious pharyngitis: Mildly hyperintense T2 edema

C-9   Retropharyngeal Space Masses on MR

Common

1. Inflammatory
    a. Reactive adenopathy: Intermediate T1, intermediate to mildly hyperintense T2
    b. Cellulitis: Intermediate T1, hyperintense T2
    c. Abscess: Hypointense or intermediate T1, hyperintense T2 with or without hypointense center
2. Malignant tumor
    a. Nodal metastases
        Nasopharyngeal squamous cell carcinoma: Intermediate T1, intermediate to hyperintense T2, inhomogeneous
    b. Nodal non-Hodgkin's lymphoma: Intermediate T1, intermediate to hyperintense T2, homogeneous
    c. Direct invasion from primary squamous cell carcinoma of the posterior wall: Intermediate T1, intermediate or mildly hyperintense T2, inhomogeneous

Uncommon

1. Benign tumor
    a. Lipoma: Hyperintense T1, hypointense T2, homogeneous
    b. Hemangioma: Hypo- to isointense T1, very hyperintense T2, hypointense T2, phleboliths
2. Pseudotumor
    a. Tortuous carotid artery: Usually hypointense flow void
    b. Lymphedema or phlebedema secondary to venous or lymphatic obstruction: Poorly defined hyperintense T2

C-10   Pearls in the Differential Diagnosis of Neck Cysts

1.   Sialocele:* Intra- or periparotid location

2.   Thyroglossal duct cyst: Elliptical

3.   Ranula: Minor salivary gland or floor of mouth (plunging ranula/sublingual space)

4.   Hygroma: Multiloculated, neck or periscapular

5.   Branchial cleft cyst

   a.   First arch: Communicates with external auditory canal

   b.   Second arch: Communicates with palatine tonsil

   c.   Third arch: Communicates with pyriform sinus

   d.   Fourth arch: Communicates with subglottic esophagus

6.   Mucocele: Related to paranasal sinuses

7.   Laryngocele:† Related to pyriform sinus appendix

* Can have hyperintense T1 and T2 signal due to hemorrhage and/or protein.
† Often black signal (air-filled) on T1 and T2.

C-11   Tumor Findings: Extension Through the Foramen Ovale

1.   Homogeneous thickening of the third branch of the trigeminal nerve
2.   Concentric expansion of the foramen ovale by intermediate T1 signal
3.   Replacement of the normal hypointense trigeminal cisternal CSF signal by isointensity on T1
4.   Atrophy of the masticator muscles

C-12   Findings in Hemifacial Spasm *

1.   Vascular flow void secondary to loops or aneurysms of PICA, vertebral artery or cochlear artery
2.   Linear or rounded flow void due to prominent or anomalous veins or arteriovenous malformation
3.   T2 hyperintensity associated with cerebellopontine angle neuroma
4.   T2 isointensity associated with cerebellopontine angle meningioma

* Hemifacial spasm is related to compression of the facial nerve at the anterior caudal aspect of its root exit from the brain stem and is most commonly seen in middle-aged women on the left side.

C-13   Pearls in the Assessment of Bell's Palsy

1. Enhancement on C+ MR of the facial nerve from the labyrinthine portion to the descending canal (85%); cisternal segment enhancement is rare

2. Enhancement at the genu and just posterior to it is normal and due to venous plexus, but mild enhancement on C+ MR in the distal canalicular facial nerve (25%) is always abnormal

3. MR indicated
   a. Facial palsy greater than two months' duration
   b. Slowly progressive or worsening palsy
   c. Facial spasm
   d. Recurrent palsy
   e. Excessive pain
   f. Multiple cranial neuropathy

4. Secondary Bell's palsy etiologies
   a. Facial or acoustic neuroma
   b. Brain stem tumor
   c. Parotid malignancy
   d. Otomastoiditis or cholesteatoma
   e. Multiple sclerosis
   f. Temporal bone trauma
   g. Sarcoidosis
   h. Lyme disease
   i. Radiation therapy

5. Idiopathic Bell's palsy
   a. Most commonly caused by herpes simplex I and varicella-zoster viruses
   b. The virus usually lies dormant in the geniculate ganglion

6. Any idiopathic or viral Bell's palsy exhibits remission in 50% by one month and 70% undergo eventual complete remission

7. Bell's palsy involves the lower motor neuron of the 7th cranial nerve (hemifacial palsy includes forehead)

C-14   Enhancing Intracanalicular Masses (Less than 5 mm)

Common
1. Small acoustic neuroma
2. Vascular labyrinthine loop
3. Petrosal vein

Uncommon
1. Hemangioma
2. Tumefactive neuritis
3. Intracanalicular meningioma
4. Carcinomatosis
5. Lymphoma
6. Labyrinthine

C-15   Nasosinus Disease on MR

1. Normal nasal cycle
   a. Mucoperiosteal T1 isointensity and T2 hyperintensity limited to the nasal septum, nasal cavity and ethmoid sinuses (< 2-3 mm mucosal thickness)
   b. Frontal, maxillary and sphenoid sinuses are spared
   c. Alternating fullness of right and left turbinates during day (frequent unilateral prominence, transient)
2. True nasosinus inflammation: Isointense T1 and hyperintense T2 with frontal, maxillary or ethmoid sinus involvement (> 2-3 mm mucosal thickness)
3. Mucus retention cyst or mucocele
   a. Serous type: Hypointense T1, hyperintense T2, homogeneous
   b. Mucoid type: Hyperintense T1, hyperintense T2, homogeneous
   c. Inspissated type: Hyperintense T1, hypointense T2
4. Nasosinus polyp: Isointense T1 and hypointense center on T2, peripheral enhancement
5. Squamous cell carcinoma or other malignancy: Mixed T1 intensity, intermediate T2 isointensity, inhomogeneous enhancement
6. Rhinolith: Hypointense T1, hypointense T2
7. Fungus ball/mycetoma: Intermediate T1, hypointense T2

C-16   Lesions of Sinus Origin: Signal Intensities

Hypointense T1, Hyperintense T2

1.   Acute infection

2.   Mucus retention cyst

3.   Mucocele

4.   Lymphoma

5.   Epidermoid

Hypointense T1, Hypo- to Isointense T2, Inhomogeneous

1.   Squamous cell carcinoma/sarcoma

2.   Polyp

3.   Inverting papilloma: Central T2 hypointensity

4.   Mucus retention cyst (inspissated type)

5.   Mucocele (inspissated type)

6.   Osteoma

7.   Sinolith

8.   Fungus ball, aspergilloma

Hyperintense T1 & T2

1.   Mucocele (mucoid type)

2.   Mucus retention cyst

3.   Hemorrhage

C-17 Chronic Nasosinus Hypointensity on MR *

Lesion	T1	Proton Density	T2
Chronic secretions			
Pastelike consistency	Low	Lower than T1	Lower than proton density or signal void
Desiccated, rocklike	Signal void	Signal void	Signal void
Mycetomas			
Cheesy consistency	Low	Lower than T1	Lower than proton density or signal void
Desiccated, rocklike	Signal void	Signal void	Signal void
Acute hemorrhage	Low	Lower than T1	Lower than proton density or signal void
Air remaining in inflamed sinus	Signal void	Signal void	Signal void
Tooth in dentigerous cyst	Signal void	Signal void	Signal void

* Adapted from Som PM, Dillon WP, Curtin HD, et al. Hypointense paranasal sinus foci: differential diagnosis with MR imaging and relation to CT findings. Radiology 176:777, 1990.

C-18   Intermediate Signal Intensity in the Upper Nasal Cavity

1.   Extracranial meningioma

2.   Hyperostotic esthesioneuroblastoma

3.   Bone forming sarcoma

4.   Fibrous dysplasia*

5.   Anaplastic sarcoma*

6.   Radiation osteitis*

7.   Chronic infectious inflammation*

8.   Lymphoepithelioma*

9.   Lymphoma

10. Chloroma

11. Nasofrontal encephalocele

* May have hyperintense signal on T2 in 60% of cases

C-19   Cavernous Sinus Lesions*

1. Primary tumors (rare)

    a. Meningioma

    b. Neurinoma

    c. Aneurysm of the cavernous carotid artery

2. Tumors from adjacent areas that may extend into cavernous sinus

    a. Meningioma

    b. Neurinoma

    c. Chordoma

    d. Chondroma

    e. Chondrosarcoma

    f. Pituitary tumor

    g. Nasopharyngeal carcinoma

    h. Esthesioneuroblastoma

    i. Nasopharyngeal angiofibroma

    j. Metastatic tumor

* Modified from Greenberg MS. Handbook of Neurosurgery, p 172. Lakeland, Florida, Greenberg Graphics, 1991.

C-20   Acute Chiasmal Syndrome on MR *

Common

1.   Compression from underneath by a suprasellar neoplasm that has undergone hemorrhage

2.   Large sellar tumor (pituitary microadenoma with suprasellar extension)

Uncommon

1.   Optic glioma: Mild T2 hyperintensity

2.   Retrochiasmatic craniopharyngioma: Hyperintensity on T1 and/or T2

3.   Extensive demyelination: Hyperintensity and swelling on T2

4.   Aneurysm with rupture: Flow void with mixed T1 hyperintensity

Rare

1.   Retrochiasmatic hemorrhage or hematoma, called blue-domed cysts or blueberry infarcts: T1 hyperintensity

* Chiasmal syndrome is characterized by mental confusion, memory disturbance and visual deficit but differs from pituitary apoplexia in that endocrine and cavernous sinus symptoms are absent.

271

C-21   Differential Diagnosis of Vertigo*

1. Meniere's disease
2. Benign (paroxysmal) positional vertigo (also cupulolithiasis)
3. Disabling positional vertigo
4. Acoustic neuroma
5. Vestibular neuronitis
6. Vertebrobasilar insufficiency
7. Multiple sclerosis

* Modified from Greenberg MS. Handbook of Neurosurgery, p 293. Lakeland, Florida, Greenberg Graphics, 1991.

C-22   Malignant Tumors of the Parapharyngeal Space & Upper Neck

Paraganglioma

T1 Image: Intermediate

T2 Image: Moderately high, usually salt-and-pepper appearance except when < 1.5 cm

Contour: Smooth

Overall: Flow voids common

Calcification, Fibrosis or Bone Fragments: Sites of fibrosis

Metastatic Vascular Tumor

T1 Image: Intermediate

T2 Image: Moderately high, salt-and-pepper appearance

Contour: Irregular

Overall: Flow voids may not be as numerous as in paragangliomas

Calcification, Fibrosis or Bone Fragments: Bone fragments possible

Hemangioma

T1 Image: Intermediate

T2 Image: High

Contour: Usually smooth, irregular in some cases

Overall: Flow voids

Calcification, Fibrosis or Bone Fragments: Central calcific phleboliths

Salivary Gland Tumor

T1 Image: Intermediate

T2 Image: High

Contour: Usually smooth, irregularity may indicate high-grade malignancy

Overall: Homogeneous

Calcification, Fibrosis or Bone Fragments: Focal calcium, fibrosis

C-22   Malignant Tumors of the Parapharyngeal Space & Upper Neck (Cont'd)

Neurogenic Tumor

T1 Image: Intermediate

T2 Image: High, salt-and-papper appearance possible

Contour: Smooth

Overall: Homogeneous

Calcification, Fibrosis or Bone Fragments: Focal calcium, fibrosis

Lymphoma

T1 Image: Intermediate

T2 Image: Moderately high

Contour: Smooth

Overall: Homogeneous

Calcification, Fibrosis or Bone Fragments: Rare

Soft Tissue Sarcoma

T1 Image: Intermediate

T2 Image: Moderately high

Contour: Variable

Overall: Homogeneous

Calcification, Fibrosis or Bone Fragments: Bone fragments

Liposarcoma

T1 Image: High

T2 Image: Moderately high

Contour: Irregular

Overall: Homogeneous

Calcification, Fibrosis or Bone Fragments: Rare

C-22   Malignant Tumors of the Parapharyngeal Space & Upper Neck (Cont'd)

Chordoma

T1 Image: Variable

T2 Image: High

Contour: Smooth

Overall: Homogeneous

Calcification, Fibrosis or Bone Fragments: Focal calcium, fibrosis, bone fragments

* Adapted from Som PM, Braun IF, Shapiro MD, et al. Tumors of the Parapharyngeal Space and Upper Neck: MR Imaging Characteristics. Radiology, 164:828, 1987.

C-23   MR Appearance of Laryngeal Tissues *

Structure	T1 Images	T2 Images
Uncalcified cartilage	Intermediate	Intermediate
Calcified cartilage	Hypointense	Hypointense
Bone marrow	Hyperintense	Intermediate
Perichondrium	Hypointense	Hypointense
Pre-epiglottic body	Hyperintense	Intermediate
Tumor	Intermediate	Intermediate

* From Kikinis R, Wolfensberger M, Boesch C, et al. Larynx: MR Imaging at 2.35 T. Radiology 171:169, 1989.

C-24   Foramina & What Passes Through Them

Cribiform Plate

Location: Medial floor of anterior cranial fossa

Transmitted structures: Olfactory nerve (I), ethmoidal arteries (anterior & posterior)

Connects: Anterior fossa to superior nasal cavity

Optic Canal

Location: Lesser wing of sphenoid bone

Transmitted structures: Optic nerve (II), ophthalamic artery, subarachnoidal space, CSF & dura around optic nerve

Connects: Orbital apex to middle cranial fossa

Superior Orbital Fissure

Location: Between lesser & greater sphenoid wings

Transmitted structures: Cranial nerves III, IV, V, VI, superior ophthalmic vein

Connects: Orbit to middle cranial fossa

Foramen Rotundum

Location: Medial cranial fossa floor, inferior to superior orbital fissure

Transmitted structures: Cranial nerve V2, emissary veins, artery of the foramen rotundum

Connects: Meckel's cave to pterygopalatine fossa

Foramen Ovale

Location: Floor of middle cranial fossa, lateral to sella

Transmitted structures: Cranial nerve V3, emissary veins form cavernous sinus to pterygoid plexus, accessory meningeal branch of maxillary artery (when present)

Connects: Meckel's cave to nasopharyngeal masticator space (infratemporal fossa)

C-24   Foramina & What Passes Through Them (Cont'd)

Foramen Spinosum

Location: Posterolateral to foramen ovale

Transmitted structures: Middle meningeal artery, recurrent (meningeal) branch of mandibular nerve, middle meningeal vein

Connects: Middle cranial fossa to nasopharyngeal masticator space (infratemporal fossa)

Foramen Lacerum

Location: Base of medial pterygoid plate at petrous apex

Transmitted structures: Meningeal branches of ascending pharyngeal artery (**not** internal carotid artery), vidian nerve and vein, emissary veins

Connects: Not a true foramen, filled with fibrocartilage in life

Vidian Canal

Location: In sphenoid bone below and medial to foramen rotundum

Transmitted structures: Vidian artery and nerve

Connects: Foramen lacerum to pterygopalatine fossa

Carotid Canal

Location: Within petrous temporal bone

Transmitted structures: Internal carotid artery, sympathetic plexus

Connects: Carotid space to cavernous sinus

Jugular Foramen

Location: Posterolateral to carotid canal, between petrous temporal & occipital bones

Transmitted structures:

Pars nervosa: Inferior petrosal sinuses (cranial nerve IX and Jacobson's nerve)

Pars vascularis: Internal jugular vein cranial nerves X, XI, nerve of Arnold, small meningeal branches of ascending pharyngeal and occipital arteries

Connects: Posterior fossa to nasopharyngeal carotid space

C-24   Foramina & What Passes Through Them (Cont'd)

Stylomastoid Foramen

   Location: Behind styloid process

   Transmitted structures: Cranial nerve VII

   Connects: Parotid space to middle ear

Hypoglossal Canal

   Location: Base of occipital condyles

   Transmitted structures: Cranial nerve XII

   Connects: Foramen magnum to the nasopharyngeal carotid space

Foramen Magnum

   Location: Floor of posterior fossa

   Transmitted structures: Medulla & meninges, spinal segment of cranial nerve XI, vertebral arteries & veins, anterior & posterior spinal arteries

   Connects: Posterior fossa to cervical spinal canal

CATEGORY C: HEAD & NECK

Section 2: TMJ   Page

C-25   Grading of Meniscal Displacement on MR *

Description

Grade 0   Posterior meniscal band position lies at 12 o'clock relative to the mandibular condyle

Grade I   Anterior meniscal displacement with the posterior meniscus band lying between nine o'clock and 12 o'clock relative to the mandibular condyle

Grade II   Complete anterior meniscal displacement relative to the mandibular condyle without meniscocondylar contiguity; the meniscus has a spherical or elliptical corrugated shape

* This meniscal grading system is performed with a closed mouth view.

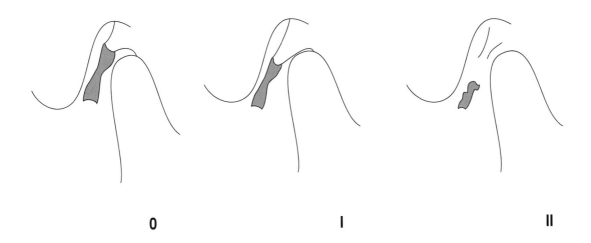

0   I   II

C-26   MR & Clinical Classifications of TMJ Disease

Early Prederangement Stage

MR   Redundant or elongated disc attachment with normal meniscal position

Clinical   Disc hesitation or joint stiffness without reproducible clicking, particularly noticeable after periods of inactivity or sleep

Reducible Anterior Disc Displacement (Partial Internal Derangement)

MR   Subcategorized by moment of meniscal reduction which can be early or late; limited condylar translation with anterior meniscal position until the condylar head overrides the posterior disc margin producing disc recapture

Clinical   Ipsilateral mandibular deviation followed by opening click followed by jaw returning to the midline with normal further opening; closing click is soft

Semipermanent Anterior Disc Displacement

MR   Episodes of intermittent disc displacement on the cine images, evidence of locking on static images

Clinical   Periods of locking and unlocking with intermittent reciprocal clicking

Permanent Anterior Disc Displacement (Complete Internal Derangement)

MR   Disc displacement without evidence of reduction (closed lock); the displaced disc usually limits condylar translation

Clinical   Variable limitation of mouth opening with lateral protrusion and deflection of opening movement toward the affected side

Terminal Anterior Displacement or Lock

MR   Anterior meniscal displacement without reduction but with stretching or perforation of ligaments, meniscal fragmentation, linear hypointense adhesions and condylar head deformity

Clinical   Severe limitation of motion with joint crepitus

C-27   American Dental Association Classification of Disc Interference Disorders

Description

Class I   Interference

Class II   Interference only with initial opening

Class III   Interference with event of translation

Class IV   Interference with spontaneous dislocation

C-28   Appearance of the Mandibular Condyle & Osteoarthritis by Stages

Description

Stage I   Pointing or tapering of the anterosuperior condyle

Stage II   Attenuation of articular cartilage thickness with areas of punctate T1 hypointensity

Stage III   Hypointense bone erosions with subarticular cysts, spur formation and bone-on-bone appearance

C-29   Criteria for Internal Derangement of the TMJ

Partial Internal Derangement

1. Closed mouth subluxation: Posterior meniscal band lies anterior to the 12 o'clock position relative to the mandibular condyle
2. Open mouth reduction: Posterior meniscal band lies behind the 12 o'clock position relative to the mandibular condyle; the intermediate zone becomes the articular surface

Complete Internal Derangement

1. Closed mouth subluxation: Posterior meniscal band lies anterior to the 12 o'clock position relative to the mandibular condyle
2. Open mouth nonreduction: Posterior meniscal band continues to lie anterior to the 12 o'clock position relative to the mandibular condyle

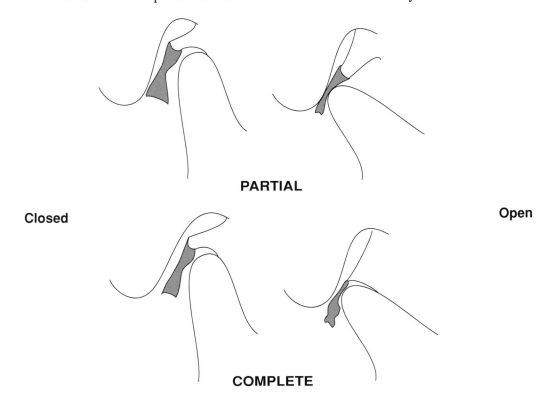

Fig. C-29.1

C-30   Etiology of Craniomandibular Disorders

Habits, Injuries

1. Acute injury or whiplash

2. Irregular sleeping habits

3. Idiosyncrasies including bruxism

Iatrogenic Trauma or Arthritic Disorders

1. Iatrogenic trauma or infection: Intubation during general anesthesia, dental extraction or cavity repair

2. Osteoarthritis or rheumatoid arthritis

3. Paranasal sinus disease or allergies

Occupational Health Hazards

1. Body or muscle fatigue

2. Mental stress

3. Orthopedic imbalance

4. Singing or playing a musical instrument

Wearing Prostheses or Previous Orthodontics

1. Wearing complete or partial dentures

2. Prior orthodontal treatment

Poor Nutrition

1. Poorly balanced dietary intake

2. Liquid intake

Mental/Emotional Health

1. Mental attitude

2. Adverse life events

3. Personality type

C-31   Factors Perpetuating Craniomandibular Disorders

Mechanical Stresses

1. Skeletal asymmetry
2. Skeletal disproportion

Muscular Stresses

1. Poor posture
2. Muscle abuse

Nutritional Inadequacies

1. Vitamin deficiencies (C, B_1, B_6, B_{12} and folic acid)
2. Mineral deficiencies (calcium, potassium and iodide)

Metabolic Disturbance

1. Hypometabolism
2. Endocrine disturbances

Psychological Disorders

1. Depression
2. Anxiety

Chronic Infections

1. Viral
2. Bacterial
3. Parasitic

Allergies

Impaired Sleep

Radiculopathy

Chronic Visceral Disorders

C-32 Organic Craniomandibular Disorders Associated with TMJ Syndrome*

Common

1. Bruxism
2. Occlusal disorders

Uncommon

1. Arthropathy
2. Trauma
3. Inflammation
4. Developmental
5. Neuromuscular
6. Ankylosis
7. Neoplasia
8. Myofascial pain
9. Phantom pain
10. Conversion hysteria

* Adapted from Lunnr, et al. Principles, concepts and practices of the management of craniomandibular diseases. Compendium of the American Equalibration Society. 20:177-227, 1987.

C-33   MR Differential Diagnosis of Masticator Space Lesions

Common

1. Inflammatory

    Odontogenic abscess: Intermediate T1, hyperintense T2, peripheral enhancement

2. Pseudotumors

    a. Benign masseteric hypertrophy: Isointense with adjacent muscles, bilateral

    b. Accessory parotid gland: Isointense with normal parotid gland

3. Malignant tumors

    a. Sarcoma: Mixed T1 and T2 signal, heterogeneous, enhances

        i.   Soft tissue

        ii. Chondrosarcoma

        iii. Osteosarcoma

    b. Malignant schwannoma: Mixed T1 and T2 signal, heterogeneous, enhances

    c. Non-Hodgkin's lymphoma: Intermediate T1, mildly hyperintense T2, homogeneous, enhances

C-33 **MR Differential Diagnosis of Masticator Space Lesions (Cont'd)**

Uncommon

1. Benign tumor

   a. Leiomyoma: Intermediate T1, intermediate to mildly hyperintense T2, well marginated

   b. Neurofibroma/schwannoma: Intermediate T1, hyperintense T2, may exhibit central fibrous hyperintensity secondary to cystic change or necrosis

2. Congenital

   a. Hemangioma: Intermediate T1, hyperintense proton density, very hyperintense T2, well marginated, enhances

   b. Lymphangioma: Hypointense T1, hypo- to isointense proton density, hyperintense T2, less well marginated

3. Inflammatory

   Mandibular osteomyelitis: Hypointense T1, mixed hyperintense T2

4. Pseudotumor

   Trigeminal nerve, mandibular division denervation atrophy: Fatty replacement yields mixed hyperintense T1

5. Malignant tumor

   a. Squamous cell carcinoma from retromolar trigone: Intermediate T1, intermediate to mildly hyperintense T2

   b. Mandibular metastases: Intermediate or mixed T1 and T2

C-34   Mandibular Condyle: Signal Characteristics*

Normal Condyle

T1 Image: Increased

T2 Image: Variable or decreased

Gradient Echo: Decreased

Early (Acute) Avascular Necrosis

T1 Image: Decreased

T2 Image: Increased

Gradient Echo: Variable or increased

Late Avascular Necrosis

T1 Image: Decreased

T2 Image: Decreased

Gradient Echo: Decreased

Osteochondritis Dissecans

T1 Image: Decreased

T2 Image: Highly variable

Gradient Echo: Highly variable

Healing

T1 Image: Decreased

T2 Image: Increased or variable

Gradient Echo: Increased or variable

* Modified from Schellhas KP, Wilkes CH, Fritts HM, et al. MR of Osteochondritis Dissecans and Avascular Necrosis of the Mandibular Condyle. AJNR 10:5, 1988.

CATEGORY C: HEAD & NECK

     C-35   Preseptal Orbital Lesions on MR...........................295
     C-36   Bony Lesions About the Orbit on MR 296
     C-37   Intraconal Lesions on MR 298
     C-38   Extraconal Lesions on MR..................................299
     C-39   Normal Orbital Tissue on MR.............................301
     C-40   Extraocular Muscle Lesions on MR.......................302
     C-41   Optic Sheath Lesions on MR 303
     C-42   Childhood Ocular Lesions on MR 304
     C-43   Adult Ocular Lesions on MR 305

C-35   Preseptal Orbital Lesions on MR

Hypointense T1, Hyperintense T2
1.   Cellulitis
2.   Basal cell carcinoma
3.   Granuloma

Hypointense T1, Hypointense T2
1.   Granuloma

Hyperintense T1, Hyperintense T2
1.   Granuloma

Lesion*	T1	T2
Basal cell carcinoma	Low	High
Cellulitis	Low	High
Granuloma	Low	Low
	or Low	High
	or High	High

* Adapted from Pomeranz, SJ. Craniospinal Magnetic Resonance Imaging, p 598. Philadelphia, WB Saunders, 1989.

C-36 Bony Lesions About the Orbit on MR

Homogeneous Hypointense T2 Signal

1. Osteoma
2. Meningioma-related hyperostosis
3. Fibrous dysplasia

Inhomogeneous Hypointense T2 Signal

1. Chondrosarcoma
2. Osteoblastic osteosarcoma
3. Fibrous dysplasia

Inhomogeneous Intermediate T2 Signal

1. Metastases
2. Fibrous dysplasia

Inhomogeneous Hyperintense T2 Signal

1. Metastatic disease
2. Giant cell tumor
3. Chondrosarcoma (cystic type)
4. Giant cell or reparative granuloma
5. Epidermoid

C-36   Bony Lesions About the Orbit on MR (Cont'd)

Lesion*	T1	T2
Chondrosarcoma	Low	Inhomogeneous, low to high
Fibrous dysplasia	Low	Homogeneous low
Giant cell tumors	Low	Low or high (cyst)
Hyperostosis 2° meningioma	Low	Homogeneous low
Metastatic	Low	Inhomogeneous, moderate to high
Osteoblastic osteosarcoma	Low	Inhomogeneous low
Osteoma	Low	Homogeneous low

* Adapted from Pomeranz, SJ. Craniospinal Magnetic Resonance Imaging, p 600. Philadelphia, WB Saunders, 1989.

C-37   Intraconal Lesions on MR

Hypointense T1, Hypointense T2

1. Vascular malformation
2. Pseudotumor
3. Optic sheath meningioma

Hypointense T1, Hyperintense T2, Homogeneous

1. Cavernous hemangioma
2. Lymphangioma
3. Lymphoma

Hypointense T1, Hyperintense T2, Inhomogeneous

1. Sarcoma
2. Carcinoma

Hyperintense T1, Hyperintense T2

1. Subacute or chronic hemorrhage

Hyperintense T1, Hypointense T2

1. Lipoma

Iso- or Hypointense T1, Hypointense T2

1. Acute hematoma

C-38   Extraconal Lesions on MR

Inhomogeneous Hypointense T1, Hyperintense T2, Hyperintense N(h)

1.   Carcinoma or sarcoma

Homogeneous Hypointense T1, Hyperintense T2, Hyperintense N(h)

1.   Hemangioma
2.   Lymphangioma
3.   Lymphoma
4.   Mixed/adenoma
5.   Granuloma
6.   Orbital varix

Hypointense T1, Hyperintense T2, Hypointense N(h)

1.   Encephalocele

Hyperintense T1, Isointense T2, Hyperintense N(h)

1.   Lipoma
2.   Dermoid
3.   Subacute hemorrhage
4.   Granuloma (rare)

Iso- to Hypointense T1, Hypointense T2, Hypointense N(h)

1.   Pseudotumor
2.   Tolosa-Hunt (cavernous sinus inflammatory disease)
3.   Arteriovenous malformation
4.   Amyloid
5.   Granuloma

C-38   Extraconal Lesions on MR (Cont'd)

Hyperintense T1, Hyperintense T2, Hyperintense N(h)

1. Late subacute to chronic hemorrhage
2. Dermoid
3. Granuloma (rare)
4. Epidermoid cyst

Lesion*	T1	T2	N(h)
Carcinoma/ sarcoma	Inhomogeneous low	Inhomogeneous high	Inhomogeneous high
Lymphoma	Homogeneous low	Homogeneous high	Homogeneous high
Hemangioma	Homogeneous low	Homogeneous high	Homogeneous high
Lymphangioma	Homogeneous low	Homogeneous high	Homogeneous high
Mixed/adenoma	Homogeneous low	Homogeneous high	Homogeneous high
Granuloma	Homogeneous low or high	Homogeneous low or high	Homogeneous low or high
Epidermoid	Low	High	Low
Encephalocele	Low	High	Low
Lipoma	High	Moderate	High
Dermoid†	High-moderate	Moderate-high	High-moderate
Amyloid	Moderate	Low	---
Tolosa-Hunt	Low	Low	Low
Pseudotumor	Low	Low	Low
AVM	Low	Low	Low
Hemorrhage (methemoglobin phase)	High	High	High

* Adapted from Pomeranz, SJ. Craniospinal Magnetic Resonance Imaging, p 601. Philadelphia, WB Saunders, 1989.

† Nondependent/dependent fluid levels.

C-39   Normal Orbital Tissue on MR *

Tissue	T1	T2	N(h)
Vitreous	Low	High	Moderate-low
Aqueous	Low	High	Moderate-low
Ophthalmic artery	Low	Low	Low
Ophthalmic veins	Low	Low	Low
Cortical bone	Low	Low	Low
Sclera	Low	Low	Low
Bone marrow	High	Moderate	High
Orbital fat	High	Moderate	High
Muscles	Moderate	Low	Moderate
Optic nerve	Moderate	Moderate	Moderate
Cornea, external layer	Moderate	High	Moderate
Cornea, mid layer	Low	Low	Low
Cornea, inner layer	High	---	High
Choroid, retina	High	---	High
Lens, external layer	High	High	High
Lens, inner zones	Low-moderate	Low	Low-moderate
Ciliary body	High	Low	High
Zonule	High	---	---
Iris	High	Low	High

* Adapted from Pomeranz, SJ. Craniospinal Magnetic Resonance Imaging, p 599. Philadelphia, WB Saunders, 1989.

C-40   Extraocular Muscle Lesions on MR

Hypointense T1, Hypointense T2

1. Thyroid ophthalmopathy
2. Orbital myositis or pseudotumor
3. Brown's syndrome (superior oblique tendon sheath syndrome)

Hypointense T1, Hyperintense T2

1. Rhabdomyosarcoma
2. Lymphoma

Lesion*	T1	T2
Brown's syndrome	Low	Low
Endocrine ophthalmopathy	Low	Low
Lymphoma	Low	High
Orbital myositis	Low	Low
Rhabdomyosarcoma	Low	High

* Adapted from Pomeranz, SJ. Craniospinal Magnetic Resonance Imaging, p 609. Philadelphia, WB Saunders, 1989.

C-41   Optic Sheath Lesions on MR

Hyperintense T2

1. Glioma
2. Radiation change
3. Optic neuritis
4. Dural ectasia

Hypo- to Isointense T2

1. Meningioma

Isointense T1

1. Meningioma
2. Radiation change
3. Optic neuritis
4. Glioma

Hypointense T1

1. Dural ectasia

Lesion*	T1	T2	C	N(h)
Glioma	Low	High	High	High
Optic neuritis	Isointense	High	High	High
Meningioma	Low-Isointense	Low-Isointense	Isointense	Isointense
Radiation	Isointense	High	High	High

C = Crossover image

N(h) = Proton density image

* Adapted from Pomeranz, SJ. Craniospinal Magnetic Resonance Imaging, p 619. Philadelphia, WB Saunders, 1989.

C-42   Childhood Ocular Lesions on MR

Hyperintense T1, Hyperintense T2

1. Coats' disease (exudative retinitis)
2. Persistent hyperplastic primary vitreous
3. Chronic hemorrhage
4. Sclerosing endophthalmitis

Hypointense T1, Hypointense T2

1. Posterior scleritis
2. Osteoma

Hyperintense T1, Hypointense T2

1. Retinoblastoma

Lesion*	T1	T2
Coats' disease	High	High
Hemorrhage	High	High
PHPV	High	High
Posterior scleritis	Low	Low
Osteoma	Low	Low
Retinoblastoma	High	Low
Sclerosing endophthalmitis	High	High

* Adapted from Pomeranz, SJ. Craniospinal Magnetic Resonance Imaging, p 620. Philadelphia, WB Saunders, 1989.

C-43   Adult Ocular Lesions on MR

Hyperintense T1, Hypointense T2

1. Primary or metastatic melanoma

Isointense T1, Hyperintense T2

1. Metastases

Hyperintense T1, Hyperintense T2

1. Subretinal effusion (may exhibit fluid-fluid levels)
2. Subacute to chronic hemorrhage

Hypointense T1, Hypointense T2

1. Phthisis bulbi
2. Glass eye

Lesion*	T1	T2
Glass eye	Low	Low
Hemorrhage (methemoglobin phase)	High	High
Melanoma	High	Low
Metastases	Moderate	Inhomogeneous high
Phthisis bulbi	Low	Low
Subretinal effusion	High	High

* Adapted from Pomeranz, SJ. Craniospinal Magnetic Resonance Imaging, p 621. Philadelphia, WB Saunders, 1989.

D-1   Evolution of Marrow Signal with Age

1. Infantile pattern: Isointense or intermediate T1 and T2 signal (red marrow) with hyperintense epiphyses and apophyses (yellow marrow)

2. Early conversion or adolescent pattern (prior to age 20): Mixed intermediate T1 signal (red marrow) and hyperintense T1 signal (yellow marrow) with hyperintense epiphyses and apophyses (yellow marrow)

3. Converted marrow or adult pattern (greater than 25 years): Diffuse T1 signal hyperintensity (yellow marrow) with islands of intermediate T1 signal (red marrow) in the skull, spine, pelvis, acetabulum, proximal femora and humeri

4. Advanced adult pattern (over age 50): Islands of intermediate T1 signal red marrow are gone (90% of patients) and marrow shows hyperintense T1 (yellow marrow) and scant iso- or hypointensity on T1 and T2 (depleted or fibrous marrow)

5. Aged or fibrous marrow (over age 65): Hyperintense T1 (yellow marrow) with mixed iso- or hypointensity on T1 and T2 (depleted or fibrous marrow), particularly prominent in the axial skeleton

Reconversion is central to peripheral while normal marrow conversion from red to yellow is peripheral to central

Red marrow reconversion is increased in extent and conspicuity in smokers

Distribution of Red Marrow in the Adult

1. Skull
2. Vertebrae
3. Ribs
4. Pelvis
5. Sternum
6. Proximal femora
7. Distal femora
8. Proximal humeri
9. Ilium
10. Proximal tibia

D-3   Idiopathic Osteoporotic Conditions on MR

1. Transient regional osteoporosis
   a. Osteoporosis of the hip: Men greater than women by a 4:1 ratio; hypointense T1 signal tends to follow a superomedial to inferolateral bony trabecular distribution; signal alteration may revert to normal in 12-16 weeks
   b. Regional migratory osteoporosis: Rapid onset of pain and swelling in a lower extremity persisting for 6-9 months; synchronous or metachronous involvement of other joints may occur; sheetlike areas of T1 hypointensity are noted
   Partial transient osteoporosis
   Zonal form: A portion of one bone is involved
   Radial form: One or two digits of the hand or foot are involved
2. Reflex sympathetic dystrophy syndrome
   a. Evidence or history of prior trauma or inciting event
   b. More commonly affects upper than lower extremities
   c. Self-limited episodes that respond to steroids or analgesics
   d. Recurrence, metachronous or synchronous joint involvement is rare
   e. MR of bone marrow may be normal or show subtle areas of patchy hypointense T1 signal

Marrow Patterns on MR

1.   Depleted: Aplasia, radiation (yellow marrow predominates and is bright white on T1)

2.   Converted: Normal yellow marrow (relatively hyperintense) begins converting at about 6 months, conversion slows at about puberty, persists more slowly until about age 55

3.   Reconverted: Pathologic, related to peripheral red cell destruction, hemolysis (gray on T1, minimally hyperintense on various water weighted sequences)

4.   Replaced: Diffuse myelophthistic replacement by tumor (gray on T1, sometimes markedly hypointense as in diffuse metastatic prostate carcinoma)

5.   Ischemic: Infarct, avascular necrosis (elliptical areas of hypointense signal usually subcortical or subcapital)

6.   Edematous: Marrow in which there is increased bulk phase water (dark on T1, bright on water weighted sequences), poorly defined margins, and which may be related to fracture, bruise, infection, reflex sympathetic dystrophy, transient osteoporosis

D-5   Lower Extremity Edema Patterns

1. Lipedema: Diffuse homogeneous large subcutaneous areas of hypointense T1, hyperintense T2 (if hypointense foci on T2, acute hemorrhage, gas, calcification)
2. Phlebedema: Fluid signal in subcutis (loss of venous flow void)
3. Lymphedema: Fluid signal between muscles and subcutis
4. Anterior tibial lipedema: Diagnosis
   a. Myxedema
   b. Erythema nodosum
   c. Weber-Christian disease
   d. SLE
   e. Polyarteritis nodosa
   f. Sarcoid
   g. TB
   h. Pancreatitis
   i. Suppurative panniculitis
   j. Fat necrosis
   k. Inflammatory bowel disease

aumatic Bone Lesions on MR

1. Bone bruise: Subtle signal hypointensity on T1 and hyperintensity on T2 that becomes less pronounced with increasing distance from the joint space

2. Stress or microfacture: Linear foci of T1 signal hypointensity millimeters in width, invisible or perceived as nominal sclerosis on conventional radiographs

3. Macrofracture: Linear hypointense line on T2 greater than 3 mm in width, usually associated with perceived fracture on conventional radiography

4. Osteochondral fracture: Macrofracture that extends from medullary bone through cortical bone and through the hyaline cartilaginous surface seen as T1 signal hypointensity in bone and cartilage

5. Osteochondral defects (OCD): A wastebasket term which includes any focal well demarcated elliptical subarticular hypointensity that may be accompanied by T1 hypointensity in the overlying cartilage

   a. Osteochrondritis dissecans: A subset of OCD with marked T1 and T2 signal hypointensity in the fragment with or without a surrounding rim of hyperintensity on fast scan or T2, cartilage signal alteration is variable, usually seen in younger patients

   b. Chondromalacia

      i. A subset of OCD which can be giant and focal or multifocal and diffuse

      ii. Signal is variable depending upon extent of chronicity, may yield T1 and T2 hypointensity with bone sclerosis or T1 hypointensity and T2 hyperintensity in medullary bone with geode formation

      iii. Hyaline cartilage thinning and hypointensity on T2 and fast scan is invariably present

      iv. Usually seen in older patients

D-7 **Growth Plate Injury: Salter-Harris-Rang-Ogden Classification****

Grade	Description
I	Fracture through the growth plate
II	Fracture through the growth plate and metaphysis
III	Fracture through the growth plate and epiphysis
IV	Fracture through the growth plate, metaphysis and epiphysis
V	Compression fracture through the growth plate
VI	Trauma to perichondrium with growth plate tethering producing a peripheral bridge
VII	Fracture through the epiphysis with associated chondral involvement
VIII	Simple metaphyseal fracture
IX	Avulsion periosteal injury

See diagram on following page.

* Salter-Harris classification of fractures involving the growth plate (I-V) with Rang and Ogden's additions (VI-IX). Adapted from Greenspan A. Orthopedic Radiology. New York, JB Lippincott, 1988.

wth Plate Injury: Salter-Harris-Rang-Ogden
assification (Cont'd)

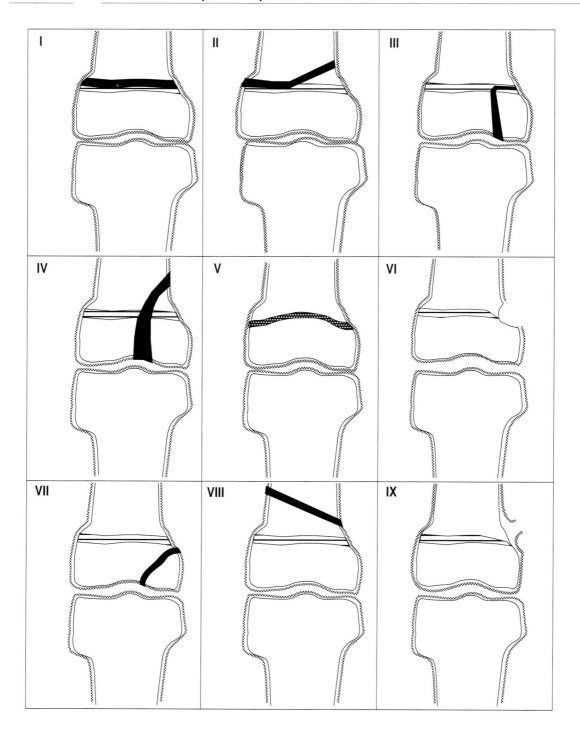

D-8   Pearls in Inflammatory Arthritis

1. Synovial redundancy or prolapse with lobular foci of intermediate T1 signal posteriorly and in the infrapatellar region
2. Joint effusion
3. Small menisci
4. Small or thin hyaline cartilage pads
5. Subchondral hypointense T1 and hyperintense T2 erosions
6. Hypertrophic epiphyses
7. Hoffa fat pad signal is hyperintense T2 and hypointense T1 (edema)
8. Synovial lining of joint enhances with IV contrast
9. Thickened

∨ial Metaplasia on MR

1. Diffuse or focal villonodular synovitis
   a. Villous or lobulated masses
   b. Intermediate T1
   c. Intermediate-hyperintense T2
   d. Effusion
   e. Capsulosynovial thickening
2. Diffuse or focal pigmented villonodular synovitis
   a. Villous or lobulated masses
   b. Intermediate-hyperintense T1
   c. Intermediate-hypointense T2
   d. Effusion
   e. Capsulosynovial thickening
3. Primary synovial chondromatosis
   a. Well-defined rounded masses
   b. Hypointense T1
   c. Hypointense T2
   d. Effusion
   e. Capsulosynovial thickening
4. Lipoma arborescens
   a. Villous or lobulated masses
   b. Uniform hyperintense T1
   c. Hypointense T2
   d. Effusion
   e. Capsulosynovial thickening

D-10   Pearls on Pigmented Villonodular Synovitis

1. Signal
   a. Variable, mixed T2 dependent hypointensity (hemosiderin)
   b. T1 and T2 hypointensity (fibrous stroma)
   c. Pigment (low T2 signal) or lipid (high T1 signal) will determine signal intensity

2. Subtype
   a. Localized and solitary lesion: Localized nodular synovitis
   b. Diffuse and villous pigmented villonodular synovitis
   c. Tendon sheath involvement (which represents extra-articular extension of primary intra-articular disease): Giant cell tumor of tendon sheath or nodular tenosynovitis

3. Average age: 30-50

4. Giant cell tumor of tendon sheath: Predilection for flexor and extensor tendons of finger

5. Bone erosion or signal alteration in 75% of foot lesions and 25% of hand lesions

6. Diffuse form of giant cell tendon sheath tumor involving multiple tendons is most common in knee or foot

7. Presentation
   a. Pigmented villonodular synovitis (80% of cases)
   b. Villonodular synovitis (10%)
   c. Localized nodular synovitis (5%)
   d. Giant cell tumor of tendon sheath (5%)

8. Intra-articular pigmented villonodular synovitis alters bone signal with the following frequency
   a. Hips: 95%
   b. Shoulders: 75%
   c. Elbows: 65%
   d. Ankles: 60%
   e. Knees: 25%

·y Versus Secondary Synovial Osteochondromatosis

Idiopathic ... mary Synovial Osteochondromatosis

1. Monoarticular
2. Male predilection
3. Peak age: Third through fifth decades of life
4. Uniform nodule size
5. Often noncalcified and invisible on conventional radiographs
6. Larger uniform fragment size
7. Normal osteocartilaginous signal
8. Loose body signal: Hypointensity on T1 and T2
9. Most common joints: Hip and knee

Secondary Synovial Osteochondromatosis

1. Monoarticular
2. Slight male predilection
3. Peak age: Second through fourth decades of life
4. Non-uniform nodule size
5. Often calcified and visualized on conventional radiographs
6. Smaller non-uniform fragment size
7. Multifocal T1 osteocartilaginous signal hypointensity
8. Loose body signal: Hypointensity on T1 and T2, or central T1 hyperintensity with peripheral rimlike hypointensity
9. Most common joints: Knee

D-12   Ringlike Skeletal Hypointensity with Central Hyperintensity

Common

1.   Osteoid osteoma

2.   Bone infarction

3.   Osteochondritis dissecans in situ (without fragment migration)*

4.   Avascular necrosis*

Uncommon

1.   Brodie's abscess

2.   Eosinophilic granuloma

Rare

1.   Melanoma metastases

* Subchondral

at Bone Ends by Signal

1. nor: Hypointense T1, hyperintense T2 (epiphyses are closed), adults

2. Chondroblastoma: Mixed hyperintensity T1, mixed isointensity T2 (epiphyses are open), children, sclerotic rim

3. Subchondral arthropathic cysts or geode: Subarticular, hypointense T1, hyperintense T2, homogeneous

4. Intraosseous ganglion: Hypointense T1, hyperintense T2; small size, does not communicate with the joint space, distal medial tibia

5. Brodie's abscess: Hyperintense T2; hypointense T1 circumferential edema (coccidiomycosis propensity for epiphyses and apophyses)

6. Pigmented villonodular synovitis: Hypointense T1, hyperintense T2 and ringlike T2 hypointensity (hemosiderin)

7. Hemophilic pseudotumor: Mixed hyperintensity T1 and T2, globular T2 hypointensity

8. Dedifferentiated chondrosarcoma (clear cell): Hypointense T1, hyperintense T2, edema

D-14   Paget's Disease: Signal Intensities

1. Cortex
    a. Diffuse symmetric circumferential T1 and T2 hypointensity (reactive sclerosis)
    b. Diffuse symmetric circumferential intermediate T1 signal and intermediate to slightly hyperintense T2 signal (fibrosis and granulation tissue)
2. Focal areas of signal hyperintensity = cystic spaces in the lytic or active phase of the disease
3. Encroachment but not invasion of the medullary bone signal, should remain hyperintense on T1 and hypointense on T2 (yellow marrow)
4. Diffuse T1 and T2 signal hypointensity = sclerotic or burned-out phase of the disease
5. Localized concentric or masslike areas of intermediate T1 and intermediate or hyperintense T2 signal = metastases or sarcomatous degeneration
6. Confluent areas of T2 hyperintensity and T1 hypointensity in medullary bone with surrounding soft tissue hyperintense edema = osteomyelitis

AL SYSTEM

Fibrous Dysplasia: MR Signal

onents: Hypointense T1 (long T1 relaxation) and hypointense T2 (short T2 relaxation)

2. Hypocellular fibrous tissue: Hypointense T1 (long T1 relaxation) and hypointense T2 (short T2 relaxation)

3. Cartilaginous islands: Isointense T1 (intermediate T1 relaxation), hyperintense T2 (long T2 relaxation) due to water component of hyaline cartilage

4. Fluid-filled cystic spaces: Hypointense T1 (long T1 relaxation) and hyperintense T2 (long T2 relaxation)

D-16   Nonossifying Fibromas: Signal Intensities & Subtypes

1. Cystic type: Hypointense T1, hyperintense T2, fibrous circumferential rim usually associated with lytic lesion on conventional radiography

2. Fibrous type: Intermediate to hypointense T1 and T2, usually lytic on conventional radiography

3. Xanthomatous type: Hyperintense T1, hyperintense T2, circumferential hypointense rim, usually lytic on conventional radiography

4. Mixed type: Any combination of above signal intensities usually associated with a mixture of fibrous signal (gray T2) and cyst signal (punctate hyperintense T2), either lytic (50%) or sclerotic (50%) on plain film

5. Healed type: Hypointense T1, intermediate or hypointense T2, uniform sclerosis on conventional radiography

...gnal in Sickle Cell Disease

..., intermediate or hypointense T2: Islands of residue of normal yellow ...

2.   Intermediate or gray signal T1, intermediate signal T2: Reconversion to red marrow (secondary to hemolysis)

3.   Hypointense T1, hyperintense T2: Ischemia, infarction or osteomyelitis

4.   Hyperintense T1, hyperintense T2: Hemorrhagic infarction

5.   Hypointense rim with central hyperintensity: Subacute infarction or avascular necrosis

6.   Pronounced hypointensity on T1 and T2: Skeletal hemosiderosis

7.   Expansile intermediate T1 and T2 signal: Extramedullary hematopoiesis

D-18   **Peripheral, Neural or Perineural Masses, Hyperintense T1 Relative to Muscle**

1. Perioperative perineural fibroblastic proliferation
2. Fibrofatty proliferation
3. Neurilemmoma
4. Schwannoma
5. Lipofibroma
6. Neurofibroma
7. Hypertrophic interstitial neuritis of Déjérine-Sottas
8. Fibrolipoma (congenital)

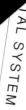

Masses by Signal

ty with Central Hypointensity

1.   ~~Neu~~
2.   Sarcoidosis
3.   Acute hematoma

Moderate to Marked T1 Hyperintensity

1.   Lipoma
2.   Hematoma
3.   Well-differentiated liposarcoma
4.   Myxoid liposarcoma or myxosarcoma

Homogeneous T1 Hypointensity

1.   Cyst
2.   Ganglion
3.   Lymphocele
4.   Hygroma
5.   Seroma

Mild T1 Hyperintensity (Relative to Muscle)

1.   Neurilemmoma or neurofibroma
2.   Hemangioma
3.   Abscess
4.   Solid malignancies (sarcomas and carcinomas)
5.   Hemorrhagic masses

D-20   Tumor or Tumor-like Conditions on MR

1. Malignant fibrous histiocytoma, synovial sarcoma, Ewing's sarcoma: Bowl of fruit mixed signal appearance

2. Arteriovenous malformation: Speckled or wormian signal void, superficial or deep

3. Epithelioid sarcoma: Mixed signal with propensity for peritendinous structures in the forearm and hand

4. Hemangioma: Intermediate T1 and hyperintense T2 signal, multifocal, round, located in the subcutaneous space

5. Pigmented villonodular synovitis: Lamellated intermediate, hyper- and hypo-intense signal, or globular hypointense signal due to calcification or hemosiderin, propensity for knee and hip

6. Hemophilic pseudotumor: Globular T2 signal hypointensity due to calcification or hemosiderin, propensity for elbow or shoulder

7. Myxoid liposarcoma: Homogeneous hyperintense T1 and T2, propensity for thigh

8. Paget's disease: Cortex thickened, hyperintense proton density and mildly hyper-intense or isointense T2, smooth, medullary stippled or striated T1 hypointensity

9. Ganglion: Peritendinous or pericapsular T1 hypointensity, T2 hyperintensity

10. Neurofibroma: Hyperintense T2 with central hypointensity

11. Fibroma: Homogeneous T1 and T2 hypointensity

12. Fibrosarcoma: Mixed intermediate T1 and T2

13. Desmoid: Homogeneous intermediate T1, intermediate or mildly hyperintense T2, subcutis, abdominal wall or retroperitoneum

ses with Lobular Hyaline Cartilage Signal

2. Fibrous dysplasia

3. Enchondroma

Uncommon

1. Chondrosarcoma

2. Chordoma

3. Parosteal chondroma

D-22   Fat-Containing Lesions by Signal

1. Soft tissue lipoma: Matches subcutaneous as a signal standard on all pulsing sequences, well-marginated

2. Intraosseus lipoma: Matches normal fat on all pulsing sequences but may contain foci of T2 hypointensity due to calcification (calcaneus propensity)

3. Hibernoma (brown fatty tumor): Matches normal fat signal but has an axillary or scapular location

4. Liposarcoma: Mixed intermediate T1 and hyperintense T1 signal, intermediate to mildly hyperintense T2 signal, circumferential edema on T2 is common

5. Myxoid liposarcoma: Relatively homogeneous T1 hyperintensity (mild to moderate), T2 hyperintensity, circumferential perilesional edema common

6. Lipoma arborescens: Mixed frondlike intra-articular hyperintense T1, hypointense T2

7. Lipoma with atypia: Well-marginated, hyperintense T1, inhomogeneous, architecture, "streaks"

8. Fatty muscle replacement: Atrophy with mixed intermediate and hyperintense T1 signal

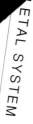

ons on MR with Profound Edema

1. stress fracture with surrounding contusion
2. Osteoid osteoma ± osteoblastoma
3. Chondroblastoma

Uncommon

1. Dedifferentiated chondroblastoma to chondrosarcoma
2. Brodie's abscess or cystic osteomyelitis
3. Benign lesion with fracture
4. Eosinophilic granuloma

D-24   Cystic Soft Tissue Masses with Marked T1 & T2 Prolongation

Common

1. Ganglion
2. Sebaceous cyst
3. Fat necrosis
4. Capsular cyst
5. Meniscal cyst

Uncommon

1. Lymphocele
2. Hygroma
3. Seroma
4. Abscess
5. Cystic neoplasm

D-25   **Fluid-Fluid Levels in Bone & Soft Tissue**

1.   Chondroblastoma
2.   Giant cell tumor
3.   Aneurysmal bone cyst (water nondependent, paramagnetic species dependent)
4.   Fibrous dysplasia
5.   Simple bone cyst (proteinaceous)
6.   Recurrent malignant fibrous histiocytoma
7.   Classic osteogenic sarcoma
8.   Soft tissue hemangioma
9.   Synovial sarcoma
10. Cystic osteomyelitis

D-26   **Common Benign Skeletal Neoplasms or Neoplasm-like Conditions***

Lesion	Common Locations	Age Range
Osteochondroma	Femur, humerus, tibia, pelvis	10-40
Fibrous dysplasia	Skull, face, ribs, femur	10-30
Giant cell tumor	Femur, tibia, radius, sacrum	20-50[†]
Osteoid osteoma	Femur, tibia, vertebrae	5-24
Aneurysmal bone cyst	Vertebrae, pelvis, tibia	10-20
Chondroma	Hand, femur, humerus, foot	10-40
Simple bone cyst	Humerus, femur, tibia	5-20
Fibrous defect	Femur, tibia	5-25
Hemangioma	Skull, vertebrae, femur	20-70
Chondroblastoma	Femur, humerus, tibia, pelvis	20-30
Osteoblastoma	Vertebrae, femur, tibia	20-40
Chondromyxoid fibroma	Tibia, femur, pelvis	20-30

* Berquist TM. MRI of the Musculoskeletal System, p 439, Berquist TH, ed. Raven Press, New York, 1990.
† After growth plate closure

D-27   Sarcoma on MR: Summary & Differential Diagnosis

1. Rule of thumb for lesions in the soft tissues: If it's not pure blood, pure water or pure fat, the lesion should be followed in 2-4 weeks or biopsied

2. Chondrosarcoma (particularly cystic/clear cell): May be cystic and demonstrate hyperintense signal on T2, frequently accompanied by hyperintense edema on T2 (matrix is hyperintense but calcium is hypointense)

3. Fibrosarcoma: A mixed, bland or gray signal on T1 and T2, sometimes completely hypointense simulating pigmented villonodular synovitis

4. Osteosarcoma: Matrix hyperintense, large mass – periosteal, classic, parosteal, telangiectatic (expansile)

5. Lymphosarcoma: Flat bone or diaphyseal, sclerotic, gray homogeneous signal T1 and T2, does not bleed, older patients

6. Ewing's sarcoma: Flat bone or diaphyseal, young, large soft tissue mass, hemorrhagic, "bowl of fruit," heterogeneous T1 and T2 signal

7. Epithelioid sarcoma: Propensity for upper extremities, grows in a peritendinous locale, demonstrates mixed gray signal ± hemorrhage

8. Malignant fibrous histiocytoma, synovial sarcoma: Demonstrates inhomogeneous bright signal on T2, may resemble the bowl of fruit sign, thigh, large muscle groups

9. Myxoid liposarcoma: Hyperintense T1 & T2 or very hypointense T1, very hyperintense T2, thigh, large muscle groups (a large myxoid component may mimic a seroma)

10. Leiomyosarcoma: Mixed cystic ± hemorrhage, uterus, abdomen

11. Soft part sarcoma: Mixed T1 & T2 signal, thigh, retroperitoneum

D-28   Osteogenic Sarcoma on MR

1.   Hyperintense peritumoral T2 signal: Edema

2.   Hyperintense T2 soft tissue signal: Edema (especially after chemotherapy)

3.   Hypointense T2 rim around extramedullary tumor: Collagenous pseudo-capsule

4.   Rounded hyperintense intratumor T2 foci: Vascular channels and necrosis

5.   Hypointense T2 foci within the neoplasm: Hemosiderin or calcium or matrix

6.   Hyperintense T1 foci: Intratumoral hemorrhage

7.   Hypointense T1 foci adjacent to tumor: Bone infarction

D-29   Tunnel Syndromes in the Upper Extremities

1. Thoracic outlet: Compression of the brachial plexus, subclavian artery or subclavian vein before separation with resultant
    a. Upper limb pain
    b. Paresthesia
    c. Vascular insufficiency and motor dysfunction
2. Anterior scalene syndrome
    a. Brachial plexus and subclavian artery compressed between the anterior and middle scalene muscles at the first rib attachment
    b. Lower brachial plexus C8 through T1 at higher risk for compression with numbness especially in fingers, hand and forearm
    c. Vascular insufficiency, paresis and atrophy of the hypothenar and interosseous muscles
3. Costoclavicular syndrome
    a. Subclavian artery, subclavian vein and brachial plexus compression passing between the clavicle and first rib
    b. Similar to anterior scalene syndrome
    c. Vascular symptoms dominate over neurological symptoms

CATEGORY E: HIP & THIGH

Page

E-1   Major Articular Components of the Hip*

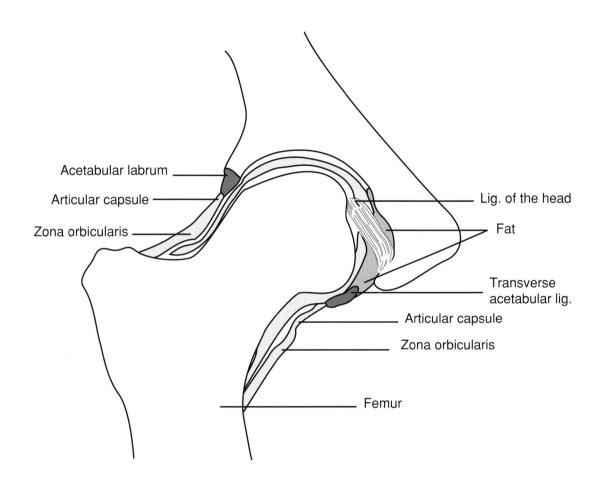

* Adapted from Berquist TM. MRI of the Musculoskeletal System, p 163. Berquist TH, ed. New York, Raven Press, 1990.

E-2   Acquisition Planes for Oblique MR Scans of the Hip

1. Oblique axial (off coronal): see diagram below

2. Oblique sagittal (off axial): see diagram below

3. Oblique coronal (off axial): see diagram below

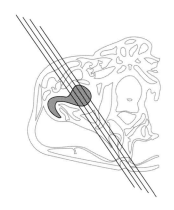

Axial scout for oblique sagittal

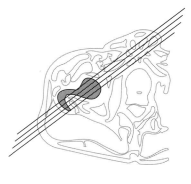

Axial scout for oblique coronal

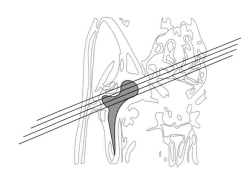

Coronal scout for oblique axial

E-3 **Pearls on Marrow Signal in the Hip**

1. Epiphyses and apophyses have no red marrow until they ossify; therefore, they are hyperintense on T1 even when the red marrow containing femoral shaft and intertrochanteric region is intermediate in signal

2. Ninety-five percent of patients under 50 years of age exhibit intermediate T1 signal due to red matter in the intertrochanteric region

3. Eighty-eight percent of patients over 50 years of age exhibit hyperintense T1 signal of yellow marrow in the intertrochanteric region

4. Premature conversion to yellow marrow in the intertrochanteric region may be an early sign of AVN

5. Normal weight-bearing trabeculae produce a linear area of signal hypointensity extending superomedial from the subcapital femoral head region to the inferolateral region, linear shape, hypointense on T1

6. Linear hypointense weight-bearing trabeculae may become more pronounced in size and lower in signal as an early sign of AVN

E-4   Pearls in Transient Marrow Edema of the Hip

1. Young or middle aged, males more often than females (originally described in the third trimester of pregnancy), usually bilateral in males but in females the left hip is often affected

2. Progresses over several weeks with clinical improvement 2-6 months

3. No risk factors (? pregnancy)

4. Lab values are normal

5. Osteoporosis on plain film is a good prognostic sign with clinical improvement usually seen 2-6 months

6. X-ray reverts to normal before MR and scintigraphy

7. Pathologic fracture of the femoral neck is rare

8. No x-ray progression to classic avascular necrosis

9. MR findings

    a. Diffuse hypointense T1 marrow edema which becomes hyperintense on water-weighted datasets including T2, T2 fast spin echo, STIR and fat-suppressed T2

    b. Vascular flow persists on both gadolinium-enhanced and bone scintigraphy flow phase and is usually hyperemic in contrast to AVN which is hypovascular

    c. Diffuse extension inter- and subtrochanteric, infrequent with AVN

    d. Small crescentic hypointense rarefactions may be present and will resolve within 2-6 months (no actual rings of hypointensity or homogeneous confluent areas of hypointensity are seen)

10. Must be differentiated from regional migratory osteoporosis which affects many joints and is likely not a disease variant but separate entity

E-5   **Bone Marrow Edema Pattern of the Hip**

1.   Transient osteoporosis of the hip
2.   Osteomyelitis
3.   Bone contusion
4.   Stress fracture
5.   Macrofracture with contusion
6.   Infiltrative neoplasm
7.   Extended pattern of avascular necrosis
8.   Reflex sympathetic dystrophy

E-6   **Reflex Sympathetic Dystrophy Versus Transient Osteoporosis**

Reflex Sympathetic Dystrophy	Transient Osteoporosis of the Hip
Minor trauma	No history of trauma
Skin and vasomotor change common	Skin and vasomotor change rare
Usually upper extremities	Usually lower extremities
Long-term disability & complications more common	Clinical improvement usually 2-6 months
Pathologic fracture uncommon	Pathologic fracture rare
Progression to avascular necrosis rare	Progression to avascular necrosis uncommon
Affects many joints	Affects only one joint

E-7   Pearls in Legg-Calvé-Perthes Disease (LCPD)

1.   Frequency: 1 in 1,000 to 1 in 5,000

2.   Males more common in a ratio of 4:1

3.   Other risk factors: Low socioeconomic class, low birth weight, inguinal hernia, genitourinary anomalies

4.   Peak age: 6-8 years

5.   More homogeneous hypointensity on T1 than with steroid necrosis which tends to be more crescentic or ring-shaped

6.   Absence of enhancement with gadolinium injection in areas of hypointense edema conveys poor prognosis

7.   Differential diagnosis

    a.   Multiple epiphyseal dysplasia (MED) which involves the humerus and hips with normal marrow

    b.   Bone contusion

    c.   Osteomyelitis

8.   Catterall classification of LCPD*

    I   Anterior epiphysis only but no metaphyseal sclerosis, sequestrum or sub-chondral fracture

    II   More severe anterior epiphyseal involvement with sequestrum and antero-lateral metaphyseal reaction, subchondral fracture line does not extend to epiphysis

    III   Entire epiphysis hypointense, femoral neck widening and posterior verti-cal fracture line

    IV   Entire head involved, flattening, mushrooming, collapse

9.   Prognosis[†]

    a.   Involvement of 20% lateral epiphyseal margin: Prognosis poor

    b.   Involvement of 50% lateral epiphyseal margin: Prognosis very poor

---

* Catterall A. The Natural History of Perthes Disease. J Bone Joint Surg [Br] 53:37, 1971.

† Green NE, Beauchamp RD, Griffin PD. Epiphyseal Extrusion as a Prognostic Index in Legg-Calvé-Perthes Disease. J Bone Joint Surg [Am] 63:900, 1981.

E-8   **Pearls in the Diagnosis of Slipped Capital Femoral Epiphysis**

1. Peak age: 10-15 years old
2. Male to female ratio 4:1
3. Bilateral: 20-25%
4. Oblique axial sections for slippage axis (slippage usually posterior)
5. Indications for MR
    a. Assess the contralateral hip
    b. Look for complicating AVN
    c. Effusion
    d. Chondrolysis
6. Other signs
    a. Calcification: Lateral to the epiphysis
    b. Gage's sign: Lateral lytic area on plain film

E-9   MR Indicators in Hip Dysplasia

1. Ultrasound is the modality of choice before 6 months of age
2. MR is the modality of choice for late presentation (5%), patients who undergo treatment failure or patients who are in a cast harness

   The following features should be evaluated on MR

   a. Infolded capsule
   b. Infolded or deformed limbus or labrum
   c. Foreshortened iliopsoas tendon
   d. Pulvinar or fat hypertrophy
   e. Avascular necrosis
   f. Chondrolysis
   g. Large effusion
3. Risk factors
   a. Family history
   b. Breech presentation
   c. Torticollis
   d. Scoliosis
   e. Metatarsus adductus
   f. Underdevelopment of anterior capsule, ligament of Bigelow or rectus muscle
4. Frequency

   20% bilateral

   50% left

   30% right
5. Dunn* Classification of Hip Dysplasia

   Type 1   Positional instability

   Type 2   Subluxation

   Type 3   Dislocation

* Dunn PM. The Anatomy and Pathology of Congenital Dislocation of the Hip. Clin Orthop 119:23, 1976.

E-10   FICAT Classification of AVN*

1. Loss of red marrow, separation of lipocytes with edema, hemorrhage & foam cells

2. Necrosis, fatty marrow

3. Medullary & trabecular necrosis

4. Necrosis, fibrosis with new bone near dead trabeculae

* Ficat RP, Arlet J. Necrosis of the Femoral Head, in Ischemia and Necrosis of the Bone, Hungerford DS, ed. Williams & Wilkins, Baltimore, 1980.

E-11   Stemberg Plain Film Classification of AVN

0	Normal bone scan and x-ray
I	Positive bone scan, normal x-ray
II	Cystic change, faint sclerosis
III	No flattening, crescent shape
IV	Flat head, normal joint space
V	Joint space narrowing, abnormal acetabulum

E-12   Avascular Necrosis (AVN) in Order of Appearance

Pattern	Description
Crescent	Subchondral crescent parallels cortical acetabular margin
Ring	Hypointense ring with normal central hyperintense T1 fat signal
Homogeneous	Homogeneous rounded T1 signal hypointensity as the ring fills in
Extended	Extension of homogeneous signal hypointensity into the cervical and intertrochanteric regions
Advanced Extended	Same as Stage IV but with collapse and fracture of the femoral head

See diagram following page

E-13   Patterns of AVN

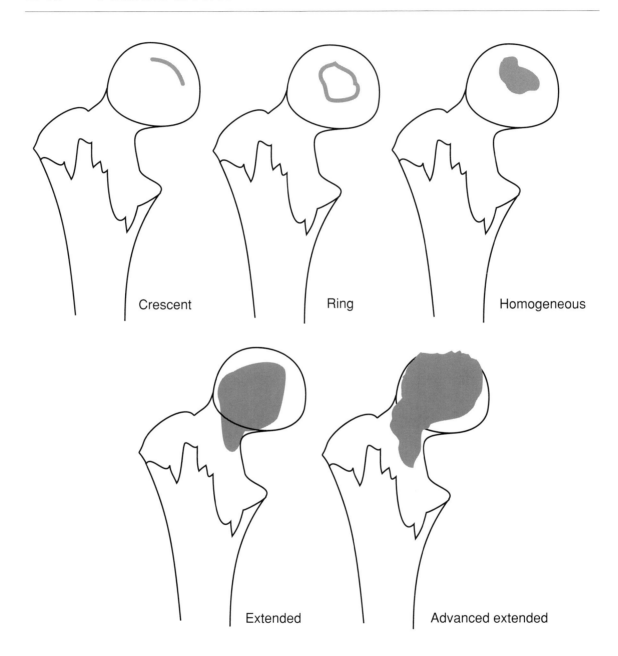

Crescent   Ring   Homogeneous

Extended   Advanced extended

E-14   **Pathologic Stages of AVN**

	Description	**MR Stage**
A	Ischemia: Red cell death (12 hours), osteocytic death (24 hours), marrow death (72 hours)	
B	Hyperemia, osteoporosis (1-3 weeks)	
C	Fat cells convert to fibroblasts with a reactive interface	Stages I–III
D	Wide reactive interface of acellularity with associated sclerosis	Early Stage IV
E	Subchondral fracture	Late Stage IV

E-15   Mitchell Classification* of AVN on MRI by Signal Intensity

	T1	**T2**
A	Hyper	Iso
B	Hyper	Hyper
C	Hypo	Hyper
D	Hypo	Hypo

* Stoller DW. Magnetic Resonance Imaging in Orthopaedics & Sports Medicine, p 58. Philadelphia, JB Lippincott, 1993.

E-16   Femoral Head AVN Versus Transient Bone Marrow Edema*

Pattern	Diagnosis	MR Features
True segmental	AVN	Thick low-signal-intensity bands with a sharp inner face, double-line sign occasionally seen on T2
Pseudosegmental	Edema	Thin, generally subchondral, low-signal-intensity bands with blurred margins, no double-line sign seen on T2
True bone marrow edema	Edema	Ill-delimited area of low signal intensity on T1 and of high signal intensity on T2 or STIR; rarely, very limited subchondral low signal intensity on T2
Pseudohomogeneous edema	AVN	Low-signal-intensity areas on T2 always present, epiphyseal collapse may be marked

* Adapted from Vande Berg, BE, Malghem JJ, Labaisse MA, et al. MR Imaging of Avascular Necrosis and Transient Marrow Edema of the Femoral Head. RadioGraphics 13:510, 1993.

E-17   Histologic Findings of AVN: Signal Intensities T1, T2 & Contrast T1*

	T1	T2	Contrast T1
Normal fatty marrow	High	Intermediate	None[†]
Early marrow necrosis w/ mummified fat	High	Intermediate	None
Advanced marrow necrosis with eosinophilic marrow & trabecular microfractures	Low	Low	None
Subchondral fractures	Low	High[‡]	None
Viable fibrous mesenchymal tissue with acellular fibrosis & bone sclerosis	Low	Low	Discrete
Viable fibrous mesenchymal tissue with predominant cellular content	Low	Intermediate	Moderate
Viable fibrous mesenchymal tissue with dilated vessels and interstitial edema	Low	High	Marked

* Adapted from Vande Berg, BE, Malghem JJ, Labaisse MA, et al. MR Imaging of Avascular Necrosis and Transient Marrow Edema of the Femoral Head. RadioGraphics 13:507, 1993.

† Enhancement needs appropriate sequence to be demonstrated

‡ The linear shape and subchondral position are other features suggestive of fracture clefts

E-18   OCD Versus AVN

Osteochondral Defect   **Avascular Necrosis**

Focal or multifocal   Usually focal

Well-defined   Less well-defined

Round with narrow radius of   Broad or elliptical
   curvature

Both sides of the joint early   One side of the joint unless late with
                                            associated arthritis

Capsular inflammation and/or   Capsulitis and effusion only late
   effusion early

Without conspicuous marrow   Marrow edema more common
   edema

No AVN risk factors   Risk factors for AVN

E-19   Pearls in the Diagnosis of Herniation Pit of the Hip

1. This phenomenon is seen on 4% of normal patients, occasionally grows but rarely symptomatic

2. Location: Subcortical anterosuperior femoral head

3. Etiology: Reaction to mechanical irritation of the adjacent hip capsule

4. Signal
    a. Cystic type: Hypointense T1, hyperintense T2 (80%)
    b. Fibrous type: Hypointense T1, hypointense T2 (20%)
    c. Sclerotic reactive new bone interface, hypointense on T1 and T2 (40-60%)

5. Differential diagnosis
    a. Intraosseus ganglion: Hypointense T1, hyperintense T2, does not communicate with the joint surface
    b. Arthropathic cyst: Evidence of cartilage or chondral abnormalities, joint effusion
    c. Metastases: Usually no well-circumscribed cystic signal
    d. Brodie's abscess: Usually associated with circumferential hypointense edema

E-20   Hip Effusion

Grade I   Thin medial slit on T2, STIR or gradient echo
               85% of normals
Grade II   Surrounds femoral head
               60% AVN cases
Grade III   Distends capsule
               50% late stage AVN

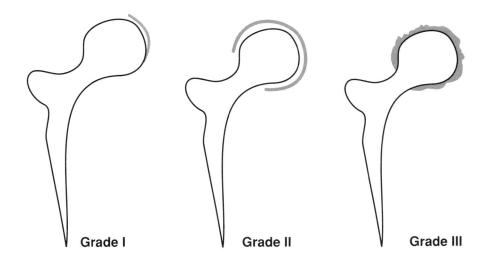

Grade I   Grade II   Grade III

E-21   Osteoarthritis: Radiograph & MR Staging

Grade	Radiograph	MR
0	Normal	Normal
1	Joint space narrowing (?), subtle osteophytes	Inhomogeneous high signal in cartilage on T2
2	Definite joint space narrowing, osteophytes & sclerosis, esp. in acetabular region	Inhomogeneity with areas of high signal in articular cartilage on T2, indistinct trabeculae or signal loss in femoral head & neck on T1
3	Marked joint space narrowing, osteophytes, cyst formation & deformity of femoral head	Criteria of stages 1 & 2 plus indistinct zone between femoral head & acetabulum, increasing subchondral signal loss on T1 & T2 due to bone sclerosis
4	Gross loss of joint space with above features plus large osteo-phytes & increased deformity of the femoral head & acetabulum	Above criteria plus deformity of femoral head

E-22   Neoplasms about the Pelvis, Hips & Upper Thighs

Bone Tumors

Malignant

Chondrosarcoma: Inhomogeneous or homogeneous/cystic

Osteosarcoma: Inhomogeneous

Lymphoma: Homogeneous, intermediate T2

Chordoma: Inhomogeneous, sacrum

Ewing's sarcoma: Inhomogeneous, hemorrhagic, flat bones

Myeloma: Expansile (?), cystic

Fibrosarcoma: Homogeneous, intermediate or hypointense T2

Post-radiation sarcoma: Inhomogeneous

Benign

Osteochondroma: Hyperintense T2, matrix cap ± calcium

Osteoid osteoma: Ring lesion with edema

Giant cell tumor: Cystic, epiphyseal, bright T2, homogeneous

Chondroma: Hyperintense T2, matrix

Chondroblastoma: Sharp hypointense rim, edema, intermediate T2

Soft Tissue Tumors

Liposarcoma: (Myxoid) homogeneous hyperintense T2, ± hyperintense T1

Desmoids: Intermediate to hypointense T2

Alveolar sarcoma: Inhomogeneous

Synovial sarcoma: Inhomogeneous, bright T2

Epithelioid sarcoma: Inhomogeneous, peritendinous growth, mixed T2

E-23   Grading for Hamstring or Tendon Injuries

Grade	Description
I	Intratendinous or myotendinous T2 signal hyperintensity
II	Intra- and peritendinous T2 signal hyperintensity with or without foci of T1 or proton density hyperintensity; intra- and peritendinous signal shape is linear
III	Same as II with homogeneous rounded or ovoid T1 signal hypointensity and T2 signal hyperintensity mass (ganglion precursor) or globular area of T1 and T2 hyperintensity (hematoma)
IV	Complete interruption in the linear hypointense tendon or myotendinous junction signal with associated pseudomass of tendon retraction and tendon defect; hematoma or ganglion formation may be present

E-24 **Fractures of the Proximal Femur**

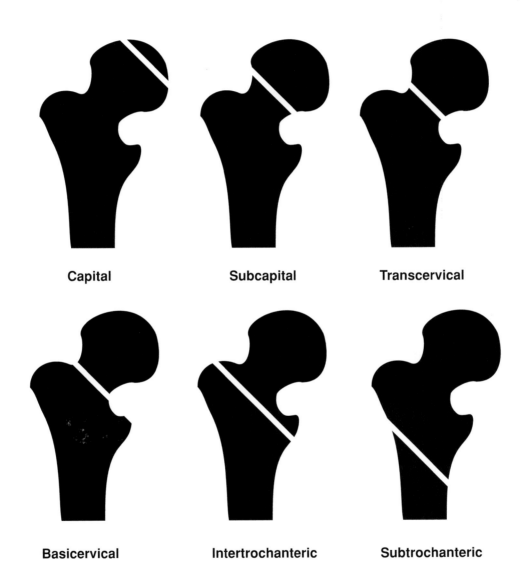

Capital

Subcapital

Transcervical

Basicervical

Intertrochanteric

Subtrochanteric

E-25   **Intertrochanteric Fractures**

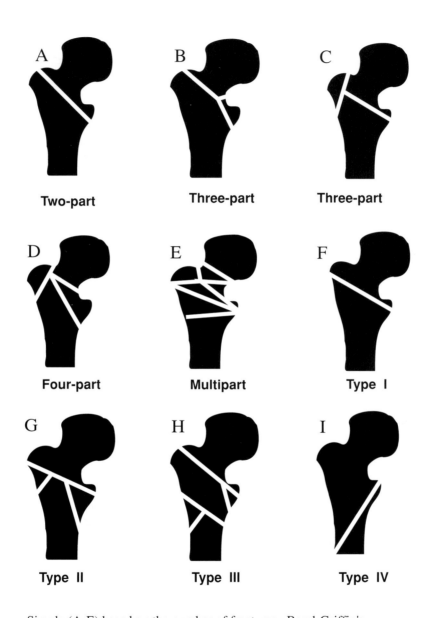

Simple (A-E) based on the number of fractures. Boyd-Griffin's (F-I) classifications of intertrochanteric fractures from Boyd HB, Griffin LL. Classification and treatment of trochanteric fractures. *Arch Surg* 58:853, 1949.

E-26   Subtrochanteric Fractures*

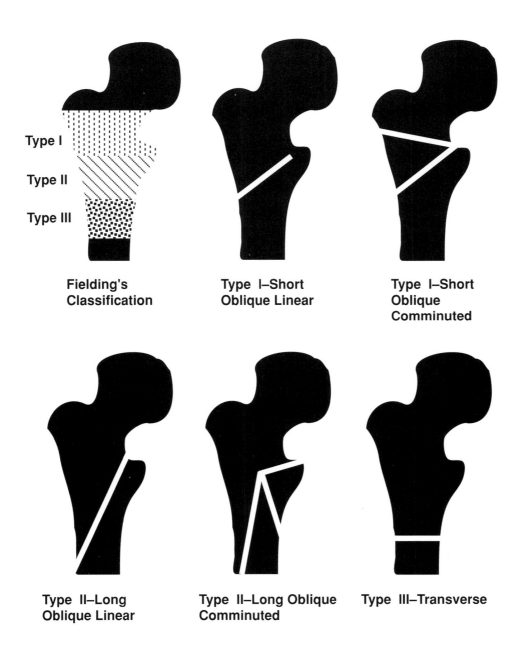

Type I

Type II

Type III

**Fielding's
Classification**

**Type I–Short
Oblique Linear**

**Type I–Short
Oblique
Comminuted**

**Type II–Long
Oblique Linear**

**Type II–Long Oblique
Comminuted**

Type III–Transverse

* Fielding's (I) and Zickel's (II-VI) classifications of subtrochanteric fractures. Adapted from Fielding JW. Subtrochanteric fractures. *Clin Orthop* 92:86, 1973 and Zickel RE. An Intramedullary Fixation Device for the Proximal Part of the Femur. *J Bone Joint Surg* 58A:866, 1976.

CATEGORY F: THE KNEE

F-1   Medial & Lateral Menisci: Anatomical Differences

1. Medial meniscus

    a. Banana-shaped, open radius of curvature

    b. Posterior horn is wider, longer and taller than the anterior horn

    c. Posterior horn is tightly attached to the medial capsule via meniscofemoral & meniscotibial ligaments making separation more common medially

    d. Myxoid Grade 2 signal more common on medial side

2. Lateral meniscus

    a. Tight C-shape

    b. Posterior and anterior horns are symmetric in size

    c. Comminutes the popliteus tendon posteriorly

    d. Separated from and loosely attached to the lateral collateral ligament

    e. The anterior horn may be hypoplastic, short or extremely thin; meniscal agenesis more common posterolateral horn

    f. Discoid meniscus & meniscal cyst more common laterally

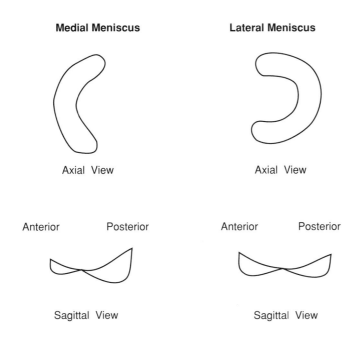

Fig. F-1.1

F-2   Determining the Position of Meniscus Tears

1. The one-third rule divides the meniscus into a posterior one-third horn, a middle one-third body and an anterior one-third horn

2. The 25-50-25 rule divides the meniscus into the inner 25% (consisting of the true anterior horn and true posterior horn) the middle 50% (consisting of the anterior and posterior body) and the peripheral 25% (consisting of the true midbody)

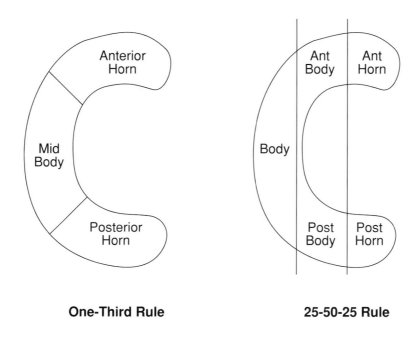

One-Third Rule   **25-50-25 Rule**

Fig. F-2.1

F-3   **Meniscal Vascularity & Good Prognosis Meniscal Tears**

1. Anterior and posterior meniscal body peripheral one-third
2. Non-full-thickness tears
3. Less than 1 cm of length
4. Knee stability with ACL intact
5. Paucity of chondromalacia
6. Younger age

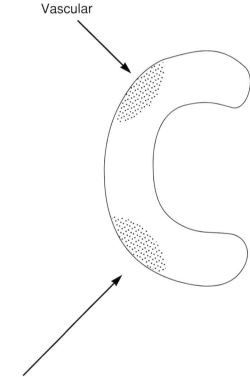

Vascular

Fig. F-3.1   Vascular

F-4   Distribution, Shape & Frequency of Meniscal Tears

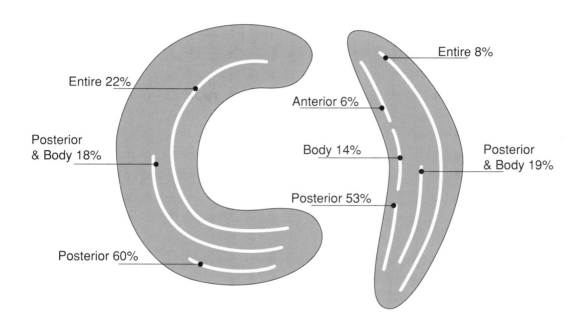

Fig. F-4.1

F-5   **Grading Meniscal Signal on MR**

Description

Grade 0   Homogeneously black meniscus

Grade I   Globular signal that does not extend to either the superior
               or inferior articular surface*

Grade II   Intrameniscal signal that is linear, not extending to an artic-
               ular surface†

Grade III   Intrameniscal signal extending to an articular surface

Grade III-A   Linear intrameniscal signal abutting an articular margin

Grade III-B   Irregular intrameniscal signal abutting an articular margin‡

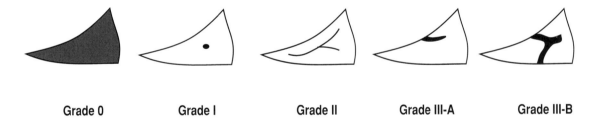

Grade 0   Grade I   Grade II   Grade III-A   Grade III-B

Fig. F-5.1

* Grade I menisci correspond to foci of myxoid degeneration located in the areas of chondrocyte deficiency.
† Grade II signal most commonly appears in the posterior medial meniscus, shaped like a Y turned on
  its side with the V shape from the Y pointed posteriorly. It often abuts the meniscocapsular junction
  and is oriented in the midplane, horizontally or with nominal anteroinferior to posterosuperior orientation. It fades in the middle and inner meniscal third. In children, Grade II menisci correspond to normal hypervascularity running along collagenous bundles, and in adults they correspond to microscopic
  areas of collagen fragmentation, chondrocyte deficiency and myxoid degeneration.
‡ An articular surface is considered the superior, inferior or inner edge of the meniscus, but not the outer
  capsular margin.

F-6   **Expanded Classification of Meniscal Injuries***

Type 0   Normal

Type I   Punctate intrameniscal signal, does not form a band, does not extend to either surface of the meniscus

Type II   Bandlike intrameniscal signal not extending to the surface of the meniscus

Type III   Unusually short meniscus with a tapered apex

Type IV   Truncated apex of the meniscus

Type V   A bandlike increased signal intensity extending to one surface of the meniscus

Type VI   Bandlike increased signal intensity extending to two surfaces

Type VII   Comminuted increased intrameniscal signal intensity extending to one or both surfaces

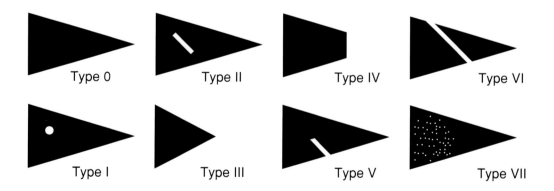

Type 0   Type II   Type IV   Type VI

Type I   Type III   Type V   Type VII

Fig. F-6.1

* Adapted from Mesgarzadeh M, Moyer R, Leder D, et al MR Imaging of the Knee: Expanded Classification and Pitfalls to Interpretation of Meniscal Tears. RadioGraphics 13:493, 1993.

F-7 **Mucoid Degeneration & True Meniscus Tear**

1. Mucinous degeneration tends to be most conspicuous in the posterior medial meniscus body and horn

2. Myxoid change has the shape of a "Y" or slingshot lying on its side

3. Myxoid change does not communicate with the superior-inferior articular cartilage

4. Myxoid change does not run in the craniocaudad or vertical direction

5. Myxoid change does not exceed the signal intensity of adjacent cartilage on the proton density (long TR, short TE) image

6. Myxoid degeneration tends not to involve the inner 1/3 of the meniscus

F-8   Risk Factors for Meniscal Tear

1. Degenerative joint disease
2. Sports
3. Prolonged kneeling or squatting
4. Soft tissue weakness or joint laxity
5. Discoid meniscus
6. Vastus medialis weakness
7. Hip disease
8. Medial, femoral or tibial shaft torsion
9. Knee fracture
10. Arthritis
11. Osteomyelitis or septic joint

F-9   Types of Meniscal Tears

1.   Longitudinal tear: Vertical shape, more common on the medial side

2.   Horizontal tear: Frequently degenerative but can be traumatic, more common laterally

3.   Radial tear: May be degenerative or traumatic, vertical, millimeters in size, often on the inner edge of the lateral meniscus, and more common than the medial meniscus; may only be seen on one or two sections and in one plane

4.   Bucket handle tear: Vertical longitudinal tear or split, more common in the medial meniscus

5.   Fish-mouth tear: A type of degenerative tear which communicates with the free edge, a subtype of horizontal tear

6.   Parrot-beak tear: Has both vertical and horizontal components occurring at the free edge of the meniscus body, usually at the junction of the body and posterior horn of lateral meniscus, better seen in the coronal projection

7.   Truncation tear: Blunting of the free edge or tip of the meniscus in either the sagittal or, more commonly, the coronal projection (probably just a large radial tear or bucket handle tear)

8.   Meniscocapsular separation: A subtype of meniscal tear in which the posterior meniscus horn pulls away from the capsule resulting in a separation of the posterior meniscal signal and the posterior tibial plateau of greater than 8-10 mm

9.   Peripheral edge tear: Any tear less than 3-5 mm in size that confines itself to a distance of less than 5 mm from the meniscus periphery

F-10   Meniscal Tears: Appearance on MR

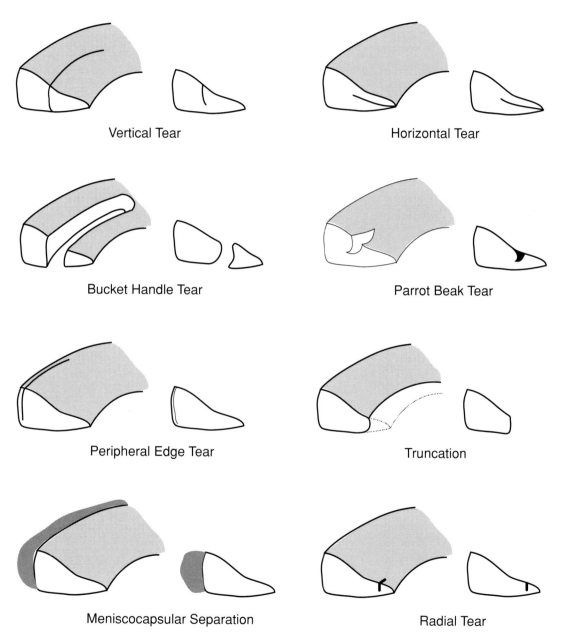

Vertical Tear

Horizontal Tear

Bucket Handle Tear

Parrot Beak Tear

Peripheral Edge Tear

Truncation

Meniscocapsular Separation

Radial Tear

Fig. F-10.1

F-11   Small Menisci on MR: Etiologies

1.   Prior meniscectomy
2.   Degenerative arthritis
3.   Rheumatoid arthritis
4.   Juvenile rheumatoid arthritis
5.   Bucket handle tear
6.   Meniscal hypoplasia

F-12   Pearls & Subtypes of Discoid Meniscus

1. Known as the snapping knee syndrome
2. Subtypes include those with intact and without intact Wrisberg ligaments, and those that are morphologically small
3. More common laterally than medially, and diagnosed when the meniscal bow tie persists on more than two or three sections in the sagittal plane on 2D, 4 or 5 mm sections (two-cut rule)
4. Signal alteration which approaches that of hyaline cartilage in a discoid meniscus always represents painful lateral meniscus tear

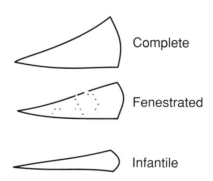

Fig. F-12.1

F-13   **Findings Associated with Discoid Lateral Meniscus**

1.   Hypoplasia of the lateral femoral condyle

2.   High fibular head

3.   Fibular muscular defects

4.   Lateral joint widening

5.   Deformed lateral malleolus

6.   Hypoplasia of the lateral tibial spine

7.   Aneurysm or ectasia of the inferior lateral genicular artery

F-14   Bucket Handle Tear: MR Appearances & Signs

1. Decreased meniscal height
2. Abnormal or bizarre meniscal shape
3. Abrupt meniscal truncation in the coronal projection
4. Separation or discontiguity of the meniscus in the coronal projection
5. Hypointense fragment within the knee notch in the coronal projection
6. Absence of normal hypointense meniscal triangle in the sagittal projection
7. The "double ACL or PCL" sign has been described as a sign of bucket handle tear with a hypointense meniscal fragment lying at the base or underneath the anterior or posterior cruciate ligaments simulating loose body

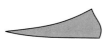

1. Decreased meniscal height

2. Abnormal meniscal shape

3. Abrupt meniscal truncation in the coronal projection

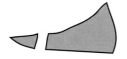

4. Separation or discontiguity of the meniscus in the coronal plane

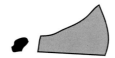

5. Hypointense fragment within the knee notch in the coronal projection

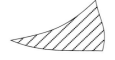

6. Absence of normal hypointense meniscal triangle in the sagittal projection

Fig. F-14.1

F-15   Diagramatic Pearls in the Assessment of Meniscus Tears

1. Meniscocapsular Separation
    a. Most common in the posteromedial meniscocapsular interface
    b. Ganglia, increased meniscocapsular fat and capsulosynovial redundancy can simulate meniscocapsular separation
    c. In true separation, the meniscus moves anteriorly
    d. Separation without associated meniscal tear, bone or cartilage injury is rare

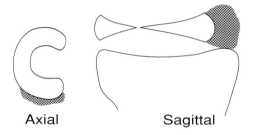

Axial   Sagittal

Fig. F-15.1

2. Pseudo Bucket Handle Tear
    a. Pseudo bucket handle tear is created by the steep concavity of the middle third and inner third of the meniscus creating the impression of meniscal separation in the coronal image
    b. Seen only on one or two slices
    c. Not associated with soft tissue or bone injury

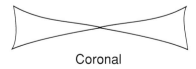

Coronal

Fig. F-15.2

F-15   Diagramatic Pearls in the Assessment of Meniscus Tears (Cont'd)

3. Meniscal Agenesis or Hypoplasia

    a. Agenesis most often occurs in the posterolateral horn and body

    b. Fluid signal completely replaces the meniscus

    c. Scant chondromalacia usually exists

    d. Hypoplasia with decreased length and height is most common in the antero-lateral horn (may simulate anterolateral horn tear)

    e. True agenesis simulates meniscectomy and vice versa

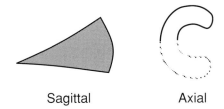

Sagittal   Axial

Fig. F-15.3

4. Meniscal Root Injuries

    a. Root tears are a pitfall by virtue of the fact that they are easily missed because they are so close to the inner aspect of the meniscal root

    b. Best seen in the coronal projection with thin sections

    c. A root tear can be simulated by enlargement of the anterolateral meniscosyn-ovial recess with associated anterolateral meniscal hypoplasia

    d. Enlarged anterolateral meniscosynovial recesses can simulate meniscal cysts

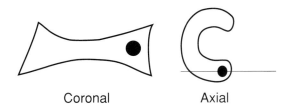

Fig. F-15.4   Coronal   Axial

**F-15   Diagramatic Pearls in the Assessment of Meniscus Tears
(Cont'd)**

5. Myxoid Change
    a. Often horizontal in shape
    b. "V" configuration in the sagittal orientation
    c. No communication with capsular surface
    d. Less conspicuous in inner one-third of meniscus
    e. Generally less intense than hyaline cartilage on T1

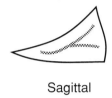

Sagittal

Fig. F-15.5

6. Wrisberg Ligament
    a. Most commonly seen in the inner aspect of the posterolateral meniscus horn simulating a posterosuperior margin tear
    b. The interface between Wrisberg and the meniscus runs from superoanterior to inferoposterior
    c. Tip-off: There is no tear visible in the coronal projection

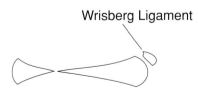

Wrisberg Ligament

Fig. F-15.6

F-15 **Diagramatic Pearls in the Assessment of Meniscus Tears (Cont'd)**

7. Ligament of Winslow

    a. The transverse ligament of Winslow courses between the two anterior menisci

    b. When prominent, this may simulate a meniscal avulsion or anterior tear

    c. The interface between the ligament of Winslow and the anterolateral horn courses from posterosuperior to anteroinferior

    d. The Winslow pitfall may simulate the folded bucket handle tear, particularly on the lateral side

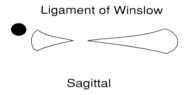

Ligament of Winslow

Sagittal

Fig. F-15.7

8. Popliteus Reflection

    a. Runs vertically or from posterosuperior to anteroinferior

    b. Perforated by the superior and inferior fascicles of the lateral meniscus

    c. Intermediate in signal on proton density and T1 (the tendon lies posterior to it and is black)

    d. On rare occasions, the vertical reflection will simulate a tear, and conversely, a vertical tear may be mistaken for the popliteus reflection

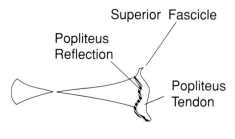

Superior Fascicle

Popliteus Reflection

Popliteus Tendon

Fig. F-15.8   Sagittal

F-16   Pitfalls in Diagnosing Meniscal Disease: Summary

1.   Myxoid change can simulate meniscal tear

2.   True intrameniscal tear can simulate myxoid change but can be identified by

   a. Involvement of the inner 1/3 of the meniscus

   b. Signal intensity equal to adjacent hyaline cartilage on single echo short TE imaging

   c. Unusual shape

3.   Transverse meniscal ligament of Winslow can simulate bucket handle tear or anterolateral horn

4.   Meniscal fibrillation: Wear and tear fraying usually seen in the inner tip near the intracondylar notch producing a fuzzy appearance to the meniscal apex (true truncation should be considered abnormal while fibrillation is usually asymptomatic)

5.   Popliteus tendon: Simulates a posterolateral meniscus vertical tear

6.   Two-tone meniscus sign: Fluid in the inner aspect of a meniscus may simulate an intact meniscus (while the fluid on short TE image is gray, the meniscus itself is black creating two tones to the meniscus appearance)

7.   Partial volume averaging: The meniscus is shaped like an arrow, and peripheral sections may volume average capsular tissue creating a sandwich of hypointense meniscus, linear intermediate signal and hypointense meniscus

8.   Meniscofemoral ligaments: The ligament of Wrisberg may simulate a posterosuperior meniscus tear separated from the meniscus by a line coursing from anterosuperior to posteroinferior

9.   Pseudo bucket handle tear: The posterolateral horn may appear separated into two parts in the coronal section due to external positioning of the knee and concavity of the lateral meniscus, less common on the medial side (there is no associated contusion or soft tissue injury)

10. Pseudohypertrophy of the anterior horn: A fragment of meniscus folded posterior to anterior creates a pseudomass anteriorly

11. Lax meniscocapsular and meniscosynovial attachments make the meniscus appear to be prolapsing out of the joint space (not uncommon with arthropathy or effusion)

F-16   Pitfalls in Diagnosing Meniscal Disease: Summary (Cont'd)

12. Vacuum phenomenon: Magnetic susceptibility from intra-articular gas may produce areas of signal void or "blooming" artifact, particularly on gradient echo images; this may simulate a meniscal injury

13. Meniscocapsular separation: A subset of meniscus tear which can be missed, displacement of the posterior horn of the medial meniscus 5 mm anterior to the uncovered tibial articular cartilage suggests the presence of detachment (detachments less than 1 cm in length are treated conservatively)

14. Curettage tracks: Post-meniscectomy areas of curettage or oversewing may persist as areas of increased signal in the meniscus for months or years. Differentiation of an oversewn track or a curette site from a retear may be made by utilizing intra-articular contrast and exercise prior to scanning. True tears will fill while successfully oversewn curettage sites will not.

15. Meniscal agenesis: Absent meniscus, usually posterolateral meniscus

16. Meniscal hypoplasia: Usually thin anterolateral horn

17. Large anterolateral meniscosynovial recess: May simulate meniscal cyst

18. Inferolateral genicular artery: May simulate anterior meniscal fragment

F-17   Pearls of Meniscal Cyst

1. Four times more common on the lateral than on the medial meniscus
2. Incidence: 1-2% of the population
3. Lateral cysts are smaller, more often symptomatic and produce lateral joint line swelling and tenderness, worsened with extension
4. Medial cysts are larger, more often nontender and asymptomatic
5. Medial cysts dissect through soft tissue planes, may migrate and become giant
6. Medial cysts may mimic popliteal cysts
7. Meniscal cysts have a 3:1 male predominance
8. Signal intensity is that of proteinaceous water, hypointense T1 and hyperintense T2
9. Ovoid shape
10. Intrameniscal signal alteration or tear is invariably present
11. Differential diagnosis
    a. Ganglion: Eccentric, pericapsular, usually not at joint line
    b. Capsular cyst: At the joint line but no meniscus tear
    c. Gastrocnemius semimembranosus bursal cyst: Posterior prolapse between tendons
    d. Pes bursitis: Extends along pes anserine

F-18   Primary Skeletal Neoplasms of the Knee

Malignant (listed in order of frequency)

Osteosarcoma: Homogeneous or storiform*

Chondrosarcoma: Homogeneous or storiform, ± cystic

Reticulum cell sarcoma: Homogeneous, intermediate T2

Fibrosarcoma: Homogeneous, intermediate or hypointense

Ewing's sarcoma: Storiform, hemorrhagic

Benign (listed in order of frequency)

Osteochondroma: Hyperintense T2 cap, hypointense calcium

Giant cell tumor: Homogeneous, hyperintense T2

Aneurysmal bone cysts: Hemorrhagic hypointense T2

Chondroma: Homogeneous

Osteoid osteoma: Circumferential edema around hypointense rim

Chondroblastoma: Hypointense rim, circumferential edema, intermediate T2

Chondromyxoid fibroma: Mixed T1 and T2 signal

  * Storiform, or pleomorphic results in an inhomogeneous appearance with mixed hyper- and
    hypointense T1 & T2 signal due to variable aged hemorrhage, calcification, myxoid material or
    fibrous tissue.

F-19   Soft Tissue Tumors of the Knee & Leg

(Listed in order of frequency)

Liposarcoma: Myxoid type, homogeneous, mildly hyperintense T1 & T2

Malignant fibrous histiocytoma: Inhomogeneous mixed hyperintensity

Fibrosarcoma: Homogeneous, intermediate to hypointense T2

Synovial sarcoma: Inhomogeneous mixed hyperintensity

Alveolar sarcoma: Inhomogeneous mixed hyperintensity

Hemangioma: T2 wormian hyperintensity with hypointense phleboliths

Rhabdomyosarcoma: Inhomogeneous mixed mild T2 hyperintensity

Hemangiopericytoma

Epithelioid sarcoma: Inhomogeneous mixed mild T2 hyperintensity

Desmoid tumor: Homogeneous T2 iso- or hyperintensity

Giant cell tumor of tendon sheath: T2 hyperintensity

F-20   Lateral Knee Masses on MR

Common

1. Ganglion: Hypointense T1, hyperintense T2, closely associated with tendons or joints but without meniscus tear, often superomedial or lateral

2. Meniscus cyst: Proteinaceous water signal, associated meniscus tear, mid-coronal plane location

3. Loculated lateral retinacular effusion: Water signal, anterior coronal plane location, communicates with patellofemoral bursal reflection under lateral retinaculum

4. Tibiofibular bursitis: Water signal, posterior coronal plane, tibiofibular interface location

Uncommon

1. Popliteus reflection cyst or rupture: Posterolateral location, proteinaceous water signal, 30% associated with popliteus tendon rupture

2. Capsular redundancy: Heterogeneous T2 signal, history of arthropathy, chondromalacia and small menisci often present

3. Hematoma: Intermixed foci of T1 hyperintensity and T2 hypointensity, may have associated fracture or rupture of the lateral collateral ligament

4. Abscess: Intermediate to hypointense T1 and hyperintense T2 signal, hypointense soft tissue and/or bone edema on T1

5. Neoplasm

F-21   Medial Knee Masses on MR

Common

1. Gastrocnemius semimembranosus bursal cyst (Baker's): Water signal, postero-medial location between medial gastrocnemius and semimembranosus tendon heads

2. Loculated effusion: Water signal, communicates with suprapatellar bursa, antero-medial location

Uncommon

1. Giant meniscal cyst: Proteinaceous water signal, associated meniscal tear

2. Ganglion: Water signal intensity, associated with joint capsule or tendons, no associated meniscal tear

3. Capsular redundancy: Signs of arthropathy including small menisci, attenuated hyaline cartilage or subchondral ulceration

4. Pes anserine bursitis: Waterlike signal, extends along the pes tendon complex (semitendinosus, gracilis, and sartorius)

5. Neoplasm

F-22   Posterior Knee Masses on MR

Common

1. Gastrocnemius semimembranosus bursal cyst: Water signal, arises between medial gastrocnemius tendon head and semimembranosus tendon head
2. Giant medial meniscal cyst with posterior extension: Associated with meniscal tear or meniscocapsular separation

Uncommon

1. Ganglion: Water signal, closely associated with joint capsule or tendons
2. Popliteal artery aneurysm: Lamellated hyper- and hypointense signal on T1 and T2
3. Soleus or gastrocnemius muscle rupture: Hyperintense T2 signal, intramuscular
4. Soleus or gastrocnemius muscle hematoma: Hyperintense T1 signal, intramuscular
5. Ruptured biceps femoris or semitendinosus muscle tendon insertion
6. Synovial or capsular redundancy: history of arthritis, small menisci, attenuated hyaline cartilage or chondromalacia

Rare

1. Herniation of the gastrocnemius muscle through the epimysium: Edema confined to one muscle group
2. Neoplasm
3. Abscess: Proteinaceous water signal mass

F-23   Knee Masses: Marked T2 Hypointensity

Rounded Shape

1.   Primary synovial chondromatosis

2.   Secondary synovial chondromatosis

Globular Shape

1.   Post traumatic myositis ossificans

2.   Periosteal osteogenic sarcoma

Circumferential or Lamellated Configuration

1.   Pigmented villonodular synovitis

2.   Hemophilia

3.   Popliteal artery aneurysm

Linear Shape

1.   Cortical bone fragment

2.   Chronic cartilaginous flake or fragment

F-24   Key Ligaments & Tendons About the Knee

1. Posterior cruciate ligament: Originates from lateral side of posteromedial femoral condyle and attaches to the extreme posterior intracondylar tibial region

2. Anterior cruciate ligament: Originates from the medial aspect of the lateral femoral condyle and inserts on the anterior tibial plateau 1 cm posterior to its most anterior margin

3. Medial collateral ligament
   a. Superficial tibial collateral ligament: Originates from the medial femoral condyle and inserts on the medial tibia 5 cm below the joint line
   b. Deep capsular ligament attaches tightly to the medial meniscal third; origin is from the femoral condyle and epicondyle; insertion is just below the tibial articular margin

4. Lateral collateral ligament
   a. Iliotibial band: Insertion is proximally into the lateral femoral condyle and distally into the lateral tibial tubercle (Gerdy's tubercle)
   b. Fibular collateral ligament: Originates from the lateral femoral epicondyle just proximal to the popliteus tendon and inserts with the biceps femoris tendon as the conjoined tendon onto the femoral head
   c. Biceps femoris tendon: Originates from the lateral aspect of the ischial tuberosity and inserts on the fibular head

5. Transverse meniscal ligament (of Winslow): Inserts along the anterior aspect of the lateral and medial anterior meniscal horns

6. Popliteus tendon: Originates from the lateral femoral condyle just below the fibular collateral ligament as the popliteus muscle inserts along the posteromedial tibia

7. Meniscofemoral ligament
   a. Wrisberg ligament originates from the posterior horn of the lateral meniscus, inserts at the lateral surface of the medial femoral condyle (behind the PCL)
   b. Humphry's ligament: Originates from posterior horn of lateral meniscus and inserts or blends with the posterior cruciate ligament (passes in front of the PCL)

F-25   Posterior Cruciate Ligament: Buckling in the Sagittal Plane

Common

1. Overextension of the knee
2. ACL laxity
3. ACL acute tear
4. ACL chronic tear
5. Oversizing of anterior cruciate ligament graft

Uncommon

1. Distal posterior cruciate ligament tear
2. Avulsion of the posterior cruciate ligament tibial insertion

Rare

1. Ehlers-Danlos syndrome
2. Marfan's syndrome
3. Cutis-Laxa

F-26   Pearls of the Posterior Cruciate Ligament

1.   More hypointense than the ACL

2.   Arcuate shape in extension

3.   Straight shape in flexion

4.   30% thicker than the ACL (16-18 mm)

5.   Two times as strong as ACL or MCL

6.   Insufficiency is associated with quadriceps tendinitis, patellar grinding and premature degenerative disease

7.   Intra-articular but extrasynovial location

8.   Accessory ligaments of Humphry in front or Wrisberg behind the PCL seen in 90% of normal studies

9.   Tears of the PCL are repaired by suturing +/- graft augmentation

10. Avulsions of the tibial insertion are repaired with screw fixation or pull-through procedures

11. Bone contusions with PCL tear are not as consistent as with ACL tear; however, meniscal injuries near the meniscal roots either medially or laterally may occur

12. Retraction of the PCL with complete tear is rare

F-27   Evaluation & Pitfalls of PCL Injuries on MR

1.   Atrophy, common with chronic injuries

2.   Even with high grade tears, PCL shape is often preserved

3.   The extent of signal and its cross-sectional involvement of the ligament allows grading

4.   Avulsion injury, particularly off the tibial end, is uncommon

Pitfalls in the Diagnosis of PCL Injury

1.   Acute blood in the PCL sheath may simulate a higher grade of injury than really exists

2.   A bone flake or avulsion injury, particularly seen in children, may be missed on MR without the plain film and is often associated with a large hemarthrosis

3.   Sheath inflammation with arthritis may obscure the PCL; this is particularly profound on T1 or proton density imaging

4.   High grade PCL tears still do not often retract

5.   Remember that a PCL tear may be profound on MR and may be missed arthroscopically, since the tibial end of the PCL is difficult to visualize with the arthroscope when the ACL is intact, regardless of the experience of the arthrographer

F-28   Direct & Indirect Signs of ACL Injury on MR

1.   Atrophy
2.   Abrupt changes in caliber
3.   Focal angulation
4.   Focal signal change
5.   Bleeding into the ACL sheath
6.   Fraying and fibrillation of ACL fibers (the "octopus" sign)
7.   Lateral femoral sulcus terminalis contusion
8.   Posterolateral tibial contusion
9.   ACL discontiguity with retraction
10. Abnormal ACL course or direction (the "laying down" sign)
11. Buckling of the posterior cruciate ligament, a sign of ACL laxity, injury or tear
12. Anterior tibial translation sign or luxation of the femur posteriorly relative to the tibia

F-29   Pitfalls in the Diagnosis of ACL Injury

1. Volume averaging of the posterior femoral cortex may simulate ACL contiguity

2. The femoral end of the ACL may be poorly visualized in the sagittal projection due to imprecise angulation, and the coronal view should be examined

3. Bleeding into the sheath of the ACL without complete tear or severe capsulosynovial thickening may obscure its visualization on proton density or T1 imaging

4. The chronically injured or torn ACL may be focally angulated, but may remain contiguous due to the presence of fibrosis and hemosiderin at the injury site

5. Avulsion of an epiphyseal or tibial spine cortical surface

    a. May not be easily seen without plain films and may be missed

    b. A large hemarthrosis is frequently present

    c. This injury is most common in children and represents the avulsion type of ACL injury

6. A reverse pitfall is the presence of a high grade or complete ACL tear with a normal arthroscopy

    a. We have seen this on several occasions, where the sheath of the ACL demonstrates no evidence of discontiguity, edema, hyperemia or bleed

    b. It is only with careful probing that the orthopedic surgeon finds the true high grade ACL tear

F-30   Angles of Acquisition Employed for ACL Evaluation

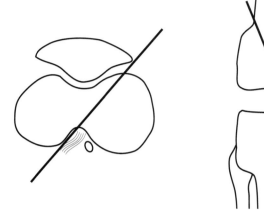

Using an axial image to obtain
correctly aligned sagittal images

Using a coronal image to obtain
correctly aligned sagittal images

Fig. F-30.1

F-31   Anatomy & Variations of the Anterior Cruciate Ligament

1. Approximately 12 mm in thickness (in the most frequently scanned position appears straight without angulation)
2. Intermediate to hypointense
3. Intermediate signal along the distal tibial end is not uncommon due to the presence of sheath thickening
4. Periligamentous tissues may be of intermediate signal, particularly if there is capsulosynovial thickening
5. Continuous and can be seen in at least two major bundles, anterolateral and posteromedial
6. Extends from posterosuperior and lateral to anteroinferior and medial
7. Can be found in the lateral aspect of the femoral tunnel
8. With knee flexion the ACL may appear lax or may not be visualized

F-32 **Pearls of the Anterior Cruciate Ligament**

1. Thinner, straighter, and less hypointense than the PCL

2. Extrasynovial intracapsular location

3. Two major fiber bundles, anteromedial and posterolateral

4. Normal width equals 10-13 mm

5. Length: 4 cm

6. Becomes buckled or poorly visualized with knee flexion or over-rotation

7. Tears are most often in the ACL midsubstance

8. Avulsion with fragments of bone usually occur at the femoral attachment

9. Postoperative graft

   a. Size approximates 12 mm

   b. Tibial tunnel 2 cm anterior to posterior cruciate tibial insertion

   c. Femoral tunnel placed as far posterior and close to posterior cortex as possible

   d. Graft may assume intermediate signal due to ingrowth of granulation tissue up to 6 months

F-33 Criteria for ACL Tear

Complete ACL Tear

Direct Criteria

1. Complete midsubstance discontiguity
2. Abnormal cruciate course (ligament does not attach to its normal posterosuperior femoral site or anteroinferior tibial site)
3. Midsubstance intracapsular hematoma pseudomass
4. Cruciate ligament corrugation or buckling

Indirect Criteria

1. Buckling of the posterior cruciate ligament
2. Posterior femorotibial subluxation (MR drawer sign)

Incomplete ACL Tear

1. ACL thinning (less than 10 mm)
2. Periligamentous hematoma pseudomass with intact fibers
3. Increased intraligamentous signal with residual intact fibers

F-34   Grades of Medial Collateral Ligament Injury

Description

Grade I
Capsular injury with intermediate T1 signal deep to the hypointense tibial collateral ligament

Grade II
Intermediate T1 signal deep and superficial to the tibial collateral ligament with associated fiber attenuation

Grade III
Intermediate T1 signal in the capsule and replacing the tibial collateral ligament with associated ligamentous retraction or corrugation

Grade IV
Same as Grade III with associated micro- or macrofracture and meniscal tear

F-35   Medial Collateral Ligament Injury by Grade

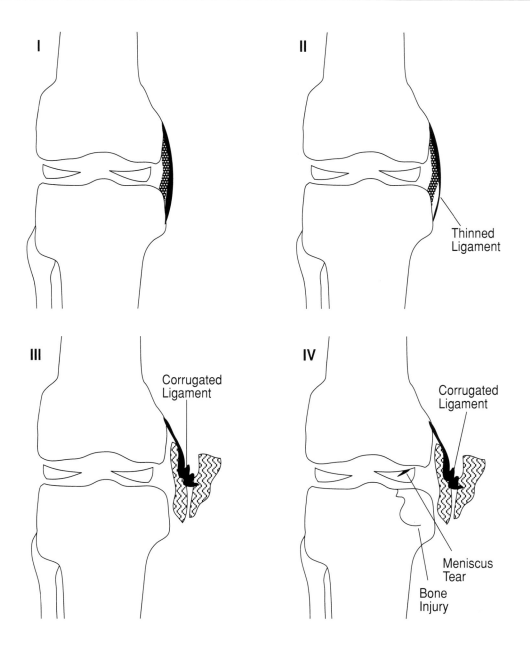

Fig. F-35.1

F-36   Anatomy of the Lateral Capsular Ligament

1. Anterior division: Anterior capsule plus anterior iliotibial band

2. Middle division: Midcoronal capsule and iliotibial band as far back as the fibular collateral ligament (the strongest portion of the lateral complex)

3. Posterior division (arcuate complex): Fibular collateral ligament (FCL), arcuate ligament, and musculotendinous aponeurosis of the popliteus muscle

    a. FCL arises from the lateral epicondyle of the femur and joins the biceps femoris tendon to insert on the fibular head as the conjoined tendon

    b. The popliteus tendon passes deep to the FCL, perforating the posterolateral meniscus, becoming muscular along the posterior tibia

    c. The arcuate ligament arises from the fibular styloid with lateral limb attachment to the femur and popliteal tendon and medial limb attachment to the posterior horn of the lateral meniscus

F-37   The "Terrible Pentad" of Hyperextension Injury of the Knee

1. Meniscus tear

2. Medial collateral ligament tear

3. Anterior cruciate ligament tear

4. Hyaline cartilage edema, fissure or fragmentation (thickened hyaline pad on T1 with inhomogeneous hyperintense signal on fast scan)

5. Bone contusion, edema, or microfracture (hypointense T1)

F-38   Evaluating the Patella with Flexion

Features which can be assessed with 10° of flexion on axial MR

1.   Articular facet size and shape of the patella
2.   Size of the femoral ridges
3.   Trochlear depth
4.   Sulcus angle
5.   Congruence angle
6.   Patellar signal
7.   Cartilaginous thickness and signal
8.   Lateral patellar subluxation or displacement
9.   Plical thickness

F-39   The Patellofemoral Joint: Morphologic Indices

Axial View

1.   Trochlear facet angle (E' TI') An angle greater than 145° is abnormal.

2.   Trochlear depth (E' I': TH'). An indication of sulcus retentiveness with higher ratios indicating a propensity toward subluxation and poor retentiveness. Normal range is 4.2-6.5.

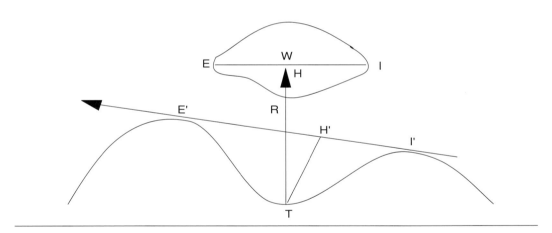

Modified from Ficat RP, Hungerford DS. Disorders of the Patellofemoral Joint. Baltimore, Williams & Wilkins, 1977.

Fig. F-39.1

F-40   Normal Tilting Angle

The normal tilting angle B'BA is 8° (Diagram 1) and is open to the lateral side. With tilt, the angle closes and is now open on the medial side (Diagram 2) and -8° of tilt exists.

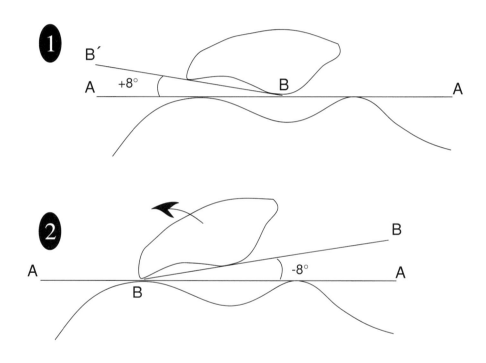

Fig. F-40.1

F-41 The Patella: Measuring Subluxation & Tilting

1. Tilting angle: An angle (a) created by the line AB that courses from the edge of the lateral to the medial patellar facet and the line LM that courses across the lateral and medial femoral condylar ridges

2. Lateral shift or subluxation: Determined from the degree of patellar displacement lateral to a line perpendicular to the lateral femoral ridge apex (CL)

   a. The percent of patella lying lateral to this line is the degree of lateral shift, = AC/DC X100 (%)

   b. The degree of lateral subluxation = % of patella lying lateral to this line (AC)/transverse patellar line (AB); the latter is more commonly used to determine the degree of MR lateral patellar displacement

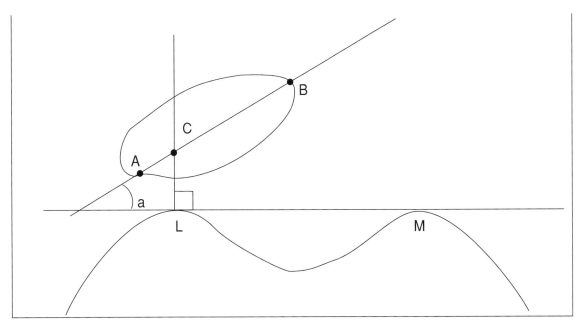

A –lateral edge of the facet
B –medial edge of the facet
M–highest point of the medial condyle
L –highest point of the lateral condyle
C –crossing of the transverse patellar line (AB) and the perpendicular line from L
a –tilting angle

Methods for measuring lateral shift (as a percentage) and tilting angle (in degrees) from the CT image at the middle part of the patella. Lateral shift = AC/BC x 100 (%). Tilting angle = a degrees.

Adapted from Sasaki T, Yagi T: Subluxation of the patella. Int Orthop (SICOT) 10:116-120, 1986.

Fig. F-41.1

F-42   Patella Alta on MR

Insall-Salvati index: At 30° of flexion, the ratio of the patellar tendon length to that of the greatest diagonal length of the patella is calculated (normal < 1.2).

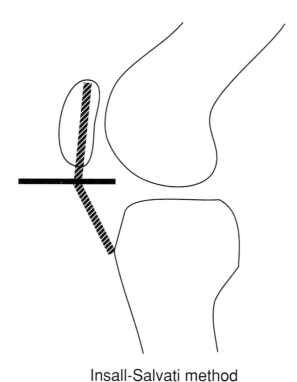

Insall-Salvati method

Fig. F-42.1

F-43   Patella Alta & Baja

Patella Alta (High Patellar Position)

1.   Recurrent subluxation
2.   Chronic chondromalacia and degenerative arthropathy
3.   Larsen-Johansson disease
4.   Cerebral palsy
5.   Quadriceps atrophy

Patella Baja (Low Patellar Position)

1.   Poliomyelitis
2.   Achondroplasia
3.   Juvenile rheumatoid arthritis
4.   Long-standing rheumatoid arthritis

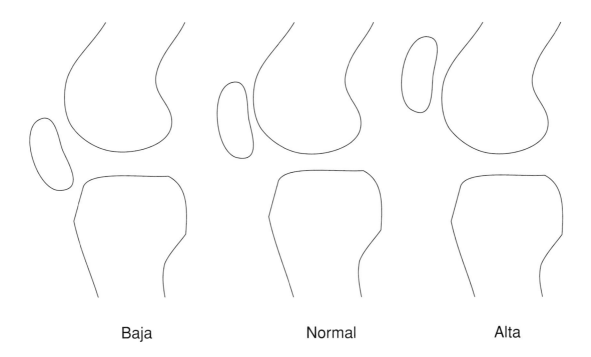

Baja   Normal   Alta

Fig. F-43.1

F-44   The Patella: Measuring the Congurence Angle

The congruence angle is measured by bisecting the sulcus angle (I' TE') with reference line TO and then projecting a second line (RT) from the sulcus (T) to the lowest point on the articular ridge of the patella (R). The congruence angle (TOR) is negative if R is medial to reference line TO and positive if it is lateral to reference line TO. The angle TOR is expressed in +/- degrees, with the normal range being 0° to -8°.

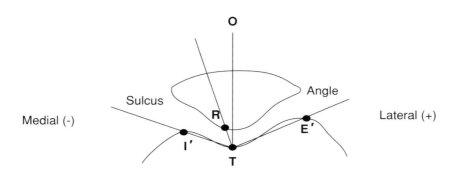

Fig. F-44.1

F-45   **The Patella: Types of Subluxation**

Description

Type I	Subluxation without tilt
Type II	Subluxation with tilt
Type III	Tilt without subluxation

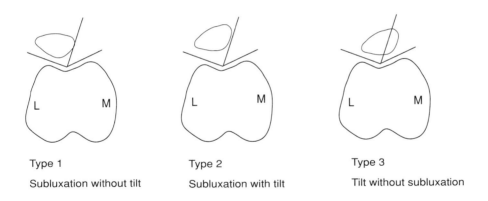

Type 1

Subluxation without tilt

Type 2

Subluxation with tilt

Type 3

Tilt without subluxation

From Minkoff J and Fein L. The Role of Radiography . In Henry J, ed. *Clinics in Sportsmedicine*, April 1989.

Fig. F-45.1

F-46   Normal Patellar Measurements & Angles

1. Patellar tilt angle: Greater than 6° (open angle)
2. Congruence angle: -6° to +6°
3. Insall-Salvati Index: 0.9 to 1.10 (+/- 2 SD)
4. Sulcus angle: 135° to 145° (+/- 2 SD)
5. Lateral shift: Less than 5%
6. Lateral displacement: Less than 5%
7. Trochlear depth: 4.2:6.5

F-47   Pearls in the Diagnosis of Bi- and Tripartite Patella

1. Thought to be congenital and usually asymptomatic
2. Patella ossifies by age five, ossification centrifugally
3. Chondral osseous separation may occur during development
4. Male:female ratio = 9:1
5. Decreases for women in jumping sports, may be acquired variation
6. 50% unilateral
7. 5% superior pole, 20% lateral, 75% superolateral
8. It is critical to exclude fracture in patients with acute anterior knee pain in tripartite patella (peripatellar and infrapatellar edema should be sought)

F-48   Pearls of Plica Syndrome

1. A post-traumatic or post-inflammatory syndrome producing anterior knee pain

2. A normal embryologic septation, crescent-shaped, extending from the infrapatellar fat pad medially, looping around the femoral condyle and crossing under the quadriceps tendon in the suprapatellar region to pass laterally over the lateral femoral condyle

3. Clinical syndrome: Pain, progressively worse with sitting and knee flexion, aggravated by the first 8-10 steps of walking, and subsequently ameliorates

4. Associated with atony of the articularis genu muscle, which is slow in extracting the plica from the patellofemoral joint

5. Fibrotic plica produces popping or snapping on flexion and extension

6. MR findings
    a. Thickened linear hypointense band medial or inferior to the patella (> 3 mm)
    b. Hypointense band with circumferential T2 hyperintensity
    c. Hypointense band adjacent to patellar spur
    d. Joint effusion

7. Other associated findings
    a. Quadriceps atrophy
    b. Hamstring shortening

F-49   Hoffa Fat Pad Sign: Etiologies

1.   Trauma with hemarthrosis
2.   Rheumatoid arthritis
3.   Extensive degenerative arthritis
4.   Juvenile rheumatoid arthritis
5.   Hemophilia
6.   Pigmented villonodular synovitis
7.   Lyme arthritis

F-50   Pearls in Hoffa's Disease

1. Irregular signal hypointensity in the infrapatellar fat pad with variable T2 signal

2. Enlargement or bulging of the fat pad so that the infrapatellar tendon is pushed anteriorly

3. Ninety-five percent of all cases are secondary to prior trauma or surgery, with idiopathic Hoffa's disease rare

4. Secondary intermediate infrapatellar tendon signal alteration (20%)

5. Hypointense foci secondary to calcification or increased calcific density on plain film (10%)

6. Atrophy of the quadriceps musculotendinous complex (5%)

F-51   Pearls in the Diagnosis of Osgood-Schlatter Disease

1. Most common in puberty
2. Usually inactive with regard to pain after age 15
3. Tendinitis associated with incomplete fusion of the tibial apophysis originally thought to be osteochondrosis but more likely traumatic in nature
4. Males predominate 3:1
5. Bilateral 40%
6. Irregularity of the apophyseal fragments results in secondary inflammatory edema
7. Localized pockets of fluid or cystic T2 hyperintensity may be present
8. Treatment: Injection of localized cysts of fluid signal with anesthetic and steroid

F-52   Tendon Injuries About the Knee

(Listed in descending order of frequency)

1. Quadriceps

    a. Suprapatellar: More common in patients under 40

    b. Infrapatellar: More common in patients over 40

2. Gastrocnemius rupture

    a. Either at the insertion site or associated with intramuscular hematoma formation

    b. May also be associated with compartment syndrome and Type III tibial stress syndrome

3. Plantaris rupture

    a. Has a far better prognosis than that of gastrocnemius tendon rupture, although the two look alike clinically

    b. With plantaris rupture, the return to active physical duty and active sports is much quicker than with gastrocnemius rupture

    c. Plantaris rupture is easily diagnosed, since the length of involvement extends all the way from the knee down to the distal leg

    d. In contrast, gastrocnemius rupture and hematoma is localized to a few centimeters and is intramuscular within the confines of the gastrocnemius

4. Popliteus rupture: Rare unless there is severe internal derangement

F-53   **Spectrum of Tendon Injury on MR**

1. Tendinitis: Linear striated areas of intermediate T1 or proton density signal with minimal T2 hyperintensity
2. Partial tear: More discrete and conspicuously hyperintense on T2
    a. Chronic: Associated with tendon hypertrophy
    b. Acute: Associated with normal sized or edematous tendon
    c. Tendon tear associated with tendon atrophy or decreased size is uncommon

Tendon injury should be assessed with regard to the following:
-   Location in tendon or myotendinous junction
-   Hemorrhage
-   Fluid
-   Ganglion formation
-   Retraction
-   Status of smoothness or roughness of the torn edges
-   Presence or absence of muscular atrophy or fatty replacement

F-54   Pearls in the Diagnosis of Quadriceps Tendinitis

1. Quadriceps tendon components
    a. Rectus femoris
    b. Vastus lateralis
    c. Vastus medialis
    d. Vastus intermedius
2. Tendinitis often a precursor of tendon rupture
3. Avulsion at patellar insertion more common than midsubstance tear
4. Anisotropic rotation or magic angle (55°) phenomenon produces false intratendinous signal
5. Complete rupture is associated with tendon discontiguity
6. Tendinopathy may be associated with hypertrophic or enlarged tendon with intermediate T1 and hyperintense T2
7. Lamellated appearance to the tendon consisting of alternating bright and dark signal on T1 imaging is related to interposition of fat between layers of the quadriceps tendon (layers of bright signal may be 1, 2, 3 or 4 in number)
8. Focal signal at the infrapatellar teno-osseous junction is known as "jumper's knee" and is seen in volleyball and basketball players

F-55   Pearls of Quadriceps Mechanism Injury

1. Quadriceps tendon anatomic contributions: Rectus femoris, vastus medialis, intermedius and lateralis

2. Three quadriceps layers

   a. Superficial layer rectus femoris

   b. Middle layer vastus lateralis and medialis

   c. Deep layer vastus intermedius

3. Normal patellar tendon length should approximate patellar bone length

4. Mechanism of injury

   a. Elderly patients descending stairs or jumping

   b. Abrupt deceleration in a highly trained athlete

5. Sites of involvement in order of frequency

   a. Muscle/tendon junction

   b. Intratendinous

   c. Tendon/bone junction (above or below patella)

   d. Tibial tubercle insertion

6. Presdisposing conditions

   a. Gout

   b. Systemic lupus erythematosus

   c. Diabetes mellitus

7. Frequency of tears by age

   a. Intratendinous central anterior tear predisposed in elderly patients

   b. Patellar intratendinous tears predisposed in younger athletes

8. MR criteria for complete tear

   a. Complete diastasis of tendon anatomy or tendon/osseous separation

   b. Intermediate T1 signal and hyperintense T2 signal at injury site

F-56   Magic Angle Versus Patellar Tendon Injury or Tendinitis

Magic Angle
Abrupt cut-off margins
Signal alterations occur at sites of signal
    angulation that are oriented 55° from
    the main magnetic field
Occurs at sites of tendon undulation
Less conspicuous on T2 long TE images
The tendon caliber is normal

Tendon Injury or Tendinitis
Zones of transition are indistinct
Tendinitis and tendon injury signal is
    not dependent on tendon angulation

Unrelated to tendon undulation
May persist on T2 or water weighted images
Tendon caliber may be increased (rarely,
    decreased)

F-57   Variable MR Appearance of the Quadriceps Tendon

1.   Lamellated with three layers of alternating fat and tendon (56%)

2.   Lamellated with two layers of alternating fat and tendon (30%)

3.   Poorly lamellated with appearance of one central tendon (8%)

4.   Four lamellations of alternating fat and tendon (6%)

The layered configuration of the quadriceps tendon is related to fusion of the muscular layers of the vastus intermedius, vastus lateralis, vastus medialis and rectus femoris.

Zeiss J, Saddemi SR, Ebraheim NA. MR Imaging of the quadriceps tendon: normal layer configuration and its importance in cases of tendon rupture, AJR: 159, 1031-1034 1992

F-58   Patellar Bursitis & Tendinitis by Location

1. Prepatellar bursitis: Hyperintense T2 signal, located between the skin and outer surface of the patella or upper half of the patellar tendon; known as housemaid's knee or lover's knee

2. Deep infrapatellar bursitis: T2 signal hyperintensity located between the infrapatellar tendon and the tibia just above the tibial tubercle and within the caudal aspect of the Hoffa fat pad

3. Superficial infrapatellar bursitis: T2 signal hyperintensity located just anterior to the inferior or tibial insertion of the patellar tendon; association with Osgood-Schlatter disease may be present

4. Quadriceps tendinitis: Intermediate T1 and mild to moderate hyperintense T2 signal in the suprapatellar tendon

5. Infrapatellar tendinitis
   a. Subpatellar: Called jumper's knee with intermediate T1 signal at the inferior patellotendinous attachment; may be associated with Larsen-Johansson disease
   b. Tibial insertion: Intermediate intratendinous T1 signal associated with acute injury in athletes or with Osgood-Schlatter disease

F-59   Pearls in the Diagnosis of Iliotibial Band Syndrome

1. Friction or overuse syndrome producing lateral knee or thigh pain
2. Long distance runners, cyclists, football players or weightlifters
3. Etiology: Friction of the iliotibial band of the lateral femoral condyle
4. Changes in the iliotibial band caliber with thickening or focal thinning associated with perilesional hyperintense T2 edema

F-60   Pearls in the Diagnosis of Bone Contusion

1. Lateral side more common than medial, 8:1

2. Lateral side bruise associated with MCL or ACL tear

3. Medial side bruise associated with LCL injury

4. Resolution of signal in 2-4 weeks for small lesions, up to 8-10 months for large lesions

5. Arthroscopic examination of the femoral condylar cartilage is normal

6. Vague, poorly defined T1 signal hypointensity becomes less pronounced as one moves farther away from the joint surface

7. Epiphyseal or epimetaphyseal location in all cases

8. No evidence of linear hypointensity unless macrofracture is concomitantly present

9. T2 signal is variable depending upon contusion age and may be hyperintense (edema), isointense (mixed edema and hemorrhage), or hypointense (hemorrhage)

F-61   Spectrum of Stress-Related Bone Injury

Classification According to Detmer

Grade I   Classic stress fracture consisting of edema in bone with sparing of the periskeletal tissues such as periosteum and soft tissues. Injury to bone can occur in overuse of normal bone (as in marathon runners) or with insufficiency fractures in patients with abnormal bone, as in osteomalacia. Bone scan is hot in all three phases, and usually demonstrates fusiform longitudinal or horizontal increased uptake.

Grade II   Periosteal inflammation or edema on MR, most conspicuous on T2 and/or fat saturated sequences. This has also been referred to as the soleal syndrome, since commonly the periosteum deep to the soleus muscle is involved.

Grade III   There is involvement of bone, periosteum and/or one of the muscular compartments, either anterior, lateral, medial or posterior. Muscular hemorrhage, hematoma, and edema is apparent on T2 and fat saturated water weighted sequences.

F-62   Pitfalls in Bone Evaluation of the Knee

1. Red marrow, more common in smokers, may simulate a mass and is hypointense on T1 and slightly hyperintense on T2 (distal and proximal femurs, proximal tibia, sternum, iliac crest, proximal and distal humeri are common locations)

2. Tibial pit is an irregularity in the proximal tibial surface in between the tibial spines or adjacent to them which can simulate an osteochondral defect (such lesions remain hypointense and are poorly visualized in other projections)

3. The normal physis may be volume averaged in the axial projection to simulate a macrofracture line

4. Cortical desmoid

    a. Normal periosteal reaction resulting in enthesopathic traction of the adductor magnus on the posteromedial femur

    b. Biopsy of this lesion may reveal proliferation of new bone and simulate neoplasia

    c. The desmoid remains relatively hypointense on all pulsing sequences

5. Nonossifying fibroma

    a. A common eccentric distal femoral bone lesion

    b. Well marginated with narrow zone of transition

    c. Hypointense fibrous content, a potential hyperintense T2 cystic content, and potential hypointense T1 and T2 sclerotic content

    d. A dark, hypointense rim may be present

    e. When less than 2 cm in size, it is referred to as a fibrous cortical defect; from 2-4 cm, a fibrous endosteal defect, and greater than 4 cm, a fibrous medullary defect or nonossifying fibroma

    f. Such lesions do not enhance with gadolinium and enhance faintly or not at all on bone scintigraphy

    g. With fat content these are referred to as fibroxanthomatous lesions of bone (on MR we subcategorize these lesions as nonossifying fibromas of the fibrous, sclerotic, cystic or xanthomatous type)

    h. Eccentric location and narrow zone of transition in the posteromedial femur are the keys to diagnosis

F-62   Pitfalls in Bone Evaluation of the Knee (Cont'd)

6.   Stippled epiphysis or small foci of persistent hypointensity, punctate in size, do not demonstrate T2 hyperintensity

7.   Nonossified epiphysis is of intermediate signal intensity on T1 and demonstrates no hyperintense T1 marrow

8.   Irregular or fragmented epiphysis is common in the nonweight-bearing portion of the femur and may simulate osteochondritis dissecans (this process is symmetric and not associated with surrounding edema or soft tissue signal alteration)

F-63   Osteochondritis Dissecans: Sites of Predilection

Medial Femoral Condyle

1. Classic (69%): Lateral aspect of medial femoral condyle on the nonweight-bearing surface

2. Inferocentral (10%): Weight-bearing surface of the medial femoral condylar apex

3. Extended classic (6%): Weight-bearing and nonweight-bearing surface of the medial femoral condyle

Lateral Femoral Condyle

1. Inferocentral (13%): Apex of the lateral femoral condyle

3. Anterior (2%): Anteropatellar portion of the femur

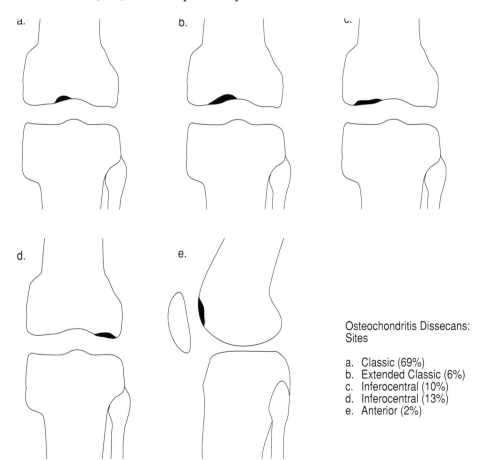

Osteochondritis Dissecans:
Sites

a. Classic (69%)
b. Extended Classic (6%)
c. Inferocentral (10%)
d. Inferocentral (13%)
e. Anterior (2%)

Fig. F-63.1

F-64   **Classification of Osteochondritis Dissecans**

Grade	Description
I	In situ bone fragment without evidence of displacement
II	In situ bone fragment without migration but migrated irregular cartilaginous fragment
III	In situ bone fragment with migrated irregular cartilaginous fragment
IV	Migrated bone and cartilage fragment

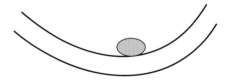

Grade I: In situ bone fragment without evidence of displacement

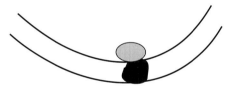

Grade II: In situ well-demarcated bone & cartilage fragments without migration

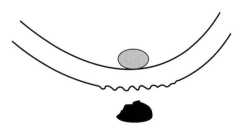

Grade III: In situ bone fragment with migrated irregular cartilaginous fragment

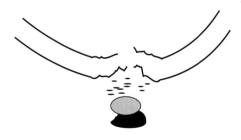

Grade IV: Migrated bone & cartilage fragments

Fig. F-64.1

F-65   Osteochondral Defects & Loose Bodies

1.   Lateral aspect, medial femoral condyle most common (69%)
2.   Sequestered elliptical, subcortical signal hypointensity
3.   The degree of signal hypointensity varies with age of injury
4.   Criteria for fragment instability or loosening
    a. Size greater than 1 cm
    b. Hypointense perilesional rim greater than 3 mm in thickness
    c. Hyperintense fluid signal on fast scan or T2 between the lesion and the overlying femur
5.   Signal intensity of osteochondritis dissecans or loose bodies
    a. Hypointense on T1 and T2 (65%)
    b. Hyperintense centrally with hypointense rim on T1 (30%)
    c. Hypointense or hyperintense on T1 and hyperintense on T2 (5%)

F-65   Osteochondral Defects & Loose Bodies (Cont'd)

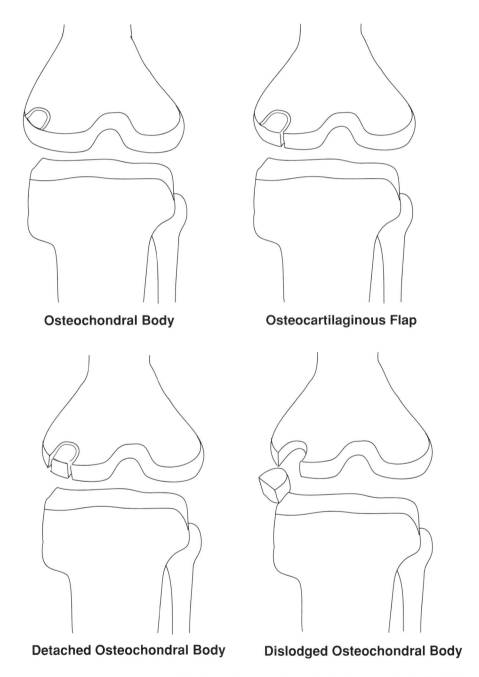

Osteochondral Body   **Osteocartilaginous Flap**

Detached Osteochondral Body   **Dislodged Osteochondral Body**

From Greenspan A. *Orthopedic Radiology: A Practical Approach*. Philadelphia, JB Lippincott, 1988.

Fig. F-65.1

F-66   Pearls in Spontaneous Osteonecrosis of the Adult

1. Occurs in elderly women (3:1 female to male ratio)
2. A specific history of trauma or an acute pain syndrome is often elicited clinically (80%)
3. Joint effusion (90%)
4. Associated medial meniscus tear (40%)
5. Location: Apex of the medial femoral condyle–weight-bearing surface
6. Attenuation or thinning of the hyaline cartilage pads on T1 or fast scanning (50%)
7. Signal: Hypointensity on T1 and T2–confluent, crescentic, and subarticular

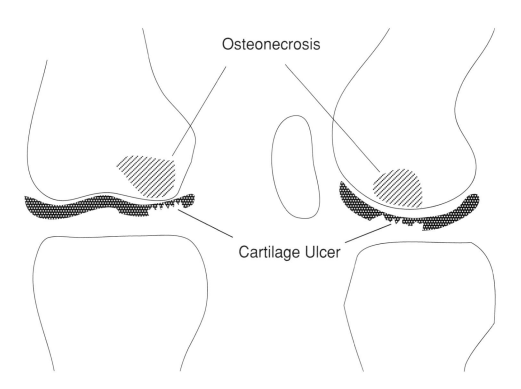

Fig. F-66.1

F-67   Tibial Plateau Fractures: Hohl's Classification*

Description

Grade I   Nondisplaced vertical sagittal split

Grade II   Local central depression

Grade III   Displaced vertical sagittal split and associated depression with or without fibular head fracture

Grade IV   Displaced total medial plateau depression without comminution

Grade V   Nondisplaced anterior or posterior local vertical split oriented coronally without depression

Grade VI   Displaced comminuted fractures involving both plateaus with or without fibular head fractures

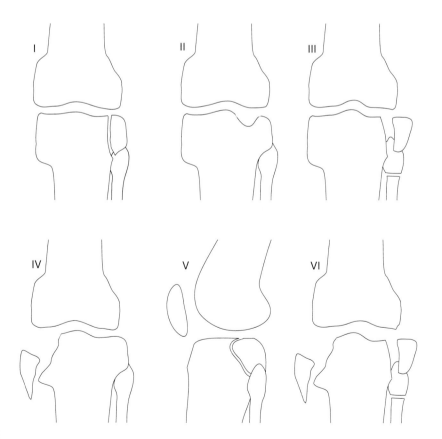

Fig. F-67.1

* Modified from Hohl, 1967.

F-68   Tibial Plateau Fractures: Muller's Classification

Description

Grade I	Nondisplaced wedge or vertical split (A, B)
Grade II	Localized central depression on either plateau (C, D)
Grade III	Displaced vertical wedge with local central depression and fibular fracture (E)
Grade IV	Displaced comminuted fractures involving both plateaus with fibular fracture (F)

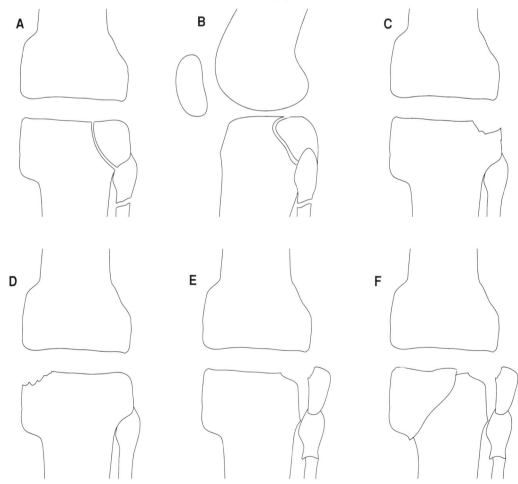

Fig. F-68.1

* Modified from Muller, 1970.

F-69   **Grades of Chondromalacia on MR**

Description

Grade I   Intrameniscal hypointense signal on T1, N(h) and T2 (or fast scan)

Grade II   Intracartilaginous hypointensity with deformity or blistering of the cartilaginous surface

Grade III   Broad-based hypointense signal extending from superficial surface to bony surface but with normal underlying bone signal

Grade IV   Deep or fissured intracartilaginous hypointense signal with underlying skeletal hypointensity on T1 and hyperintensity on T2 (edema and geode formation) or marked hypointensity on T1 and T2 (subchondral sclerosis)

CATEGORY G: FOOT & ANKLE

G-1   Tendons & Vascular Structures About the Ankle (Axial)

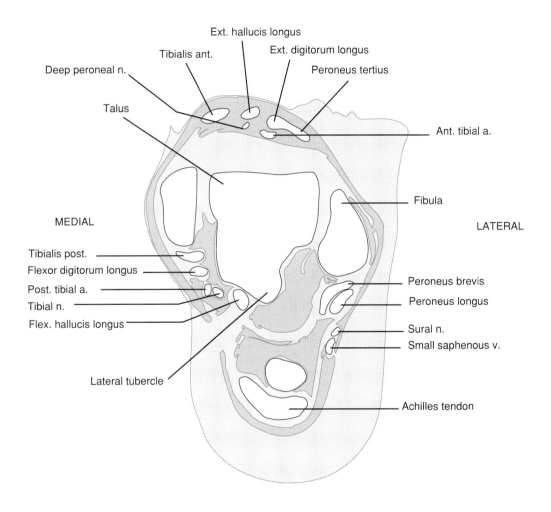

Fig. G-1.1

* Adapted from Berquist TM. MRI of the Musculoskeletal System, p 294. Berquist TH, ed. New York, Raven Press, 1990.

G-2   Muscles & Tendons in the Foot (Short Axis)

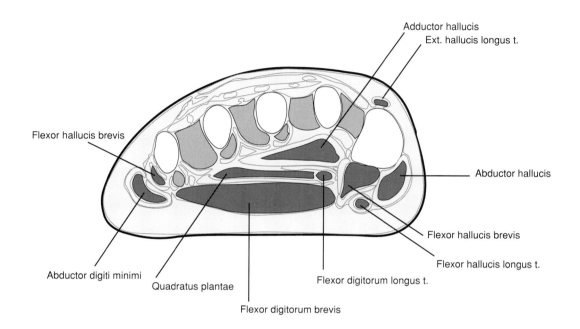

Fig. G-2.1

* Adapted from Berquist TM. MRI of the Musculoskeletal System, p 281. Berquist TH, ed. New York, Raven Press, 1990.

G-3   **Calcaneal Bursae**

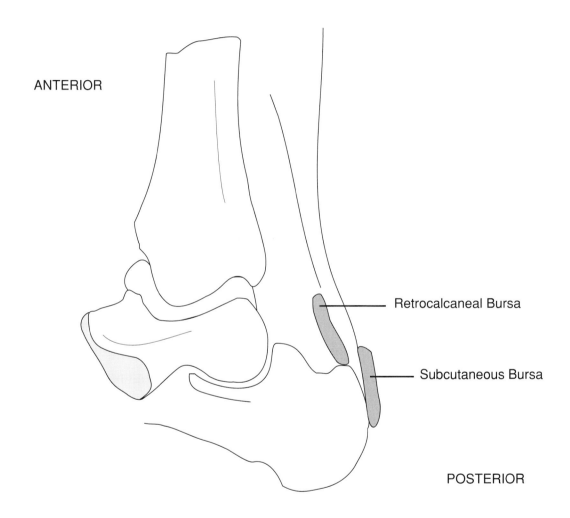

ANTERIOR

Retrocalcaneal Bursa

Subcutaneous Bursa

POSTERIOR

* Adapted from Berquist TM. MRI of the Musculoskeletal System, p 297. Berquist TH, ed. New York, Raven Press, 1990.

G-4   Pearls on Tendon Ruptures of the Foot

1. The most commonly affected tendons are Achilles and tibialis posterior followed by peroneus brevis and longus, flexor hallucis and tibialis anterior

2. Most tears are longitudinal and appear as a thin slit of signal alteration in the tendon

3. Definitive tears are not diagnosed unless signal alteration persists on T1 and T2

4. Tears with atrophic tendons have a much poorer prognosis than hypertrophic tendon tears

5. The tibialis anterior tendon is the only one in the foot with its own synovial sheath; therefore, in arthritides such as rheumatoid it may exhibit isolated involvement

6. Peroneus sheath degeneration, inflammation and subsequent tear may occur from calcaneofibular ligament rupture and extravasation of capsular content into the peroneus sheath complex

7. Flexor hallucis tendon ruptures may not be seen on MR due to the tight surrounding sheath that keeps the tendon fibrils opposed to one another as the tendon courses around the medial side of the ankle joint

8. Accessory muscle may masquerade as tendon disease
   a. Accessory soleus may simulate Achilles tendinopathy
   b. Peroneal calcaneal or peroneus quartius may simulate peroneus tendinopathy

9. The risk factors for tear include
   a. Prior tendinopathy
   b. Ballet dancing (flexor hallucis longus and Achilles)
   c. Soccer players (tibialis anterior)
   d. Basketball players (Achilles tendon)
   e. Accessory muscles (peroneus and Achilles tendons)
   f. Calcaneal fracture or calcaneofibular ligament tear (peroneus longus and brevis)
   g. Spastic flatfoot, subtalar arthritis or sinus tarsi syndrome (tibialis posterior tendon)

G-5   **Frequency of Tendon Injury or Tendinopathy**

1.   Achilles tendon: 41%

2.   Tibialis posterior tendon: 32%

3.   Peroneus brevis: 14%

4.   Peroneus longus: 4%

5.   Flexor hallucis longus: 3%

6.   Other (tibialis anterior, flexor hallucis longus, flexor digitorum, etc.): Less than 5%

G-6   Grading of Tibialis Posterior Tendon Rupture

Description

Grade I   Enlarged or globular tendon with peritendinous but no intratendinous signal alteration on T2

Grade II-A   Intratendinous T1 or proton density intermediate signal persisting on T2 but tendon shape is normal

Grade II-B   Intratendinous T1 or proton density intermediate signal with mild morphologic tendon alteration on T2

Grade II-C   Attenuation at tear site with tendon enlargement proximal and distal to the tear

Grade III-A   Tendon gap with complete transection

Grade III-B   Tendon retraction

Grade III-C   Hyperintense synovial fluid on T2 at retraction site with flatfoot, heel valgus, talar plantar flexion and forefoot adduction

G-7 Projections for Tibialis Posterior Tendon Evaluation

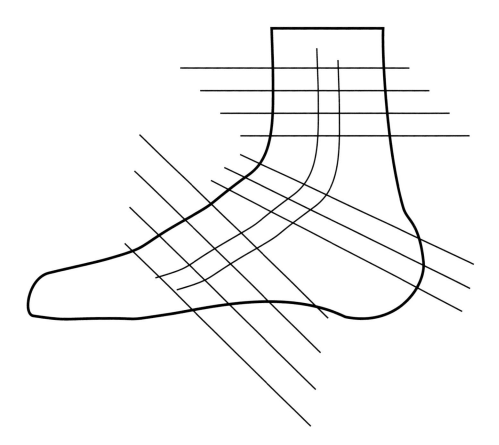

G-8   Tibialis Posterior Tendon Injury: Associated Findings

1.   Flatfoot
2.   Hindfoot/subtalar arthritis
3.   Erosion at the sinus tarsi angle (sinus tarsi geode)
4.   Peritendinous inflammation or tenosynovitis
5.   Forefoot eversion
6.   Tarsal tunnel inflammatory change

G-9   Achilles Tendon Tear on MR

1. Retrocalcaneal bursitis: Hypointense T1
2. Tendinitis
3. Ganglion of the Achilles or posterior ankle joint: Hypointense T1
4. Posterior talofibular or tibiofibular rupture or injury
5. Hindfoot or sinus tarsi syndrome
6. Subtalar joint arthropathy or capsular cyst
7. Accessory soleus muscle: Isointense with muscle
8. Hypercholesterolemic xanthoma: Variable hyperintense T1
9. Kagel's fat pad hypertrophy: Hyperintense T1
10. Mass
11. Hematoma: Hyperintense T1

G-10   Pearls in the Diagnosis of Achilles Tendon Injury

1. Occurs in jumping sports and in athletes who practice sudden changes in direction (nearly always preceded by prior tendinopathy)
2. Hypertrophic tendon size implies chronic tendinopathy and disease
3. More distal tears have a poorer prognosis while very proximal tears at the myotendinous junction ("tennis leg") have an excellent prognosis nonsurgically
4. Myxoid cyst formation
    a.. Diagnosed with focal hyperintensity on T1 and T2
    b.. Small or moderate in size
    c. Not associated with transection which does not respond to conservative treatment
    d. Treated with curettage of the myxoid cyst and subsequent immobilization

G-11   Achilles Tendon Rupture: Predisposing Factors

1. Increased frequency or severity of athletic training (hill climbing, stair climbing, running on rough terrain)
2. Acute trauma with excessive forefoot pronation
3. Chronic renal failure
4. Gout
5. Rheumatoid arthritis
6. Systemic steroid administration
7. Prior localized steroid injection
8. Heredofamilial connective tissue disease

G-12   Features of Achilles Tendon Injury To Be Addressed in Standard Dictation

1. Signal on T1 and T2 and relative change in signal between sequences
2. Tendon size (hypertrophy versus atrophy)
3. Peritendinous inflammation or masses
4. Extent of retraction (and potential apposition in the plantar flexion position)
5. Status of torn edges
6. Presence or absence of hematoma
7. Proximal or distal extent of tear
8. Status of proximal musculature
9. Status of hindfoot, ankle joint and subtalar space

G-13   **Achilles Tendon Injury: Subtypes**

1. Tendinitis: Linear or subtle foci of intermediate T1 signal with normal tendon size or slight hypertrophy, relatively inconspicuous on T2

2. Chronic tear: Usually associated with tendon hypertrophy

3. Acute tear: Associated with edema and surrounding inflammatory change that is moderate to marked, tendon size may be normal provided there is no prior chronic inflammation or tear

4. Partial tear: Focal area of intermediate T1 and increased T2, most commonly seen in deep tendon surface without complete transection, signal must persist and increase on T2, tendon size may be normal (acute) or hypertrophied (chronic or acute superimposed on chronic)

5. High grade partial tear: Same criteria as partial tear; however, area of involvement in the short axis view is greater than 50% of the tendon

6. Complete tear: Complete Achilles transection with or without retraction or maceration of the tendon ends

G-14   **Signs of Sinus Tarsi Syndrome & MR Findings**

1. Sinus tarsi is filled with fluid and granulation tissue
2. Posterior subtalar joint arthritis, sclerosis and erosive change
3. Erosion involving the overlying talus and calcaneal angle
4. Hindfoot arthropathy and subtalar arthritis
5. Calcaneal fluid or capsulosynovial thickening in subtalar space
6. Sinus tarsi ligament may be intact or torn
7. Everted foot
8. Spastic flatfoot
9. Tibialis posterior tendon disease, tear, tendinopathy
10. Sensation of hindfoot instability & pain = sinus tarsi syndrome

G-15   Tarsal Tunnel Syndrome on MR

Common

1. Idiopathic: Fibrosis
2. Post-traumatic: Fibrosis or spur
3. Inflammation: Tenosynovitis, ankylosing spondylitis
4. Metabolic: Diabetes, pregnancy, myxedema, acromegaly
5. Autoimmune: Rheumatoid arthritis, amyloid, sarcoid, dermatomyositis, gout, scleroderma
6. Hindfoot malformation or malalignment: Abductor hallucis hypertrophy, posterior talar process

Rare

1. Neoplastic soft tissue masses: Ganglion, neurilemmoma, cysts, neurofibroma
2. Vascular: Varicose veins, excessive standing, vascular insufficiency

G-16   Osteochondral Lesions About the Ankle Joint

1. Arthropathic cyst or geode: Hypointense T1 and hyperintense T2, multifocal, hypointense T1 and T2 sclerosis, loss of hyaline cartilage thickness or chondrolysis, joint effusion common, often communicates with joint space

2. Talar avascular necrosis: Crescentic and confluent T1 hypointensity and variable T2 signal, talar dome predilection followed by talar neck, may exhibit double ring sign with T2 hypo- and hyperintensity around the lesion, no evidence of chondrolysis or osteochondral depression

3. Osteochondritis dissecans: Eccentric location, superomedial talus location, usually isolated, associated with focal cartilaginous signal alteration only, joint effusion

4. Intraosseus ganglion: Rare before age 15 to 20, eccentric location, hypointense T1 and hyperintense T2, gelatinous consistency, most common location is the medial distal subarticular tibia, joint effusion uncommon, does not communicate with the joint space, overlying hyaline cartilage thickness is normal, patient is usually physically active in running or aerobic sports

G-17   Pearls in Osteonecrosis of the Foot

1. The talus is most commonly affected bone with body and dome involvement more common than neck
    a. Revascularization is a good prognostic sign and is seen as areas of hyperemia on bone scintigraphy and edema on MR with osteoporosis on plain film
    b. The Hawkins' sign (the presence of a linear subcortical zone of radiolucency in the talar dome following fracture of the talus–a sign of intact blood supply) suggests a good prognosis
    c. As opposed to osteochondritis dissecans, AVN is more diffuse with a wider zone of transition, has a broad base and a subcortical distribution (the differential diagnosis includes osteomyelitis and regional migratory osteoporosis)
2. Navicular avascular necrosis is spontaneous and is seen in women, frequently bilateral (by contrast, osteochondrosis or Köhler's disease is usually asymptomatic and seen in children)
3. Metatarsal osteonecrosis most common in the second metatarsal head known as Freiberg's disease
    a. More common in women 13-18 years of age (before epiphyseal closure)
    b. The differential diagnosis includes gout, diabetes mellitus, CPPD and rheumatoid arthritis

G-18   Pearls in the Diagnosis of Stress Fracture

1. Two basic types
    a. Fatigue fracture seen in military recruits, basketball players and long-distance runners
    b. Insufficiency fractures in patients with abnormal bone: Most common sites include
        i.   Calcaneus
        ii. Second and third metatarsals
2. Best pulsing sequence includes long axis oblique either sagittal or coronal with favored sequences including
    a. T1 spin echo
    b. Fat suppression T2 or T2 fast spin echo
    c. Short time inversion recovery
3. Callus may present as an ovoid intermediate signal intensity pseudomass surrounding an area of linear or localized bone edema
4. MR findings
    a. Horizontal discrete T1 hyperintensity
    b. Periosteal or periskeletal T2 hyperintense edema
    c. Above plus diffuse myoedema or hemorrhage

G-19   Muller's Classification of Pilon Fractures

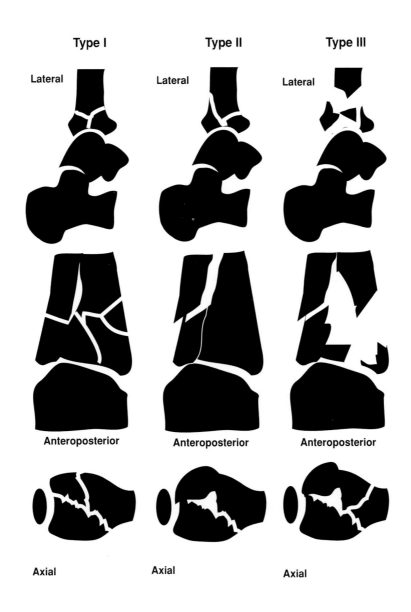

Type I   Type II   Type III

Lateral   Lateral   Lateral

Anteroposterior   Anteroposterior   Anteroposterior

Axial   Axial   Axial

Adapted from Muller et al, 1979.

Fig. G-19.1

G-20   Sesamoiditis (Sesamoid Pain) *

1. Fracture: Bone edema (hypointense T1, hyperintense water-weighted or T2)

2. Bursitis: Water signal (hypointense T1, hyperintense T2, perisesamoid)

3. Degenerative joint disease: Hypertrophic bone change with or without peri-sesamoid edema

4. Osteochondritis dissecans: Hypointense T1 & T2

5. Osteonecrosis: Diffuse hypointensity T1, variable hypointensity T2 (usually seen in females 10-30 years of age)

6. Infection: Intraskeletal and periskeletal water signal with extension into subcutis space

7. Turf toe: Sprain of plantar capsule/ligamentous complex of the metatarsal phalangeal joint of the great toe, most common in athletes with flexible shoes on rigid surface, high grade injuries lead to edema in volar capsule with secondary involvement of cartilage and bone

* The first digit sesamoids are the structures being emphasized here. Inserting on them are the flexor hallucis brevis medial and lateral heads as well as the intersesamoid ligaments.

G-21   Pearls in the Diagnosis of Posterior Tibiotalar Impingement Syndrome (PTTIS)

1. Etiology: Seen in those with excessive or recurrent plantar flexion (e.g., soccer players) leading to crush of soft tissue in the tibiocalcaneal pliers

2. Causes: Anatomic

    a. Bone: Fracture or hypertrophy of the posterolateral tibiotalar facet, os trigonum or os trigonum bipartition

    b. Osteocartilaginous

    c. Soft tissue: Capsular inflammation, flexor hallucis longus impingement or inflammatory disease

3. Anatomy

    a. Tibiocalcaneal pliers which equals the posterolateral tibiotalar and posteromedial tibiotalar facets

    b. Posterolateral talar process which equals posterolateral tibiotalar facet *

4. MR findings

    a. Posterior tibiotalar capsular cyst

    b. Pericapsular edema or phlegmon

    c. Prominent lateral or medial tibiotalar process or spur

    d. Posterior bone fragment, hypertrophy or irregularity of os trigonum or os trigonum bipartition

    e. Deformity of the posterior tibial facet secondary to prior fracture

---

* The flexor hallucis longus muscle and tendon is surrounded by the posterolateral and posteromedial tibiotalar facets. The posterior talofibular ligament inserts on the posterolateral tibiotalar process. Normally, the myotendinous junction of the flexor hallucis longus sits above the posterior talar process.

G-22   Common Accessory Muscles of the Foot by Frequency

1.   Accessory soleus: Inserts on calcaneus or Achilles tendon
2.   Peroneus quartius or peroneal calcaneal muscle: Begins on lower peroneus brevis and inserts on peroneal calcaneal tubercle
3.   Accessory flexor digitorum: Rare

G-23   Bone Tumors of the Foot & Ankle

Malignant

Osteogenic sarcoma: Inhomogeneous, hypointense bone matrix

Ewing's sarcoma: Heterogeneous, hemorrhagic

Chondrosarcoma: May be cystic ± hypointense calcification

Hemangioendothelial sarcoma: Inhomogeneous, hemorrhagic

Fibrosarcoma: Mixed T2 hypointense

Lymphoma: Homogeneous, intermediate signal

Adamantinoma: Distal tibia, diaphysis, destructive, edema

Multiple myeloma: Expansile, well-marginated, bright T2

Desmoplastic fibroma: Expansile, intermediate signal, destructive

Benign

Osteochondroma: Hyperintense T2 matrix cap ± hypointense calcification

Nonossifying fibroma: Hypointense rim, eccentric, mixed internal signal

Osteoid osteoma: Ring lesion with profound edema

Giant cell tumor: Hypointense T1, hyperintense T2, cystic, bone end

Aneurysmal bone cyst: Fluid-fluid levels, hypointense T2, expansile, ± bone end

Simple bone cyst: Calcaneus, hypointense T1, hyperintense T2

Enchondroma: Hyperintense T2 with hypointense calcium

Chondromyxoid fibroma: Mixed T2 hypointensity, expansile

Chondroblastoma: Intermediate T2, hypointense rim, edema, bone end

Osteoblastoma: Mixed T1 and T2 hypointense with perilesional edema

Fibrous histiocytoma: Heterogeneous signal

Lipoma: Calcaneus, hyperintense T1, hypointense central calcium

G-24 **Ovoid Lesions of the Heel**

1. Fibroma: Hypointense on T1 and T2

2. Desmoid: Hypointense T1, mixed T2

3. Nodular fasciitis (rare): Hypointense on T1, moderately hyperintense on T2

4. Juvenile aponeurotic calcifying fibroma: Isointense on T1, hypointense on T2

5. Granuloma: Variable T1 & T2

6. Localized fibromatosis, tumefactive: Isointense T1, mild hyperintense or hypointense T2*

* Increased T2 suggests increased cellularity and increased aggressiveness.

G-25   Soft Tissue Masses About the Foot

Common

1. Morton's neuroma (perineural fibroma): Mild hyperintensity or intermediate T2 signal with central hypointensity due to abundant fibrosis with female predilection between the third and fourth metatarsal heads

2. Neuroma: Mild to moderate T2 hyperintensity with occasional mixed central T2 hypointensity

3. Post-amputation neuroma: History of trauma or amputation and low or intermediate T2 signal

4. Ganglion: Homogeneous hypointense T1 and hyperintense T2 signal with peritendinous or pericapsular predilection

5. Giant cell tumor of tendon sheath: Mixed T2 hyperintensity and hypointensity, may be infiltrative with involvement or destruction of cortical or medullary bone

Uncommon

1. Implantation epidermoid: Hypointense T1, hyperintense T2 with a subcutaneous location

2. Implantation granuloma: Intermediate T1 and slightly hyperintense T2 signal, central hypointensity

3. True neoplasm: Signal varies with lesion histology (especially synovial sarcoma)

G-26   Soft Tissue Tumors: Signal Homogeneity

Fibrohistiocytic tumors (inter. malignancy)	Inhomogeneous
Glomus tumor	Inhomogeneous
Synovial sarcoma	Inhomogeneous
Clear cell sarcoma	Homogeneous
Epithelioid sarcoma	Inhomogeneous
Liposarcoma	Homogeneous* or Inhomogeneous
Angiosarcoma w/ & w/o lymphedema	Inhomogeneous
Rhabdomyosarcoma	Inhomogeneous
Hemangiopericytoma	Homogeneous or Inhomogeneous
Glomangioma	Homogeneous or Inhomogeneous
Alveolar sarcoma (soft part)	Inhomogeneous
Fibromatoses	Homogeneous
Extraskeletal Ewing's sarcoma	Inhomogeneous
Glomangiomyoma	Inhomogeneous
Giant cell tumor (tendon sheath)	Homogeneous

* Myxoid and well-differentiated histology more homogeneous.

CATEGORY H: THE SHOULDER

Page

H-1   Glenohumeral & Acromioclavicular Joints

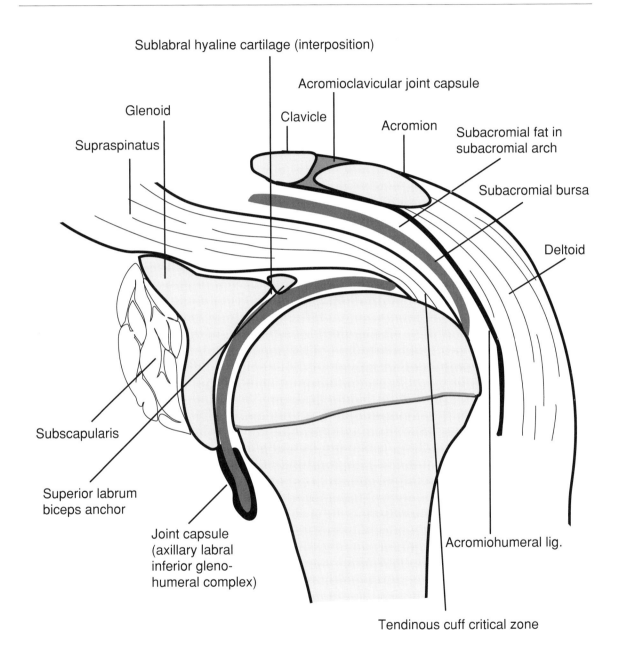

Sublabral hyaline cartilage (interposition)

Acromioclavicular joint capsule

Glenoid

Clavicle

Acromion

Subacromial fat in subacromial arch

Supraspinatus

Subacromial bursa

Deltoid

Subscapularis

Superior labrum biceps anchor

Joint capsule (axillary labral inferior gleno-humeral complex)

Acromiohumeral lig.

Tendinous cuff critical zone

* Adapted from Berquist TM. MRI of the Musculoskeletal System, p 163. Berquist TH, ed. New York, Raven Press, 1990.

H-2   Muscles of the Shoulder & Arm

Intrinsic

Deltoid

Origin: Lateral clavicle, acromion, scapular spine

Insertion: Deltoid tuberosity humerus

Action: Abduction of humerus

Innervation: Axillary nerve (C5, C6)

Supraspinatus

Origin: Supraspinous fossa of scapula

Insertion: Greater tuberosity superiorly

Action: Abduction of humerus

Innervation: Suprascapular nerve (C5, C6)

Infraspinatus

Origin: Infraspinous fossa of scapula

Insertion: Posterior inferior greater tuberosity

Action: External rotation of humerus

Innervation: Suprascapular nerve (C5, C6)

Teres minor

Origin: Lateral midscapular border

Insertion: Lateral inferior facet, greater tuberosity

Action: External rotation of humerus

Innervation: Axillary nerve (C5, C6)

Subscapularis

Origin: Subscapular fossa

Insertion: Lesser tuberosity

Action: Internal rotation of humerus

Innervation: Subscapular nerves (C5-C7)

H-2   Muscles of the Shoulder & Arm (Cont'd)

Teres major

Origin: Inferior lateral scapula

Insertion: Medial intertubercular groove

Action: Internal rotation, adduction, extension of humerus

Innervation: Subscapular nerve (C6, C7)

Extrinsic

Trapezius

Origin: Ligamentum nuchae, thoracic spinous processes

Insertion: Distal clavicle, acromion, scapular spine

Action: Retraction and elevation of scapula

Innervation: Spinal accessory C2, C3

Latissimus dorsi

Origin: Spinous processes T6-T12, lumbar, upper sacrum

Insertion: Medial intertubercular groove

Action: Adduction, internal rotation and extension of humerus

Innervation: Thoracodorsal nerve (C6-C8)

Levator scapulae

Origin: Posterior tubercles, C1-C4 transverse processes

Insertion: Upper medial scapula

Action: Elevation of medial scapula if neck fixed; if shoulder fixed, the levator scapulae inclines neck to same side

Innervation: Cervical plexus (C3-C4), spinal nerves C3, C4; from C5-dorsal scapular nerve

H-2   Muscles of the Shoulder & Arm (Cont'd)

Rhomboideus major

Origin: Spinous processes, second through fifth thoracic vertebral and supraspinous
   ligaments

Insertion: Posterior medial scapula

Action: Retractor of scapula

Innervation: Dorsal scapular nerve (C5)

Rhomboideus minor

Origin: Ligamentum nuchae, C7 & T1 spinous processes

Insertion: Posterior medial scapula at base of scapular spine

Innervation: Dorsal scapular nerve

Serratus anterior

Origin: Anterior ribs 1-9

Insertion: Anterior medial scapula

Action: Protraction, anterior drawing of scapula

Innervation: Long thoracic or pectoral nerve (C5-C7)

Pectoral Region

Pectoralis major

Origin: Inferomedial clavicle, sternum & costochondral junctions

Insertion: Lateral intertubercular groove

Action: Adduction of humerus

Innervation: Medial & lateral anterior thoracic or pectoral nerves (C5-T1)

Pectoralis minor

Origin: Anterior ribs 2-5

Insertion: Coracoid of scapula

Action: Depresses angle of scapula

Innervation: Medial pectoral nerve (C8-T1)

H-2   Muscles of the Shoulder & Arm (Cont'd)

Subclavius

Origin: Anteromedial first rib

Insertion: Midinferior clavicle

Action: Stabilization of sternoclavicular joint

Innervation: Medial pectoral nerve (C8-T1)

* Adapted from Berquist TM. MRI of the Musculoskeletal System, p 163. Berquist TH, ed. New York, Raven Press, 1990.

H-3   Brachial Plexus: Muscle Innervation

Radial Nerve
> Triceps
>
> Brachioradialis
>
> Extensor carpi radialis brevis & longus
>
> Supinator

Axillary Nerve
> Teres minor
>
> Deltoid

Musculocutaneous Nerve
> Coracobrachialis
>
> Biceps
>
> Brachialis

Dorsal Scapular Nerve
> Rhomboids major & minor
>
> Levator scapulae

Suprascapular Nerve
> Supraspinatus
>
> Infraspinatus

Subscapular Nerve
> Teres major
>
> Subscapularis

Thoracodorsal Nerve
> Latissimus dorsi

Long Thoracic Nerve
> Serratus anterior

* Adapted from Greenberg MS. Handbook of Neurosurgery, p 345-347. Lakeland, Florida, Greenberg Graphics, 1991.

H-4   Criteria for Complete Rotator Cuff Tear

Major Criterion

T2 signal hyperintensity extending through the entire cuff substance and communicating with the subacromial or subdeltoid space

Minor Suggestive Criteria

Intratendinous signal hyperintensity with any three of the following

a. T1 effacement of the subacromial fat space

b. T1 effacement of the subdeltoid fat space

c. T2 signal hyperintensity in the subacromial bursa

d. T2 signal hyperintensity in the subdeltoid bursa

H-5   Increased Signal in the Rotator Cuff*

1.   Rotator cuff tear
2.   Partial rotator cuff tear
3.   Tendinitis
4.   Myxoid or mucoid change
5.   Eosinophilic degeneration
6.   Magic angle effect
7.   Volume averaging of myotendinous muscle slips
8.   Fatty metamorphosis at the myotendinous junction
9.   Suture granuloma
10.   Distal capsulitis

* Kjellin I, Ho TC, Cervilla V, et al. Alterations in the Supraspinatus Tendon and MR Imaging: Correlation with Histopathologic Findings in Cadavers. Radiology 181: 837-841, 1991.

H-6   Rotator Cuff Disease on MR

Short TE (Proton Density & T1)

Clinical	MR Appearance
Normal	Black
Mild	White
Severe	White
Tear	White

Long TE (T2)

Clinical	MR Appearance
Normal	Black
Mild	Black
Severe	Gray
Tear	White

H-7   Surgical Classification of Partial Rotator Cuff Tears*

Grade I   Less than 3 mm deep

Grade II   3-6 mm deep

Grade III   Greater than 6 mm

Partial tears may be simulated by areas of myxoid degeneration

* Zlatkin MB. MRI of the Shoulder. New York, Raven Press, 1991.

H-8   **Pitfalls in Diagnosing Rotator Cuff Tear**

1. Anterior rotator cuff interval: An area of anterior intermediate signal intensity where the vertical portion of the biceps takes its turn; the biceps tendon and coracohumeral ligament lie in an interval between the superior subscapularis and the anterior edge of the supraspinatus

2. Interdigitated cuff: Alternating signal of hypointensity (tendon) and intermediate signal (muscle or capsule) or bright signal (fat) on T1 give a striped or stippled appearance to the cuff

3. Mucoid degeneration: Mild hyperintensity in the critical zone of the cuff which is less conspicuous on T2 and may simulate tear (the shape and margins of this lesion are amorphous and poorly defined)

4. Magic angle phenomenon: Increased signal on a short TE image when tendon and tropocollagen is angled 55° to the main magnetic field axis or bore

5. Fluid in the biceps tendon sheath as it crosses the superior humerus may simulate small rotator cuff tear

6. Isolated subscapularis tear (visualized axially) or infraspinatus tear (visualized sagittally) may be missed on conventional coronal sections

H-9   Shoulder Pain: Failed Rotator Cuff Surgery

Common

1. Capsulitis and inflammatory disease: Diffuse intermediate signal capsular thickening, deep to the cuff, mild to moderately hyperintense on T2

2. Cuff degeneration and atrophy: Usually concomitant with capsulitis but with decrease in cuff caliber and irregular cuff morphology

3. Retear
   a. Often requires gadolinium on T1 coronal and sagittal MR for confirmation
   b. Sine qua non is persistent cuff defect that is conspicuously hyperintense on T2 through the full thickness of the remaining cuff tissue
   c. Extravasation of hyperintense gadolinium on T1 imaging after intra-articular injection is confirmatory

Uncommon

1. Deltoid muscle atrophy
2. Supraspinatus muscle atrophy and fatty replacement or metamorphosis
3. Periscapular muscle weakness and dysfunction
4. Infection
   a. Capsular thickening
   b. Synovial thickening
   c. Joint effusion
   d. Soft tissue hyperintense edema
5. Suture granuloma: Local rounded hyperintensity usually arising from the superficial peripheral cuff margin, may be indistinguishable from high grade bursal side partial tear

H-9   **Shoulder Pain: Failed Rotator Cuff Surgery (Cont'd)**

Rare

1.   Localized regional osteoporosis or reflex sympathetic dystrophy

     a.   Clinical sympathetic dysfunction including pilomotor signs

     b.   Hypointense T1 bone edema with subtle or pronounced hyperintensity on water-weighted images

     c.   Occasionally no obvious bone edema but marbelized or heavily trabeculated bone appearance

2.   Osteomyelitis, extensive bone edema, hypointense on T1 and hyperintense on T2 with periosteal and soft tissue edema

H-10   Biceps Tendon Abnormalities on MR

Common

1. Peritendinous inflammation: Fluid signal in the biceps tendon sheath with associated clinical point tenderness
2. Tendinitis
   a. Hypertrophy non-degenerative type: Tendon enlarged with intratendinous signal on short TE imaging, barely conspicuous on spin echo T2
   b. Atrophic degenerative: Severe tendon thinning
3. Rupture: Tendon transection anywhere along the course from the superior tubercle of the glenoid to the distal brachium
   a. Descending portion tears: May retract as hypo- or hyperintense pseudomass in the lower or upper brachium, absent hypointense tendon in the bicipital groove in the short axis view
   b. Horizontal portion tears: May be associated with tear or rupture of the hypointense labral anchor
4. Partial: Intrasubstance, first echo hyperintensity that persists as discrete hyperintensity on T2 dataset

Uncommon

1. Biceps dislocation: Usually medial
   a. With intact subscapularis
   b. With torn subscapularis

H-11   Types of Anterior Acromion Shape*

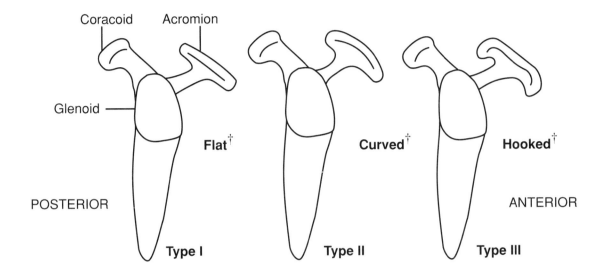

Coracoid   Acromion

Glenoid

Flat[†]   Curved[†]   Hooked[†]

POSTERIOR   ANTERIOR

Type I   Type II   Type III

* Bigliani
† Inferior surface of acromion

H-12   Clinical Stages of Impingement

Stage I

1. Excessive overhead use in sports
2. Patients under 25 years old
3. Edema and hemorrhage in cuff, tendons
4. This type of impingement is usually reversible

Stage II

1. Fibrosis and thickening of subacromial, subdeltoid bursa and/or tendon
2. Frank rotator cuff tendinitis
3. Athletes over 25 years old
4. Less common than Stage I
5. Conservative therapy 18 months is the more common treatment
6. Surgery: Coracoacromial ligament transection or bursal stripping (not usually necessary)

Stage III

1. The most common stage of impingement
2. Most often seen in patients over 40 years old
3. Degeneration and inflammation of biceps long head tendon with rotator cuff tear
4. Secondary bone erosion and arthropathy of coracoacromial arch

H-13   Classification of Subacromial Arch Stenosis

Description

Grade I   Encroachment on the subacromial arch (by acromioclavicular pan-
               nus or spur or acromion spur) without cuff signal alteration

Grade II   Subacromial arch encroachment with T2 cuff signal hyperintensity

Grade III   Subacromial arch encroachment with cuff discontinuity or transec-
               tion but without gaping retraction (< 1 cm), cuff atrophy or
               upward humeral migration

Grade III-A   Subacromial arch encroachment with cuff transection and retrac-
               tion greater than 1 cm

Grade III-B   Subacromial arch encroachment with transection, retraction, cuff
               atrophy and upward humeral migration

H-14   Glenoid Labral Variations & Their Frequency

1.   Pointed (30%)
2.   Round (25%)
3.   Cleaved or undercut (20%)
4.   Notched or serrated (15%)
5.   Flat or hypoplastic (10%)

H-15   Labrum Configurations

1.   Triangular labrum
     Anterior 45%
     Posterior 73%
2.   Rounded labrum
     Anterior 19%
     Posterior 12%
3.   Cleaved labrum
     Anterior 15%
     Posterior 0%
4.   Absent labrum
     Anterior 6%
     Posterior 8%
5.   Notched labrum
     Anterior 8%
     Posterior 0%
6.   Flat labrum
     Anterior 7%
     Posterior 6%

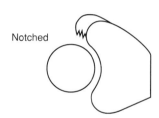

Notched

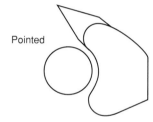

Pointed

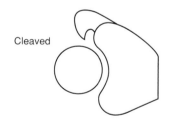

Cleaved

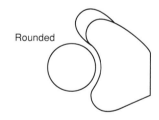

Rounded

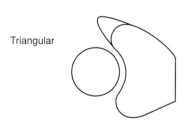

Triangular

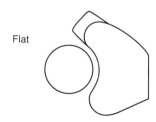

Flat

H-16   Pearls in the Diagnosis of Anterior Labral Tear

1. Most tears are distributed in the anteroinferior quadrant of the labrum
2. Isolated midlevel tears are not uncommon due to degenerative changes of aging
3. Hyaline interposition, hyaline undercutting or sublabral foramen can be differentiated from true tear by the fact that it does not communicate with the most anterior surface of the anterior labrum or the most superior surface of the superior labrum (see diagram following page)

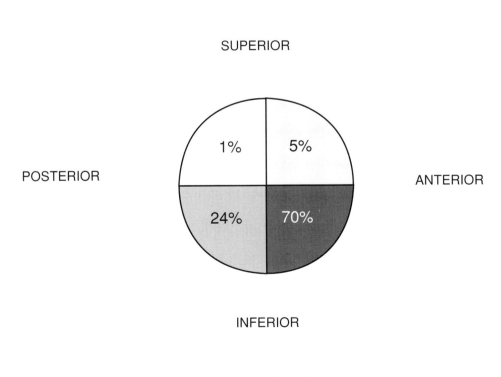

Locations of labral tears
by frequency
SAGITTAL VIEW

H-16   Pearls in the Diagnosis of Anterior Labral Tear (Cont'd)

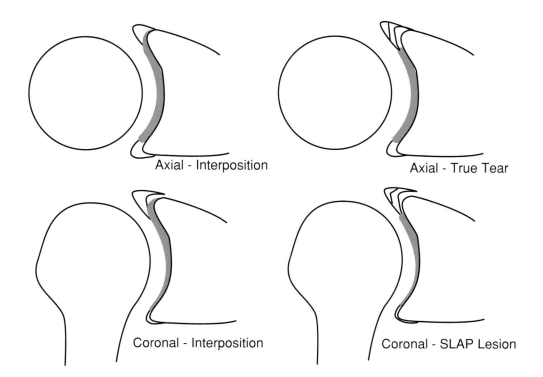

Axial - Interposition

Axial - True Tear

Coronal - Interposition

Coronal - SLAP Lesion

H-17   Types of SLAP Lesions

Superior labral tear anterior to posterior (SLAP)

Type I   Superior labral fraying (wear and tear, normal variation?)

Type II   Superior labral & biceps fraying

Type III   Labral detachment

Type IV   Labral & biceps detachment

Etiology

1.   SLAP occurs as throwing injury or fall on outstretched arm

2.   Usually young patients

3.   Coronal view most effective

4.   Beware of hyaline interposition or labral undercutting (sublabral foramen simulating a tear)

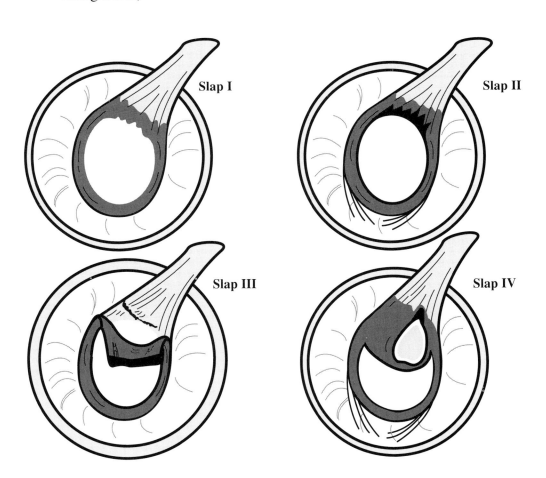

H-18   Pitfalls in the Diagnosis of Shoulder Labral Disease

1. Myxoid degeneration within the labrum: More conspicuous on gradient echo images, does not extend to the articular surface

2. Anterior and superior labral hyaline interposition or undercutting

3. Sublabral foramen

4. Glenohumeral ligament simulating a pseudomass or avulsion

5. Labral fibrillation: A wear-and-tear phenomenon

6. Absence of the labrum (common in the posterosuperior labrum and 8% of posterior mid and posterior inferior labrum)

H-19   Shoulder Capsule Types

Type I (Tight capsule)

    47%   *Anterior*

    100% *Posterior*

Type II (Capsule inserts on scapular ridge)

    50%   *Anterior*

    0%   *Posterior*

Type III (Capsule is stripped or redundant, inserts on medial scapular ridge)

    4%   *Anterior*

    0%   *Posterior*

H-20   Morphologic Summary of Capsular Attachments

1.   Anterior: Type I-II (97%)

        Type I   Dominates superior (96%)

        Type II   Dominates mid and inferior (62%)

        Type III   Uncommon (4%)

2.   Posterior: Type I (100%)

3.   No intershoulder correlation with capsular types from one shoulder to the other

Anterior Capsule Attachments

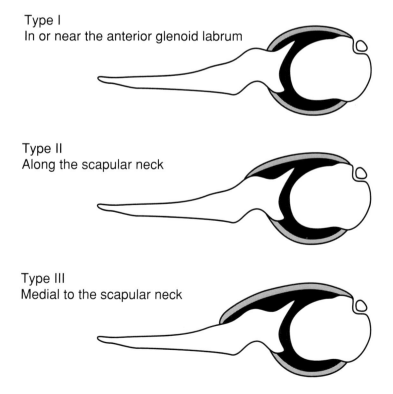

Type I
In or near the anterior glenoid labrum

Type II
Along the scapular neck

Type III
Medial to the scapular neck

* Adapted from Berquist TM. MRI of the Musculoskeletal System, p 337. Berquist TH, ed. New York, Raven Press, 1990.

H-21   Classification of Acromioclavicular Separation

Description

Grade I   Minimal widening of the AC joint (width less than 1 cm), coracoclavicular distance less than 1 - 1.3 cm, ligaments intact

Grade II   AC joint space 1 -1.5 cm, coracoclavicular distance 1.3 - 2 cm, ligament injury, thickening or edema but no complete tear

Grade III AC joint space greater than 1.5 cm and coracoclavicular distance greater than 2 cm, cephalad displacement of the distal clavicular end; the conoid and trapezoid ligaments are discontinuous

H-22   Skeletal Neoplasms of the Shoulder

Lesion	Percentage
Benign	
Osteochondroma	19
Chondroma	13
Chondroblastoma	25
Giant cell tumor	4
Osteoid osteoma	4
Hemangioma	4
Osteoblastoma	2
Malignant	
Myeloma	7
Lymphoma	12
Chondrosarcoma	16
Dedifferentiated chondrosarcoma	23
Osteosarcoma	11
Ewing's sarcoma	15
Fibrosarcoma	11

* Adapted from Berquist TM. MRI of the Musculoskeletal System, p 353. Berquist TH, ed. New York, Raven Press, 1990.

H-23   Hemorrhage or Hemosiderin-Laden Signal in the Shoulder

Common

1.   Hemarthrosis (trauma)

Uncommon

1.   Hemophilic pseudotumor
2.   Pigmented villonodular synovitis
3.   Amyloidosis

H-24   Water Signal Masses About the Shoulder

Common

1. Effusion in the subscapularis or subcoracoid bursa
2. Capsular cysts
3. Suprascapular ganglion
4. Subdeltoid bursitis

Uncommon

1. Suprascapular bursitis
2. Subacromial bursitis
3. Abscess
4. Giant synovial cysts
5. Cystic neoplasm (cystic chondrosarcoma, giant cell tumor, aneurysmal bone cysts, unicameral bone cysts, etc.)
6. Remote hematoma

H-25   **Lateral Axillary Hiatus (Quadrilateral Space) Syndrome**

1. Pearls in anatomy
    a. The quadrilateral space is formed by the long head triceps medially, the humerus laterally, the teres minor superiorly and the teres major inferiorly
    b. The triangular space is medial to the long head of triceps which serves as its base with the superior border of teres minor and inferior border teres major
    c. The triceps long head divides a triangular space that is bounded by the teres major inferiorly and teres minor superiorly with the humerus laterally forming the base of the triangles
        i. The medial axillary hiatus or triangular foramen medial to long head triceps contains the circumflex scapular artery which passes through the medial hiatus
        ii. The lateral axillary hiatus or quadrilateral space contains the axillary nerve and posterior circumflex humeral artery (the axillary nerve supplies the deltoid and teres minor muscles and the posterolateral shoulder skin and upper arm via the lateral cutaneous branch)
2. Etiology
    a. Fracture of the humerus or scapula or shoulder location via organizing hematomas or callus may produce hiatus encroachment
    b. Abduction during sleep
    c. Teres hypertrophy in paraplegics
    d. Fibrous bands
3. Clinical symptoms and signs
    a. Paresthesias and hypesthesias about the shoulder and upper arm
    b. Deltoid atrophy
4. Treatment
    a. Immobilization in adduction
    b. Physical therapy
    c. Local cortical steroid injection
    d. Surgery after 4-6 months conservative therapy failure

H-26   Lateral Axillary Hiatus (Quadrilateral Space)*

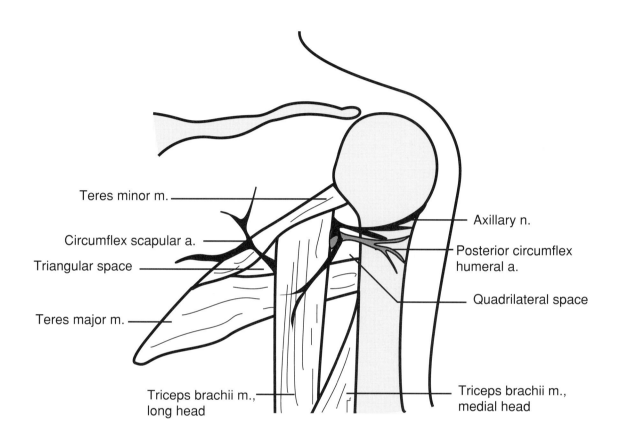

Teres minor m.

Circumflex scapular a.

Triangular space

Teres major m.

Triceps brachii m., long head

Axillary n.

Posterior circumflex humeral a.

Quadrilateral space

Triceps brachii m., medial head

* Drawing adapted from Pecina MM, Krmpotic-Nemanic J, Markiewitz AD. Tunnel Syndromes, p 28.
Boca Raton, Florida, CRC Press, 1991.

H-27   Fractures of the Proximal Humerus

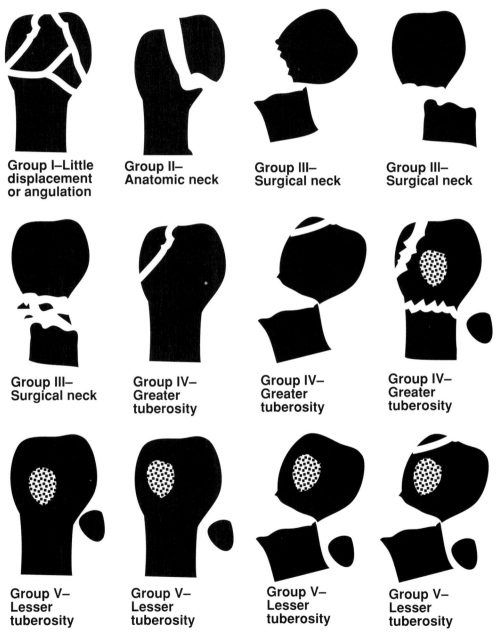

Group I–Little displacement or angulation

Group II– Anatomic neck

Group III– Surgical neck

Group III– Surgical neck

Group III– Surgical neck

Group IV– Greater tuberosity

Group IV– Greater tuberosity

Group IV– Greater tuberosity

Group V– Lesser tuberosity

Group V– Lesser tuberosity

Group V– Lesser tuberosity

Group V– Lesser tuberosity

Adapted from Neer CS. Displaced proximal humeral fractures. Part I. Classification and Evaluation. *J Bone Joint Surg* 52A-1077, 1970.

CATEGORY J: HAND, WRIST & ELBOW

CATEGORY J: HAND, WRIST & ELBOW

J-1   **Injuries & Abnormalities of Tendons in the Wrist by Frequency**

1.   Compartment 1 (60%): Abductor pollicis longus, extensor pollicis brevis (De Quervain's stenosing tenosynovitis)
2.   Compartment 6 (25%): Extensor carpi ulnaris
3.   Compartment 3 (7%): Extensor pollicis longus
4.   Compartment 5 (< 5%): Extensor digiti minimi
5.   Compartment 4 (< 5%): Extensor communis and indicis
6.   Compartment 2 (< 5%): Extensor carpi radialis longus & brevis

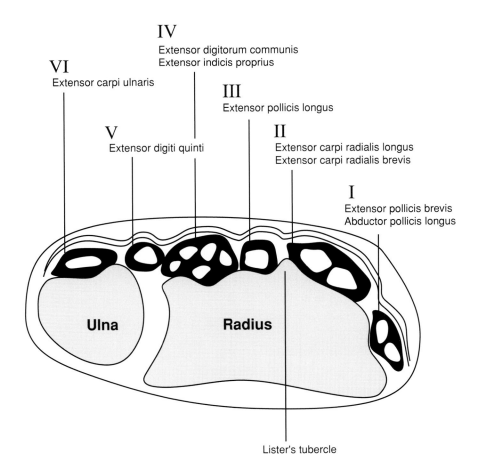

* Drawing adapted from Berquist TM. MRI of the Musculoskeletal System, p 411. Berquist TH, ed. New York, Raven Press, 1990.

J-2   Ligaments of the Wrist*

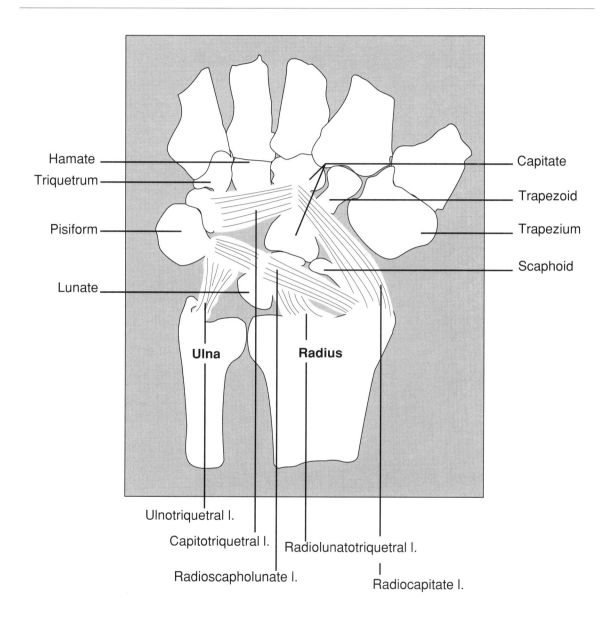

Hamate

Triquetrum

Pisiform

Lunate

Ulna   Radius

Capitate

Trapezoid

Trapezium

Scaphoid

Ulnotriquetral l.

Capitotriquetral l.

Radiolunatotriquetral l.

Radioscapholunate l.

Radiocapitate l.

* Adapted from Berquist TM. MRI of the Musculoskeletal System, p 412. Berquist TH, ed. New York, Raven Press, 1990.

J-3   Compartments of the Wrist*

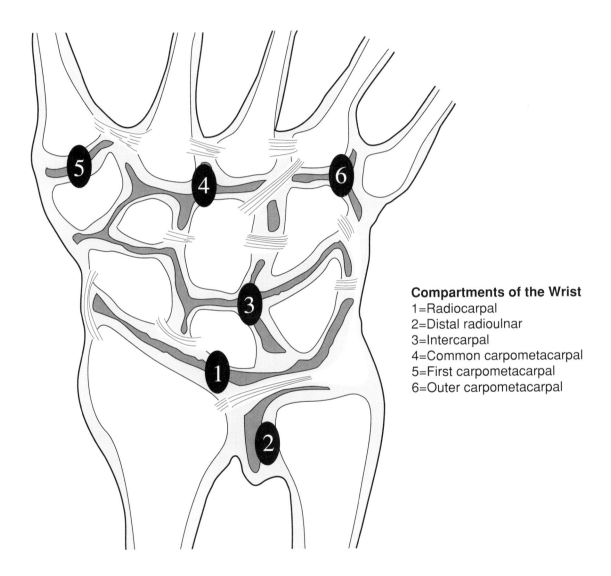

Compartments of the Wrist
1=Radiocarpal
2=Distal radioulnar
3=Intercarpal
4=Common carpometacarpal
5=First carpometacarpal
6=Outer carpometacarpal

* Adapted from Berquist TM. MRI of the Musculoskeletal System, p 413. Berquist TH, ed. New York, Raven Press, 1990.

J-4   Gamekeeper Thumb: Pearls & Differentiation of Unstable Injury*

1.   Ulnar collateral ligament (UCL) injury accounts for 6% of ski injuries

2.   Superficial displacement of the ulnar collateral ligament relative to the adductor pollicis aponeurosis = Stener lesion for which surgical repair is advocated

3.   UCL rupture that remains deep to the adductor aponeurosis is considered a non-displaced tear and, like medial collateral ligament tears of the knee, is not treated surgically

4.   Tears of the UCL usually occur distally near its insertion at the proximal phalanx

5.   A Stener lesion is usually present when there is a displaced, avulsed bone fragment

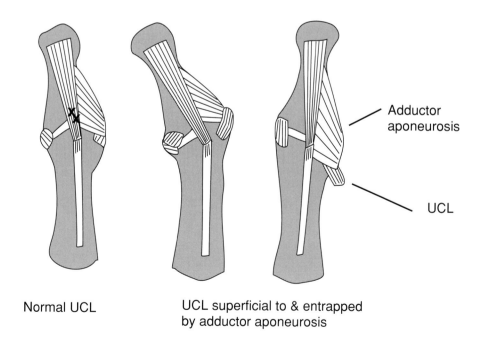

Normal UCL   UCL superficial to & entrapped
                            by adductor aponeurosis

Adductor aponeurosis

UCL

* Spaeth HJ, Abrams RA, Bock GW, et al. Gamekeeper Thumb: Differentiation of Displaced and Nondisplaced Tears of the Ulnocollateral Ligament with MR Imaging. Radiology 188: 553-556, 1993

J-5   **Pearls in Osteonecrosis of the Wrist**

1. The most common sites for osteonecrosis are scaphoid and lunate followed by capitate and greater multangular

2. The diagnosis of osteonecrosis is best made utilizing T1 spin echo and either a T2-appearing or fat saturation water weighted image such as STIR or T2 frequency selective presaturation

3. Coronal and oblique sagittal projections for assessment of lunate and scaphonecrosis

4. Avascular necrosis (AVN) occurs predominantly in areas with fatty or yellow marrow because this site has the slowest sinusoidal blood flow (this is also true in the hips)

5. Red cells and their precursors are most sensitive to ischemia, necrosing after six to 12 hours; osteocytes fail after 12 to 48 hours, and yellow marrow after two to five days

6. In the early phase of ischemia, MR may demonstrate subtle patterns of edema on T1 and STIR imaging

7. In the healing phase, radiographs demonstrate osteopenia, scintigrams demonstrate increased uptake, and MR continues to demonstrate evidence of bone edema

8. Later stages of necrosis result in persistent T1 and T2 hypointensity

9. Advantages of MR over bone scintigraphy and plain films include:
    a. Anatomic specificity in grading the site and extent of necrosis
    b. Greater specificity than bone scintigraphy or plain films
    c. Greater specificity in the diagnosis and staging of articular collapse and intercarpal arthropathy
    d. Tomographic visualization of carpal malalignment
    e. Indirect assessment of numerous volar and dorsal ligaments

J-6   Pearls in the Diagnosis of Scaphonecrosis

1. Scaphoid fractures account for 60% of all carpal bone fractures

2. The scaphoid waist and middle third of the scaphoid account for 50% of scaphoid fractures, while proximal fractures account for 20%

3. Frequency

    a. Scaphonecrosis occurs in 10-15% of all scaphoid fractures

    b. Proximal scaphoid fractures increase scaphonecrosis risk

4. Conventional radiographic evidence of sclerosis in 30%

5. Osteonecrosis: T1 homogeneous signal hypointensity on T1 and T2

    a. With nonunion, a cleft of T1 hypointensity and T2 hyperintensity exists

    b. With fibrous malunion, a cleft of T1 and T2 hypointensity exists

6. Osteonecrosis goes on to nonunion in 40% of patients, and the incidence of bone graft failure is 30%

7. Treatment: Matte-Russe graft with resection of fibrotic and sclerotic bone and insertion of autogenous corticocancellous bone

8. Potential pitfall: A healed fracture line may persist at the injury site for 1-2 years after the initial insult on MR and is hypointense on T1 and T2 (it is always less than 2 mm in thickness)

9. Technique

    a. Orthogonal coronal and sagittal oblique images (tangent or parallel to the long axis of the scaphoid)

    b. Include T1-appearing and T2-appearing sequences utilizing T1 spin echo and T2-appearing fast scan in two planes

J-7   Pearls in Lunatonecrosis (Kienböck's Disease)

1. Male-to-female ratio 2:1
2. Age: 20 to 40 years
3. Blood supply
    a. 80% nutrient vessels palmar and dorsal
    b. 20% nutrient vessels palmar only
    c. Proximal pole is relatively avascular
4. 80% of patients have negative ulnar variance, association with Madelung's deformity
5. Stages

    I   Normal or linear signal hypointensity

    II   Subtle signal hypointensity with or without alteration in height at the radial aspect of the lunate

    III   Signal hypointensity on T1 with lunate collapse and elongation in the sagittal projection; the capitate migrates proximally

    IIIA   No fixed rotatory subluxation of the scaphoid

    IIIB   Associated rotatory subluxation of the scaphoid

    IV   Same as III with arthropathy and hypointensity of adjacent carpal bones

6. Fibrous malunion: T1 and T2 hypointensity
7. Nonunion: T1 hypointensity and T2 hyperintensity
8. Differential diagnosis: Carpal instability, arthritis, occult fracture, ulnar impingement, ganglion cysts
9. Treatment
    a. Early stage: Lunate unloading (radial shortening) or immobilization
    b. Late stage: Salvage procedures (grafting) or arthrodeses

J-8   Pearls in Triangular Fibrocartilage Tear

1. Function: Stabilizes the radioulnar joint and prevents ulnar/lunate compressive forces and osteochondral injury (ballottement under arthroscopy = "trampoline sign" in normal TFC

2. Anatomy of the triangular fibrocartilage (TFC) complex

    a. Articular fibrocartilage: The ulnar-carpal meniscus

    b. Ulnar collateral ligament, extensor carpi ulnaris tendon and the dorsal and volar radioulnar ligament provide axial stability

    c. Central portion of disc is avascular

3. Location

    a. Most common (degenerative) tear site is the ulnolunate interface or center portion (central perforations are treated with closed procedures)

    b. Peripheral radial side tears

        i.   Occur in athletes with acute injury

        ii. Are uncommon

        iii. Result in loss of trampoline sign

        iv. Are treated with open procedures

4. MR findings

    a. Intermediate T1 signal communicating with an articular surface on T1

    b. Hyperintense signal on gradient echo or T2-appearing fast scan images communicating with a joint/articular surface

    c. Increased T2 or T2-appearing signal in the radioulnar joint region

    d. Synovitis with increased articular surface T2 signal and T1 thickening

    e. Erosive change of hyaline cartilage

5. Associated wth positive ulnar variance

6. Isolated central perforations of the TFC are usually asymptomatic

7. Degenerative TFC tears are five times as common as acute perforations

8. TFC perforations are rare before age 20 and common after age 50

9. Central perforations are usually degenerative, eccentric tears often traumatic

10. The significance of TFC perforations in the presence of negative ulnar variance should be questioned since nontraumatic dehiscence and congenital gaps in the TFC are common, especially in the elderly

J-9   **Components of Triangular Fibrocartilage Complex (TFCC)**

1. Dorsal & volar radioulnar ligaments
2. Ulnar collateral ligaments
3. Meniscus homologue
4. Articular disc or TFC
5. Extensor carpi ulnaris subsheath

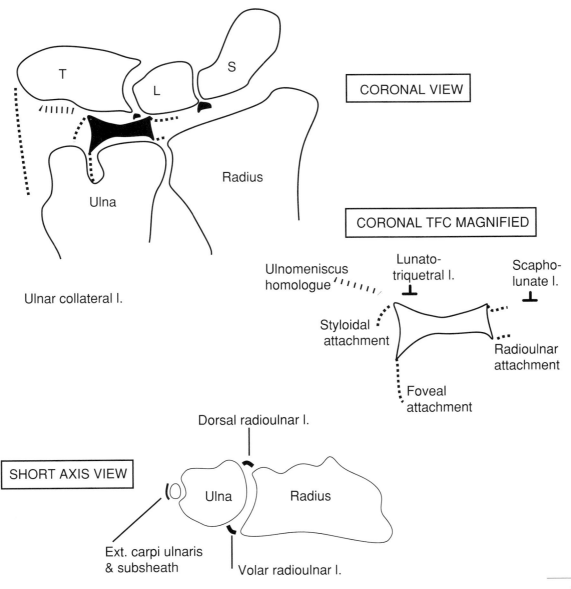

J-10 Congenital Fenestration or Degenerative Perforation Versus Traumatic TFC Tear *

Tear	Fenestration/Degeneration
Tends to run vertically or involve the attachments	Has a more horizontal course
May be associated with positive ulnar variance	Not associated with positive ulnar variance
May be associated with bony osteochondral defect and/or bone edema	Not associated with osteochondral defect or bone edema
May be associated with distal radioulnar joint fluid	Not associated with joint fluid
May be associated with thickening of the attachments	Not associated with thickening of the attachments
May be associated with thickening or disruption of the volar or dorsal radioulnar ligament	Not associated with disruption of the volar or dorsal radioulnar ligament
May be associated with fluid or thickening of the extensor carpi ulnaris subsheath	Not associated with fluid or thickening of the extensor carpi ulnaris subsheath

* Over the age of 50, asymptomatic perforations or fenestrations of the triangular fibrocartilage occur in at least 50-60% of the population.

J-11   Pearls in the Diagnosis of Ulnolunate Impingement

1. Positive ulnar variance may result in ulnolunate impingement
2. Because of its lengthened configuration, the distal ulna is impacted against the lunate
3. TFC may become thinned or degeneratively torn exhibiting signal hyperintensity
4. Ulnar and lunate hyaline cartilage becomes degenerated, thinned and destroyed, frequently accompanied by a degenerative lunate cyst

Ulnolunate Impingement Syndrome w/ Advanced Arthritis but w/o SLAC

1. Slight positive ulnar variance with destruction of the ulnolunate hyaline cartilage, deformity of the lunate and deformity of the TFC
2. TFC contains gray signal due to chronic degenerative tear on T1
3. The hyaline cartilage at the radiocarpal interface is diffusely destroyed particularly in the radioscaphoid interface
4. The capitate does not migrate proximally, and the lunate does not appear elongated or collapsed (there is severe arthritis without SLAC but with evidence of ulnolunate impingement)
5. Fibro-osseous cysts at the base of the triquetrum and lunate are apparent as areas of hypointensity on T1 and hyperintensity on T2

J-12   Dorsal Intercalated Segmental Instability (DISI) &
**   Scapholunate Dissociation (SLD)**

1. Dorsal tilting of the lunate without volar shift (capitate is dorsally displaced relative to the radius)

2. Of the types of wrist and carpal instabilities, DISI and SLD are the most commonly observed and frequently coexist (if a patient falls on an outstretched hand, lunate/perilunate dislocation, scaphoid or radius fracture may result)

3. Even without these injuries, the radioscaphocapitate or sling ligament, radioscapholunate ligament and radial collateral ligament, dorsal radiocarpal ligament or scapholunate interosseous ligament may be injured (tear may be partial or complete)

4. The weakest links between the radius and proximal and distal carpal rows are the radioscapholunate and radioscaphocapitate ligaments respectively

5. The scapholunate is the strongest interosseous ligament (usually when this is torn, other ligaments have torn with it), the radiotriquetral is the strongest volar intracapsular ligament, and the radioscaphoid is the most elastic

6. In some patients, the radioscapholunate and radioscaphocapitate ligaments can be disrupted and will not be visible

7. There is thickening and injury to the dorsal capsule

Remember that ulnar deviation of the wrist may simulate DISI in the sagittal projection. Great care should be taken when positioning the wrist in the scanner.

J-13   Pearls in Scapholunate Advanced Collapse (SLAC)

1.   A dreaded sequela of lunatonecrosis: The proximal row of carpal bones are destroyed and are surrounded by areas of pannus formation and hypointense granulation tissue

2.   Most common cause of wrist arthritis

3.   Rotatory subluxation of scaphoid results in degenerative joint disease (rapid in onset and progression)

4.   Proximal capitate migration with ulnar translocation of lunate and elongation of the lunate in the sagittal projection produces draping of the flexor tendons and median nerve over the proximal carpal bones, resulting in secondary carpal tunnel syndrome and severe arthropathy

5.   Severe hyaline cartilage loss is directly appreciated on T1 spin echo and gradient echo fast scan images

J-14   Pearls in Volar Intercalated Segmental Instability (VISI)

1. VISI is more uncommon than DISI
2. Commonly associated with ulnar wrist pain and may simulate TFC tear clinically
3. Midcarpal and medial carpal instability are accompaniments
4. There is frequent disruption of the palmar V ligament, particularly its ulnar limb
5. Painful clunk with ulnar deviation and pronation is experienced clinically

Remember that radial deviation of the wrist may simulate VISI in the sagittal projection. Great care should be taken when positioning the wrist in the scanner.

DISI: Tilting of the lunate dorsally without evidence of volar displacement but with apparent capitate malalignment

VISI: Tilting of the lunate ventrally without dorsal lunate displacement and with apparent volar displacement of the capitate

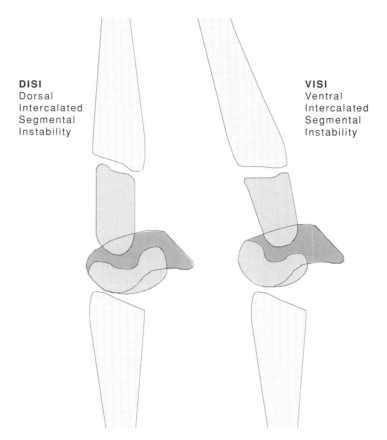

DISI
Dorsal
Intercalated
Segmental
Instability

VISI
Ventral
Intercalated
Segmental
Instability

J-15   Ulnar Variance

1.   Positive ulnar variance is associated with TFC tear or ulnolunate impingement
2.   Negative ulnar variance is associated with lunatonecrosis

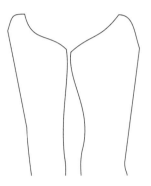 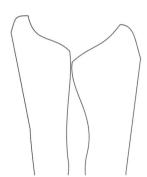 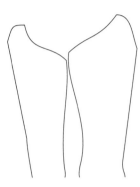

Neutral Ulnar Variance   **Positive Ulnar Variance**   **Negative Ulnar Variance**

J-16   Distal Radius Fractures

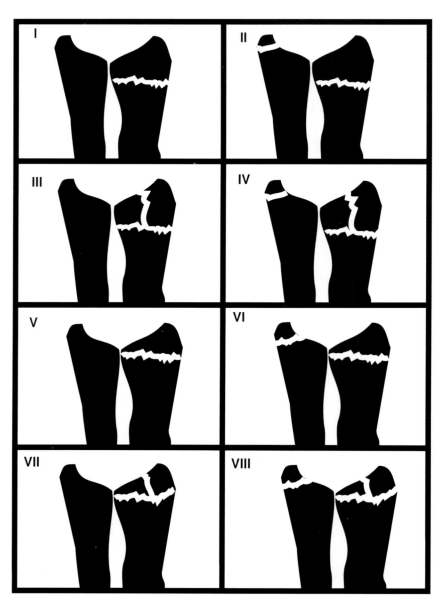

Frykman's classification of distal radius fractures. III through VII are intra-articular. Higher classifications = a worse prognosis. From Palmer AK. The distal radioulnar joint. In: Lichtman DM, ed. *The Wrist and Its Disorders*. Philadelphia, WB Saunders, 1988:220-231.

J-17   **Distal Humerus Fractures**

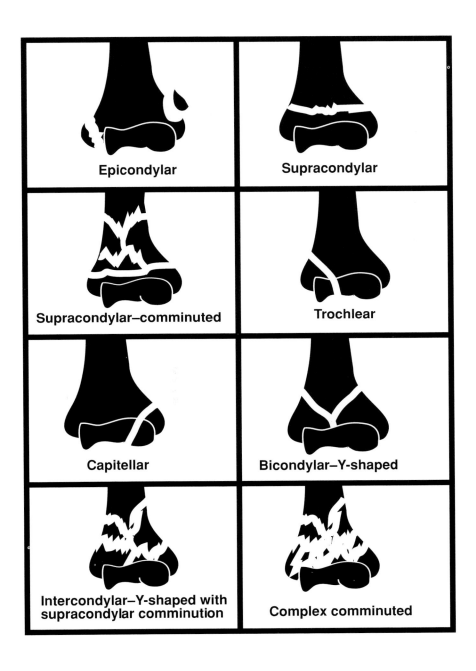

Epicondylar

Supracondylar

Supracondylar–comminuted

Trochlear

Capitellar

Bicondylar–Y-shaped

Intercondylar–Y-shaped with
supracondylar comminution

Complex comminuted

J-18   Pearls in the Diagnosis of Carpal Tunnel Syndrome

Anatomy

1.   The carpal tunnel is a confined structure which encases the median nerve and flexor tendons

2.   It is bounded by the carpal bones dorsally, medially and laterally

3.   The volar boundary is formed by the transverse carpal ligament or flexor retinaculum which attaches to the distal carpal row between the tubercle of the trapezium and hook of the hamate

4.   Secondary attachments occur between the scaphoid tuberosity and the pisiform

Clinical Symptoms

1.   Nocturnal hand discomfort

2.   Finger paresthesia

3.   Median nerve/thenar muscle weakness and/or atrophy

Demographics

1.   Most common in the 4th-7th decade

2.   Dominant hand most commonly affected

3.   Bilateral: 20%

4.   Women:men = 3:1

5.   More common in occupations that include strain or twisting and low frequency vibration (10-40Hz) such as jackhammer operators

MR Findings

1.   Dilated median nerve with T2 hyperintensity at the level of the pisiform and median nerve compression at the level of the hamate hook with variable sized effusion and bowing of the flexor retinaculum

2.   T2 median nerve hyperintense edema or paradoxical hypointense median nerve fibrosis with variable sized effusion and bowing of the flexor retinaculum

3.   Thenar muscle atrophy

J-19   Etiologies of Carpal Tunnel Syndrome

Common

1. Idiopathic: Dilated median nerve with T2 hyperintensity at the level of the pisiform and median nerve compression at the level of the hamate hook with variable sized effusion and bowing of the flexor retinaculum

2. Occupational: T2 median nerve hyperintense edema or paradoxical hypointense median nerve fibrosis with variable sized effusion and bowing of the flexor retinaculum

Uncommon

1. Rheumatoid arthritis: T2 hyperintensity joint capsule, enhances, effusions, erosions ± tenosynovitis

2. Hypothyroidism: Intermediate signal fills tunnel

3. Acromegaly: Intermediate signal fills tunnel with musculotendinous hypertrophy

4. Myeloma

5. Amyloid: Intermediate signal

6. Diabetes

7. Lunate dislocation

8. Anomalous lumbrical: Muscle signal

9. Trauma

10. Hemophilia: Mixed T1 and T2 signal

11. Lipoma: Hyperintense T1, hypointense T2, homogeneous

12. Ganglion: Hypointense T1, hyperintense T2, homogeneous

13. Vascular tumor: Mass with flow void (AVM) or intermediate T1, hyperintense T2 (hemangioma)

14. Menopause

15. Paget's disease

16. Thrombosis of ulnar artery or vein

J-20   Carpal Tunnel Surgery Failure: MR Findings & Etiologies

Common

1.   Median nerve neuritis (nerve swelling with T2 hyperintensity)

2.   Capsular inflammation (intermediate signal filling the intertendinous carpal tunnel space with enhancement as T2 intertendinous hyperintensity)

Uncommon

1.   Tumefactive fibrogranuloma or fibrolipogranuloma (mixed intermediate hyperintense and hypointense T1 signal)

2.   Neuroma or post-traumatic perineural fibroma (intermediate T1 and intermediate to slightly hyperintense T2)

3.   Nerve injury or transection (nerve edema and/or discontinuity)

4.   Postsurgical aneurysm or vascular thrombosis (more common in the ulnar vascular bundle, seen as an area of tubular hyperintensity)

J-21   Criteria for Carpal Tunnel Syndrome

Direct Signs

1.   Segmental nerve root swelling or increased contour proximal to the carpal tunnel
2.   Diffuse nerve root sausage-like swelling within and proximal to the tunnel
3.   T2 signal hyperintensity within the carpal tunnel median nerve itself
4.   Nerve root encased by hypointense fibrosis or paradoxical neural hypointensity
5.   A narrowed transverse dimension of the median nerve

Indirect Signs

1.   Swelling of flexor tendon sheaths and tendons
2.   Ventral or volar buckling and convexity of the flexor retinaculum
3.   Capsular thickening or T2 hyperintensity

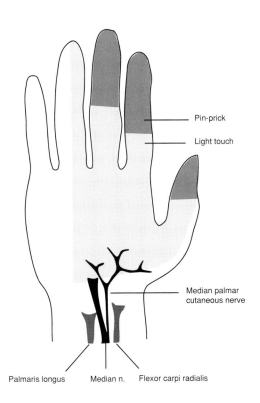

* Adapted from Greenberg MS. Handbook of Neurosurgery, p 352. Lakeland, Florida, Greenberg Graphics, 1991.

J-22   Pronator Teres Muscle Syndrome

1. Anatomy
   a. The median nerve passes between the two heads of the pronator teres and under the tendinous arch of the flexor digitorum superficialis
   b. After leaving the pronator teres, the median nerve gives rise to the anterior interosseous nerve
   c. The median nerve runs between the flexor digitorum superficialis and profundus, then between the flexor carpi radialis and palmaris longus
   d. The median nerve supplies all wrist and hand flexors except the flexor carpi ulnaris and the ulnar portion of the flexor digitorum profundus before entering the carpal tunnel
   e. The median nerve gives rise to the palmaris branch then innervates the thenar eminence and radial portion of the wrist
2. Etiologies*
   a. Myositis (irritating nerve)
   b. Fibrous band
   c. Forearm trauma (can lead to Volkmann's contracture)
   d. Dynamic relationship of the nerve and muscles in the forearm
   e. Anatomical (at the aponeurosis of the FDS and biceps brachii)
3. Clinical
   a. Carpal tunnel syndrome involves just the muscles of the thenar eminence, but pronator teres syndrome also involves wrist and finger flexors
   b. Sensory disturbance involves volar and dorsal surface of the hand, palm and several fingers
   c. Any involvement of sensation in the palm indicates compression proximal to the carpal tunnel
4. MR findings
   a. Compression in leaves of pronator teres
   b. Hyperintensity between leaves of pronator teres

J-22   Pronator Teres Muscle Syndrome (Cont'd)

5. Treatment

    a. Forearm immobilization in the neutral position

    b. Local steroid injection

    c. Surgical decompression after 6 months of conservative therapy in which tendinous arch between origins of the flexor digitorum superficialis are sectioned with release of the humeral head of the pronator teres from its radial insertion

* Adapted from Pecina MM, Krmpotic-Nemanic J, Markiewitz AD. Tunnel Syndromes, p 32. Boca Raton, Florida, CRC Press, Inc., 1991.

J-23   Anterior Interosseous Kiloh-Nevin Syndrome

1. Anatomy
   a. The anterior interosseous nerve is a motor branch of the median nerve in the cubital region
   b. The anterior interosseous or palmaris nerve is an exclusively motor nerve
   c. Dives deep to the flexor digitorum superficialis running in the interosseous membrane between it and the flexor pollicis longus laterally and the flexor digitorum profundus medially

2. Etiology
   a. Median nerve tumors
   b. Fibrous anomalies of the FPL or FDS
   c. Trauma

3. Clinical
   a. Inability to pinch between thumb and index finger (pin sign)
   b. Inability to flex wrist
   c. Inability to clench fist
   d. Dull pain in the proximal third of the forearm aggravated by radial pressure at the tendinous arch of the FDS

4. Treatment
   a. Conservative therapy for six months
   b. Surgical decompression
   c. Fibrous band transection
   d. Tendon release or removal of anomalous muscles or neurolysis

5. MR findings
   a. T1 & T2 hypointensity due to interosseous calcification or remote hematoma
   b. T2 interosseous hyperintensity secondary to trauma, inflammation or neoplasm

J-24   Supinator Syndrome

1. Anatomy
    a. After perforating the lateral intramuscular septum, the radial nerve passes from posterior to anterior in the brachial sulcus entering the sulcus cubitalis radialis (between brachialis and brachioradialis)
    b. At the capitellum, the radial nerve gives off branches to brachialis, brachioradialis, extensor carpi radialis longus, the periosteum of the lateral epicondyle, the humeral radial joint and the annular ligament
    c. In the radial cubital sulcus, it divides into two branches
        i. Deep or profundus branch
        ii. Superficial or superficialis branch
    d. Deep branch enters distal to the origin of the extensor carpi radialis brevis (ECRB) in the supinator canal, and the ECRB may dynamically compress the deep branch during pronation
    e. At the distal supinator muscle edge, the deep branch of the radial nerve divides in two
        i. Muscular branch to the extensor carpi ulnaris, extensor digitorum communis and extensor digiti minimi
        ii. Posterior interosseous nerve to the abductor pollicis longus, extensor pollicis longus, extensor pollicis brevis and extensor indicis
        iii. This nerve also supplies ligaments in the wrist capsule
    f. Superficial radial nerve branch provides sensation to the dorsum of the hand, first two fingers and radial half of the third finger
2. MR findings
    a. T2 hyperintensity around radial nerve superficial to supinator muscle
    b. Mass or mass effect in or superficial to the supinator muscle

J-24   Supinator Syndrome (Cont'd)

3.   Etiology*
   a.   General trauma
        Radial subluxation
        Monteggia fracture
        Distal humeral fracture
        Violent motion
   b.   Tumors
        Fibromas
        Lipomas
        Ganglions
   c.   Inflammation
        Neuroma
        Bursitis
        Rheumatoid arthritis
   d.   Anatomical position
        Dynamic compression (conductors, balloonists, violinists)

4.   Clinical
   a.   Deep pain, posterior dorsum of the forearm
   b.   Gradual fist weakness and local pain on compression distal to the lateral humeral epicondyle
   c.   No sensory deficits
   d.   May simulate lateral epicondylitis or tennis elbow

5.   Treatment
   a.   Physical therapy or local corticosteroid injection
   b.   Immobilization
   c.   Surgical decompression if immobilization fails within three to four months
   d.   Supinator tunnel decompression when lateral epicondylitis is resistant to conservative therapy

* Adapted from Pecina MM, Krmpotic-Nemanic J, Markiewitz AD. Tunnel Syndromes, p 37. Boca Raton, Florida, CRC Press, Inc., 1991.

J-25   Sulcus Ulnaris Syndrome

1. Anatomy
    a. Fibro-osseous tunnel between medial epicondyle and olecranon covers the ulnar nerve (this ligament prevents subluxation of the ulnar nerve with fore-arm motion)
    b. The ulnar nerve branches to supply motor innervation of these structures
        i.   Flexor carpi ulnaris
        ii.   Ulnar component of the flexor digitorum profundus
        iii. Hypothenar muscles
        iv.   Interossei muscles
        v.   Ulnar lumbricals
        vi.   Adductor pollicis
        vii. Deep head of flexor pollicis brevis
    c. Sensory branches of the fingers and hand originate distal to the sulcus
2. Etiology
    a. Trauma
    b. Rheumatic changes of the medial epicondyle
    c. Cubitus valgus
    d. Patients who chronically lean on their elbows
    e. Microtrauma from repetitive stretching (baseball players, jackhammer operators, boxers, javelin throwers)
    f. Supracondylar, distal humeral, elbow fractures or dislocations with excessive callus formation
3. Clinical
    a. Paresthesia, hyperesthesia, hypesthesia and pain in the ulnar nerve sensory dermatome
    b. Paresthesias and pain proximally near the shoulder with increased progression
    c. Tinel's sign over the ulnar sulcus
    d. Muscle wasting in the webbed space between the first and second metacarpals followed by interossei and hypothenar wasting
    e. Claw hand appearance

J-25   **Sulcus Ulnaris Syndrome (Cont'd)**

4.   Treatment
     a.   Conservative
     b.   Steroid injection
     c.   Surgical ligament release, epicondylectomy or anterior transposition of the ulnar nerve
5.   MR findings
     a.   T2 hyperintensity in or about sulcus ulnaris
     b.   Linear hypointense thickening of epicondylar-olecranon ligamentous complex

J-26   Pisohamate Hiatus Syndrome*

1. Deep branch of the ulnar nerve is compressed as in Guyon's ulnar tunnel syndrome, motor variant; however, the adductor digiti muscle is spared

2. Anatomy
    a. Pisiform bone and hamate bone form the ulnar and radial walls
    b. Pisohamate ligament forms the floor
    c. The tendinous arch forms the roof
    d. Deep branch of the ulnar nerve gives motor fibers to the hypothenar muscles (except the palmaris brevis which is innervated by the superficial branch)
    e. Also innervated are the interossei, two ulnar lumbrical muscles, adductor pollicis muscle and deep head of flexor pollicis brevis muscle

3. Etiology
    a. Ganglion cyst
    b. Anomalous muscle
    c. Intraneural cysts
    d. Carpal bone and hamate fractures
    e. Ulnar artery anomalies and disease
    f. Chronic wrist trauma
    g. Occupational neuritis

4. Clinical
    a. Absence of paresthesia or hypesthesia (i.e., no sensory component)
    b. Palmaris brevis and abductor digiti minimi are spared

5. Diagnosis
    a. Motor form of ulnar tunnel syndrome
    b. Progressive spinal atrophy
    c. Lateral amyotrophic sclerosis
    d. Juvenile amyotrophy

6. MR findings
    a. Mass encroachment, aneurysm or bone fragments in or about Guyon's canal
    b. Hyperintense edema or nerve swelling, fusiform in Guyon's canal

* Syndrome of the deep branch of the ulnar nerve

J-27   Ulnar Tunnel (Guyon's Canal) Syndrome

1. Anatomy
   a. Roof equals insertion of flexor carpi ulnaris
   b. Floor: Transverse carpal ligament
   c. Ulnar and radial borders: Pisiform and hamate bones
   d. Contents include blood vessels, superficial and deep palmar branches of the ulnar nerve (the dorsal branch is spared in ulnar tunnel syndrome)
   e. Superficial portion of palmar branch innervates palmaris brevis, palmar skin of the fifth finger and ulnar skin of the fourth finger
   f. Deep branch innervates hypothenar muscles, two lateral lumbricals, all of the interossei, adductor pollicis and deep head of flexor pollicis brevis
2. Clinical
   a. Hypothenar atrophy
   b. Uncertainty in hand movements
   c. Pain aggravated by wrist extension
   d. Numbness
   e. Tingling
   f. Paresthesia
   g. Night pain (third, fourth and fifth fingers)
   h. Phalen's sign: Paresthesia in 4th and 5th fingers with forced palmar flexion
   i. Wormser's signs (dorsal flexion causes paresthesia in the 4th and 5th fingers)
   j. Adduction of the 5th finger and abduction and adduction of the thumb and other fingers are unimpaired
3. Etiology
   a. Ulnar nerve compression
      i. Upper form: Proximal compression preventing any ulnar nerve innervation
      ii. Motor dysfunction only: Compromise of the deep branch infers deep branch compression distal to the hypothenar muscle branch
      iii. Middle form: Compression proximal to the hypothenar muscles produces primary sensory symptoms since the superficial branch is compromised

J-27   Ulnar Tunnel (Guyon's Canal) Syndrome (Cont'd)

Etiology (Continued)

      b. Trauma

          i. Fractures of the hook of the hamate

          ii. Riding bicycles

      c. Anomalies (such as passage of fourth finger flexor tendon through the tunnel)

      d. Ganglia

      e. Occupational compression

      f. Vascular disturbance

      g. Pisotriquetral arthritis

      h. Bursitis adjacent to pisiform bone

      i. Giant cell tumor of tendon sheath

      j. Inflammatory disease including rheumatic disorders

      k. Edema

      l. Aberrant muscles

      m. Idiopathic

      n. Ulnar artery aneurysm

      o. Thromboangiitis obliterans

      p. Idiopathic hypertrophy of the flexor carpi ulnaris muscle

4. MR findings

      a. Mass encroachment, aneurysm or bone fragments in or about Guyon's canal

      b. Hyperintense edema or nerve swelling, fusiform in Guyon's canal

**J-28   Syndrome of Lateral Antebrachial Cutaneous
(Musculocutaneous) Nerve**

1. Anatomy
   a. Supplies motor branches to the coracobrachialis, biceps brachii and brachialis muscles
   b. Sensory branches to portions of forearm and wrist
   c. Stays lateral to the axillary artery
   d. Spreads to form palmar and dorsal branches to the radial forearm, thenar eminence, posterior distal 1/3 of the forearm and first metacarpal base

2. Etiology
   a. Biceps aponeurosis nerve compression against brachial fascia in elbow extension
   b. Exaggerated by pronation
   c. Most common in the dominant hand
   d. Acute or chronic trauma with forced elbow extension and forearm pronation
   e. Repeated pronation, recurrent tennis backhand practice, excessive screwdriving
   f. Thoracobrachialis muscle hypertrophy

3. Clinical
   a. Resembles epicondylitis (both may occur with tennis playing)
   b. Anterolateral elbow pain often burning in nature
   c. Patients avoid elbow extension and forearm pronation

4. Treatment
   a. Rest, abstinence from sports
   b. Splinting
   c. Cortical steroid injection
   d. Surgical decompression

J-29   Pearls in the Diagnosis of Cubital Tunnel Syndrome

1. Nerve anatomy
   a. Isointense to muscle on T1, mildly hyperintense to muscle on T2
   b. The nerve lies posterior to the medial humeral epicondyle and runs with the ulnar collateral vessels in a fibro-osseous tunnel
   c. The tunnel is bounded superficially by the arcuate ligament which bridges the two heads of the flexor carpi ulnaris muscle

2. Subtypes of cubital tunnel
   a. Physiologic
   b. External compression syndrome
   c. Chronic syndrome

3. Clinical
   a. Exacerbated by physiologic flexion
   b. Associated with various athletic activities
   c. Paresthesia: Symptoms include paresthesia, hypesthesia and positive Tinel's sign leading to atrophy, wasting and claw hand

4. Etiology
   a. Tunnel syndrome ("sleep palsy")
   b. Trauma or fracture
   c. Neoplasm
   d. Hematoma
   e. Inflammation
   f. Osteophytosis
   g. Ectopic calcification or ossification (loose body)
   h. Cubitus valgus
   i. Old capitellar injury
   j. Congenital hypoplastic capitellum
   k. Chronic laxity of the medial collateral ligament

5. MR findings: Idiopathic cubital tunnel
   a. Hypointense thickening of the arcuate ligament
   b. Enlargement of the ulnar nerve
   c. T2 hyperintensity of the ulnar nerve

J-30   Supracondylar Process Syndrome

1. Anatomy
    a. Anatomic variation which is an atavistic bone formation that is connected to the medial epicondyle by a fibrous band usually found 7 cm proximal to the medial epicondyle on the anteromedial humeral surface distally
    b. The median nerve and brachial artery may pass through the tunnel that is bounded superficially by the fibrous band connecting process of the medial epicondyle
2. Etiology: Causes of median nerve compression
    a. Fractures of the supracondylar process
    b. Brachial artery ischemia
    c. Idiopathic
3. Clinical symptoms and signs
    a. Pain and paresthesias of the median nerve dermatome with blunt deep pain in the compressed area
    b. Pain exacerbated at night radiating to forearm, thumb and first three fingers
    c. Weakness, decreased thumb apposition and decreased flexion of first three fingers
    d. Palpated process in thin patients (Tinel's sign)
    e. Both median and ulnar nerve may be compressed and produce neuropathic symptoms
4. Treatment
    a. Immobilization of forearm in pronation with elbow in 40° of flexion
    b. Local cortical steroids
    c. Surgical decompression
5. MR findings
    a. Healing deformed fracture at supracondylar process
    b. Fibrosis and hypointense mixed granulation tissue about supracondylar process

J-31   **Masses & Pseudomasses with a Propensity for the Forearm**

Common

1. Ganglion: Hypointense T1, hyperintense T2, peritendinous
2. Biceps tendon rupture: Intermediate signal with hyperintense T2 edema or hypointense T2 hemosiderin if chronic
3. Dupuytren's fibrosing contracture: Fibrosis of the subcutis space and transverse palmar hypointensity (usually < 1-2 mm thick)

Uncommon

1. Epithelioid sarcoma: Mixed T1 and T2 signal with peritendinous growth pattern
2. Hygroma: Uniform T1 and T2 hypointensity
3. Nodular pseudosarcomatous fasciitis: Mixed T1 and T2 hyperintensity
4. Ulnar nerve neuroma: Intermediate T1, iso- to mildly hyperintense T2, tubular shape
5. Hemophilic pseudotumor: Mixed T1 & T2 hyper- and hypointense masses
6. Pigmented villonodular synovitis: Lamellated foci of mixed T1 & T2 hyper- and hypointensity
7. Radio-capitulum osteochondral defects: Intra-articular ovoid hyper- or hypointense mass with capitulum OCD

J-32   Pearls in the Diagnosis of Dupuytren's Contracture *

1. Fibrosing disorder involving palmar aponeurosis of the hand and its extensions

2. Begins as a subcutaneous nodule in the palm at the level of the distal palmar crease

3. Recurrence in 30-40% of patients

4. Mitotically active, cellular lesions have a higher incidence of recurrence (70%)

5. Increased cellularity and mitotic activity correlates with increasing T2 relaxation and increasing T2 signal intensity (lesions that are brighter than muscle on T2 have a higher recurrence rate)

* Yacoe ME, Bergman AG, Ladd AL, et al. Dupuytren's Contracture: MR Imaging Findings and Correlation Between MR Signal Intensity and Cellularity of Lesions. AJR 160:813-817, 1993.

CATEGORY K: ABDOMEN & BODY

CATEGORY K: ABDOMEN & BODY

K-1   **Hepatocellular Carcinoma & Cavernous Hemangioma**

Cavernous Hemangioma

1. Well marginated
2. Iso- or minimally hypointense T1 signal
3. T2 relaxation time greater than 80 msec
4. No fibrous pseudocapsule
5. Peak contrast enhancement greater than two minutes after injection
6. Marked peak contrast enhancement
7. Marked hyperintensity at five-minute delay on post-contrast T1
8. Variable central scar signal intensity on T1 and T2 due to clot or fibrous tissue
9. Progressive signal hyperintensity with increased T2 weighting
10. No daughter nodules
11. Intratumoral septa uncommon
12. No hepatic venous, portal venous or caval tumor thrombi

Hepatocellular Carcinoma

1. Poorly marginated
2. Iso- to minimally hyperintense T1 signal due to fat content (more common in Japanese)
3. T2 relaxation time less than 80 milliseconds
4. Pseudocapsule, hypointense T1 and T2
5. Peak contrast enhancement 10 seconds
6. Moderate peak enhancement
7. Faint enhancement at five-minute delay post contrast
8. Hypointense central scar on T1 and T2
9. Less pronounced hyperintensity with progressive T2 weighting
10. Daughter nodules indicate a more aggressive lesion
11. Intratumoral septa common
12. Intermediate signal intensity tumor thrombi in cava, portal vein or hepatic vein on T1 indicate a more aggressive lesion

K-2   Hyperintense T2 Simulators of Cavernous Hemangioma of the Liver

1. Insulinoma
2. Carcinoid
3. Pheochromocytoma
4. Somatostatinoma
5. Glucagonoma
6. VIPoma
7. Renal cell carcinoma
8. Medullary thyroid carcinoma
9. Choriocarcinoma
10. Melanoma

K-3   Liver Lesions with Circumferential Rim

Hypointense T2 Rim

1.   Chronic hematoma: Hemosiderin

2.   Hepatocellular carcinoma: Pseudocapsule 30%, rim is thin

3.   Hydatid cyst: Thick homogeneous rim, no perilesional edema

4.   Amebic liver abscess: Concentric rims; rim is made of collagen *

Hyperintense T2 Rim

1.   Metastases: Peritumoral edema with double ring pattern

2.   Liver abscess: One or two concentric rings of mixed signal intensity

3.   Subacute to chronic parenchymal hematoma: White rim also seen on T1

Absent Rim

1.   Adenoma

2.   Focal nodular hyperplasia

3.   Cavernous hemangioma

4.   Simple cyst

* With successful treatment, concentric rings will form, and hepatic edema will resolve with amebic abscess.

K-4   Signs of Liver Metastases

1.   Halo sign: Hyperintense lesion, thin hypointense rim and surrounding ring of hyperintensity on T2 indicate perilesional edema

2.   Wedge sign: Nodule with peripheral segmental T1 hypointensity and T2 hypointensity, wedge-shaped due to peripheral localized hepatic infarction

K-5   MR Appearance of Hydatid Cyst

1. Hypointense circumferential collagenous rim
2. Central T1 isointensity and stellate T2 hyperintensity
3. Multiple peripheral hypointense T1 and hyperintense T2 daughter cysts

K-6   Features of Central Scars & Primary Liver Tumors

Common
1. Cavernous hemangioma: Hypo- or hyperintense T2 (can be either inflammatory or fibrous scar)
2. Focal nodular hyperplasia: Hypointense T1, hyperintense T2 (inflammatory scar)
3. Hepatic adenoma: Variable signal
4. Fibrolamellar hepatocellular carcinoma: Hypointense T1, hypointense T2 (fibrotic repair or scar)

K-7   Pearls in the Diagnosis of Focal Nodular Hyperplasia (FNH)

1. Isointense T1 and T2 (80%)
2. Isointense T1, slight hyperintensity on T2 (20%)
3. Central scar hypointense T1 and hyperintense T2 (95%)
4. Central scar in fibrolamellar hepatocellular carcinoma is hypointense on T1 and T2 (65%)
5. Central scar in hepatocellular carcinoma is rare
6. Focal nodular hyperplasia margins are poorly defined or invisible
7. Pathologic FNH tumor composition includes hepatocytes and Kupffer's cells

K-8   Focal Nodular Hyperplasia Versus Hepatic Adenoma

Focal Nodular Hyperplasia

Hyperintense central stellate scar
Low propensity to hemorrhage
Hyperintense T1 fat uncommon
More common in females
Incidence not increased with birth
    control pills
Iso- to hyperintense on T2 spin echo

Poorly defined margins, no
    pseudocapsule

Hepatic Adenoma

No scar
High propensity to hemorrhage
Commonly contains T1 fat
More common in females
Incidence increased with birth control
    pills
Mild to moderate hyperintensity on
    T2 spin echo
Well defined margins, pseudocapsule

K-9   Wedge-Shaped Signal Alteration

T1 Hyperintensity
1.   Irregular fatty infiltration

T2 Hyperintensity
1.   Hepatocellular carcinoma with peripheral ischemia or infarction
2.   Metastases with wedge pattern of edema
3.   Primary or secondary portal infarction

K-10   Multifocal Hypointense Liver Nodules on T2

Common
1.   Regenerating nodules
2.   Multiple calcified granulomas

Uncommon
1.   Multifocal acute intrahepatic hemorrhages
2.   Gamna-Gandy bodies *
3.   Periportal vascular collaterals

Rare
1.   Osler-Weber-Rendu disease
2.   Multiple calcified parasitic cysts
3.   Portal venous gas

* Foci of pinpoint signal hypointensity (hemosiderin) are seen in patients with peripheral hemolysis. Portal hypertension may be seen in the spleen.

K-11   **Multiple Punctate Splenic Hypointensities**

Common

1.   Granulomas, calcified
2.   Gamna-Gandy bodies (punctate areas of fibrosis containing iron and calcium salts) and chronic portal hypertension

Uncommon

1.   Flow void of arteriovenous malformation
2.   Flow void in hereditary hemorrhagic telangiectasia (Osler-Weber-Rendu)
3.   Fungemia with multifocal microabscess formation
4.   Intrasplenic gas (infection or trauma)
5.   Melanoma metastasis
6.   Choriocarcinoma metastasis, hemorrhagic
7.   Amyloidosis

K-12   Diffuse Hepatic Hypointensity

Common

1.   Hemochromatosis

2.   Hemosiderosis

3.   Superparamagnetic contrast administration

Rare

1.   Wilson's disease *

2.   Hereditary hemorrhagic telangiectasia (Osler-Weber-Rendu disease) [†]

* The hypointensity seen in Wilson's disease is variable due to the presence of concomitant cirrhosis and lack of interaction between conjugated copper and mobile hydrogen protons.

[†] Dark signal in the liver in Osler-Weber-Rendu disease is secondary to flow void.

K-13   Hepatic Lesions with Fat Signal on T1

Common

1.   Fatty liver metamorphosis or replacement

2.   Hepatoma

3.   Hepatic adenoma

Uncommon

1.   Cavernous hemangioma *

Rare

1.   Metastatic liposarcoma or myxoid liposarcoma

* Due to fat signal, not hemorrhage signal.

K-14   Periportal Signal Hyperintensity

1. Obstructive jaundice
2. Cholangitis
3. Cholangiocarcinoma
4. Acute hepatitis
5. Hepatic cirrhosis
6. Hepatoduodenal ligament adenopathy

K-15   Splenic Vein Occlusion Versus Portal Vein Occlusion

Portal Vein Occlusion	Splenic Vein Occlusion
Loss of the normal flow void	Loss of normal splenic flow void
Umbilical vein recanalization & flow void via the left portal vein	Exaggerated flow void of gastroepiploid veins in the greater curvature of the stomach
Gastroesophageal & retroperitonal varices & flow void	Gastroesophageal & retroperitonal varices & flow void
Splenomegaly variable	Splenomegaly
Periportal collaterals or areas of flow void "rat-tail sign"	–

K-16   Pearls in the Diagnosis of Budd-Chiari Syndrome

1. Constriction or loss of a signal void in the intrahepatic or suprahepatic inferior vena cava

2. Loss in caliber or absence of the hepatic vein signal void

3. Comma-shaped intrahepatic hypointense collateral vessels

4. Hypointense T1 and hyperintense T2 ascites

5. Nodular liver with or without hypointense regenerating nodules

6. Caudate lobe hypertrophy due to its independent venous drainage

7. Ascites, massive

8. Subtypes

    a. Primary: Congenital web

    b. Secondary: Thrombosis due to hypercoagulability, compression or trauma

9. Predisposing factors

    a. Neoplasm: Hepatic, renal, adrenal and right atrial or caval sarcoma

    b. Intrinsic veno-occlusive disease secondary to congenital web

    c. Polycythemia vera

    d. Paroxysmal nocturnal hemoglobinuria

    e. Oral contraceptives

    f. Postpartum state

K-17   Ring Sign & Duodenal Hematoma *

1.   Peripheral T2 hypointensity: Hemosiderin

2.   Peripheral T1 hyperintensity: Extracellular methemoglobin

3.   Central T1 isointensity and T2 hypointensity: This concentric ring sign is common in hematomas 10-20 days old

* Adapted from Hahn PF, Stark DD, Vichi LG, et al. Duodenal Hematoma: The Ring Sign in MR Imaging. Radiology 159:379-382, 1986.

K-18   The Concentric Ring Sign *

Hypointense peripheral fibrous and hemosiderin rim on T1 and T2 circumscribes a ring of T1 hyperintensity (extracellular methemoglobin) with central T1 isointensity and T2 hyperintensity.

* Adapted from Hahn, PF, Saini S, Stark, DD, et al. Intra-abdominal Hematoma: The Concentric Ring Sign in MR Imaging. AJR 148:115-119, 1987.

K-19   Intermediate T2 Masses of the Adrenal Gland

Common

1. Adrenal adenoma

Uncommon

1. Pheochromocytoma, benign
2. Granuloma of histoplasmosis or tuberculosis
3. Myelolipoma
4. Subacute adrenal hematoma
5. Amyloidosis
6. Calcified metastatic disease

K-20   Pearls in the Diagnosis of Hepatocellular Carcinoma

1. Hypointense pseudocapsule, more common in the Japanese
2. Daughter or satellite lesions: Indicate a more aggressive lesion
3. Intratumoral hypointense septa
4. Hepatic vascular thrombosis: Indicates a more aggressive lesion
5. Portal vein occlusion with or without hepatic infarction
6. Intratumoral T1 hyperintensity secondary to fat, more common in the Japanese

K-21   Adrenal Signal on MR

Hyperintense T2 (Relative to Liver)

1.   Metastases
2.   Pheochromocytoma
3.   Adrenal carcinoma
4.   Cyst

Isointense T2 (Relative to Liver)

1.   Adrenal adenoma
2.   Subacute hemorrhage

Hypointense T2

1.   Tuberculous or fungal calcification
2.   Acute hemorrhage
3.   Remote calcified hemorrhage

Hyperintense T1

1.   Myelolipoma
2.   Subacute hematoma
3.   Chronic hematoma

Hypointense T1

1.   Necrotic metastasis
2.   Cyst
3.   Necrotic carcinoma

K-22   MR Criteria of Adrenal Adenoma

1.   Rough signal match with the liver as echo time is lengthened
2.   Size < 2 cm
3.   Intermediate T1 signal

K-23   Retroperitoneal Fibrosis on MR

1.   Malignant: Inhomogeneous hyperintense T2 signal
2.   Benign: Homogeneous hypointense T2 signal

K-24   MR & Robson Criteria for Staging of Renal Cell Carcinoma

	Pathology	**MR**
Stage I	Tumor confined to the renal parenchyma without capsular penetration	Relaxation prolongation, not matching that of water (cyst) with preservation of hypointense capsule and hyperintense perirenal fat on T1
Stage II	Transcapsular extension into perinephric fat but confined to Gerota's fascia	Intermediate signal mass interrupts hyperintense T1 perinephric fat
Stage III-A	Tumor thrombus within or invading the renal vein or inferior vena cava	Intermediate signal on T1 in the renal vein or cava in at least two planes
Stage III-B	Regional lymphadenopathy	Intermediate signal adenopathy greater than 1 cm in diameter
Stage III-C	Invasion of renal vein and/or cava with regional lymph adenopathy	Same findings as in III-A and III-B
Stage IV-A	Extension to adjacent organs	Invasion of adjacent organs
Stage IV-B	Spread to distant sites	Spread to distant sites

K-25   Pearls in the Diagnosis of Renal Cell Carcinoma

1. 85% are primary renal neoplasms

2. Incidence is 7.5 cases per 100,000

3. Increased frequency in Scandinavians and North Americans, low frequency in Africans and Asians

4. Peak age 50-60

5. Miscellaneous risk factors

   a. Smoking

   b. Hippel-Lindau syndrome

6. Clinical

   a. Flank pain (41%)

   b. Palpable mass (45%)

7. Paraneoplastic symptoms

   a. Fever

   b. Anemia

   c. Hypercalcemia

   d. Hepatic dysfunction

   e. Erythrocytosis

   f. Amyloidosis

8. Staging

   I   Confined to the renal capsule

   II   Through the capsule into perinephric fat but not through fascia

   III   Renal vein, caval or lymph node involvement

   IV   Adjacent organ invasion or distant metastases

9. Five-year survival post-radical nephrectomy

   I   60-82%

   II   47-80%

   III   35-51%

   IV   0%

K-25   Pearls in the Diagnosis of Renal Cell Carcinoma (Cont'd)

10.   Cystic renal cell carcinoma
    a.   Unilocular 50%
    b.   Multilocular 30%
    c.   Discrete less than 20%
11.   Bilateral 2-5%

K-26   Hypointense Renal Cortex

1. Sickle cell disease

2. Renal cortical necrosis

3. Paroxysmal nocturnal hemoglobinuria

K-27   Pearls in MR Findings of Renal Angiomyolipoma

1. Unencapsulated with blood vessels, smooth muscle and fat

2. Solitary

3. Women greater than men

4. Peak age: 40-60

5. Associated with tuberous sclerosis

    a. 40-80% develop angiomyolipoma

    b. 20% of all angiomyolipomas are multiple, bilateral and associated with tuberous sclerosis

    c. 5% are multiple and bilateral but not associated with tuberous sclerosis

6. Lesion may extend into renal vein, inferior vena cava or perinephric fat

7. T1 hyperintensity and mixed T2 hyperintensity (however, intermediate signal with scant fat signal may occur when smooth muscle predominates and simulates solid metastatic disease or primary neoplasm)

CATEGORY K: ABDOMEN & BODY

K-28   Bladder Carcinomas: TNM Classification & MR

Stage	TNM Description	MR Findings
I	In situ carcinoma	Normal
II	Includes the superficial muscular layer wall	Contour alteration of the bladder wall surface without muscular signal alteration
III-A	Infiltration of deep muscular layer within the wall	Hyperintense T2 signal in bladder wall but delineation of smooth outer bladder wall and normal hyperintense fat signal on T1
III-B	Perivesical infiltration	Outer bladder wall disruption seen in two planes with hypointense T1 signal interrupting hyperintense perivesical fat
IV-A	Infiltration of adjacent pelvic organs	Vesicle/rectal fat plane disruption and altered signal intensity of adjacent organs
IV-B	Infiltration of pelvic walls, distant metastases	Identical local findings as in IV-A

K-29   Staging of Primary Rectal & Rectosigmoid Tumors *

Description

Stage I   Intraluminal polypoid intermediate signal mass without bowel wall thick-
               ening

Stage II   Bowel wall thickening (greater than 0.5 cm) without invasion of hyperin-
               tense perirectal fat

Stage III-A   Invasion of surrounding hyperintense fat or intermediate signal intensity
               muscles or organs but sparing the pelvic sidewall

Stage III-B   Extension to the pelvic sidewall

Stage IV   Pelvic tumor with distant metastases

* Adapted from Butch RJ, Stark DD, Wittenberg J, et al. Staging Rectal Cancer by MR and CT. AJR
  146:1155-1160, 1986.

K-30   Criteria for Staging Prostate Cancer *

Stage	Digital Rectal Exam	Acid Phosphatase	Bone Scan	MR Imaging
A	Tumor not palpable	Negative	Negative	Stage A cannot be differentiated from Stage B on the basis of MR
B	Tumor confined to prostate	Negative	Negative	Tumor confined to the prostate gland, signal intensity normal or hetero-geneous
B-1	Tumor < 1.5 cm	Negative	Negative	
B-2	Tumor > 1.5 cm	Negative	Negative	
C	Locally extensive tumor (periprostatic tissue, seminal vesicles, urinary bladder, urethra)	Negative or positive	Negative	*Periprostatic fat:* Infiltrated; *Seminal vesicles:* Asymmetric size, abnormal signal; *Levator ani:* Increased signal on T2
D	Any size of local tumor, metastases	Negative or positive	Negative or positive	Pelvic lymph nodes > 1.5 cm
D-1	Pelvic lymph nodes > 1.5 cm			
D-2	Bone metastases			Bony or distant metastases

Note: Assignment of clinical stage is based on results of digital rectal examination, serum acid phosphatase and bone scanning. Staging classification of Whitmore (2) modified by Clein (1).

* Modified from Hricak H, Dumes GC, Jeffrey RV, et al. Prostatic Carcinoma: Staging by Clinical Assessment, CT, and MR Imaging. Radiology 162:332, 1987.

**K-31   Prostatic or Periprostatic Homogeneous Hyperintense T2
                 Signal**

Near Midline Lesions

1. Müllerian duct cysts: Near midline and usually cephalad to the prostate, greater
    than 1 cm in size, average age 30-40 years

2. Prostatic utricle cysts: Always midline occurring at the level of the verumon-
    tanum, less than 1 cm in size, associated with genitourinary anomalies (hypospa-
    dias, incomplete testicular descent, unilateral renal agenesis)

3. Ejaculatory duct cysts: May or may not appear midline but almost always close
    to the midline, yield spermatozoa on aspiration, may be associated with cystic
    dilatation of the seminal vesicle ipsilaterally

4. Vas deferens cyst: Posterior but near the midline

5. TURP defect: Funnel-shaped fluid collection with wide end communicating with
    the bladder and narrow end continuous with the prostatic urethra in the sagittal
    plane

Non-Midline Location

1. Benign prostatic hyperplasia with cystic degeneration: Most common cystic
    lesion of the prostate gland, associated with benign prostatic hyperplasia, most
    common in the periurethral transitional zone, small size, close association with
    hypointense calculi

2. Retention cysts: Obstructed prostatic gland ductules, never contain spermatozoa,
    1-2 cm in size, no zonal predilection

3. Prostatic abscess: History of diabetes, 50- to 60-year-old age group, signs and
    symptoms of infection or toxemia

4. Seminal vesicle cysts: Peripheral seminal vesicle location

Rare Cystic Lesions

1. Parasitic cysts (bilharziasis, echinococcus)

2. Cystic carcinoma

K-32   The Uterine Zones: Normal Anatomy, Menstrual Cycle Variations & Hormonal Effects

Normal Anatomy

1.   Myometrium: Intermediate T1, nominal T2 hyperintensity

2.   Endometrium and endocervix: Mildly hyperintense T1, hyperintense T2

3.   Junctional zone: T1 hypointensity, marked T2 hypointensity

Effect of the Menstrual Cycle on Uterine Signal

1.   Myometrial outer layer

   a.   Mild progressive signal hyperintensity with progressively poorer distinction in the latter stages of the menstrual cycle

   b.   Increased myometrial thickness and area during the first half (follicular phase) of the menstrual cycle

   c.   The second phase (luteal) results in slow increase in myometrial thickness

2.   Endometrium: Hyperintense signal throughout the menstrual cycle with threefold increase in area during the follicular phase and only slight increase in thickness and area in the luteal phase

3.   Junctional zone (inner myometrial layer): Remains hypointense throughout the menstrual cycle but becomes less distinct as the cycle progresses

4.   Cervix: Low intensity junctional zone of the cervix increases in thickness in the late luteal phase

Effect of Hormonal Stimulation on Uterine Signal

1.   Premenarchal and postmenopausal uterus: Small size and featureless with regard to zonal anatomy

2.   Reproductive age women: Distinct junctional, outer myometrium and endometrial zone anatomy with variations during the menstrual cycle as described

3.   Oral contraceptive gonadotropin releasing hormone (GRH): Endometrial atrophy or thinning in the myometrium with increased signal on T1 and T2 in women taking oral contraceptives and decreased myometrial signal in patients treated with GRH analog

K-33   Appearance of Cervical Carcinoma by Stage

	Description	MR Findings
0	Carcinoma in situ	Normal
I-A	Microinvasive carcinoma confined to the cervix	Normal or punctate T2 signal hyperintensity
I-B	Clinical invasive carcinoma confined to the cervix	Punctate T2 signal hyperintensity involving cervical myometrium
II-A	Vaginal invasion without involvement of the lower vagina	Mixed T2 signal involving cervix and vagina in the sagittal projection
II-B	Parametrial involvement	Parametrial involvement or invasion on axial T1
III-A	Lower 1/3 of vagina invaded	Hyperintensity in the cervix, upper and lower vagina
III-B	Pelvic sidewall extension or hydronephrosis	Pelvic sidewall extension on axial T1
IV-A	Invasion of the mucosa of the bladder or rectum	Bladder or rectum mucosal signal alteration on T1 in sagittal & axial projections
IV-B	Spread to distant organs	Same as IV-A

K-34   FIGO Classification of Cervical Carcinoma

Class	Description
Stage 0	*In situ*
Stage I	*Confined to the cervix*
FIGO Class I-A	Microinvasive
FIGO Class I-B	Clinically invasive
Stage II	*Extending beyond the cervix but not to the pelvic wall or lower third of vagina*
FIGO Class II-A	No parametrial* involvement
FIGO Class II-B	Parametrial involvement
Stage III	*Extending to pelvic wall or lower third of vagina*
FIGO Class III-A	No extension to pelvic wall
FIGO Class III-B	Extension to pelvic wall or ureteral obstruction
Stage IV	*Involving mucosa of bladder or rectum or extending beyond true pelvis*
FIGO Class IV-A	Spread to adjacent organs
FIGO Class IV-B	Spread to distant organs

Note: Cervical carcinoma appears as hyperintense T2 signal adjacent to or interrupting the normal low intensity cervical zone, and this signal may extend into the cardinal ligaments with parametrial involvement.

* Parametrium refers to the cardinal and sacrouterine ligaments.

K-35   FIGO Classification of Endometrial Carcinoma

Class	Description
Stage I FIGO Class I-A FIGO Class I-B	Confined to the corpus Uterine cavity is < 8 cm long Uterine cavity is > 8 cm long
Stage II FIGO Class II	Carcinoma has involved corpus and cervix but has not extended outside uterus
Stage III FIGO Class III	Carcinoma has extended outside uterus but not outside true pelvis
Stage IV FIGO Class IV-A FIGO Class IV-B	Carcinoma has extended outside the true pelvis or has invaded mucosa of bladder or rectum Spread to adjacent organs Spread to distant organs

Note: Endometrial carcinoma appears as hyperintense T2 signal interrupting the normal hypointense junctional zone with or without extension into the intermediate signal myometrium.

K-36   Common Signal Intensities in Uterine Leiomyomas

1. Intermediate T2 signal with speckled punctate foci of T2 hyperintensity (85%)

2. Rounded foci of T2 hypointensity (calcium) within the solid neoplasm (30%)

3. Irregular foci of T1 hyperintensity (myxoid degeneration or hemorrhage) on T1 (25%) *

4. Large homogeneous rounded foci of T2 signal hyperintensity (10%) with variable T1 signal greater than 2 cm in diameter (necrosis)

* Necrosis, myxoid or fatty degeneration is most commonly seen in lesions greater than 4-5 cm in diameter.

K-37   Endometrial Cysts on MR (Endometriomas)

1.   Loss of the clear T1 hyperintense periuterine fat due to periuterine adhesions and tethered appearance of the rectum

2.   Distinct low intensity thick fibrous capsules surrounding a cystic mass on T1 and T2

3.   Prominent low-intensity shading (see diagram) within the cyst or mass on T2 secondary to susceptibility effects and layering blood clots

4.   Multiloculation

5.   Serpiginous or gyriform foci of signal hypointensity on T1 and hypointensity or hyperintensity on T2 due to flow void of diffuse hypervascularity

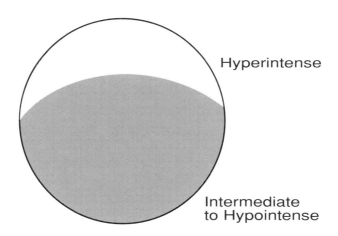

T2 Shading

K-38   Common Adnexal Masses in Women by Signal

Hyperintense T1, Hyperintense T2

1.   Endometrioma: Shading or layering*

2.   Hemorrhagic cysts: Layering or fluid-fluid level

3.   Dermoid: Layering†

4.   Cystic or sacrococcygeal teratoma

5.   Theca lutein cysts

Hyperintense T1, Isointense or Intermediate T2

1.   Endometrioma

2.   Hemorrhagic corpus luteum cyst

3.   Dermoid

Hypointense T1, Hyperintense T2 (Homogeneous–Cystic)

1.   Simple cysts

2.   Polycystic ovarian disease‡

3.   Serous cystadenoma or cystadenocarcinoma: Multiloculated, hypointense T2 punctate calcification

4.   Mucinous cystadenoma or cystadenocarcinoma: Multiloculated with protruding intermediate signal nodules

Mild Hypointense T1, Hyperintense T2 (Proteinaceous Cysts)

1.   Pelvic inflammatory disease or tubo-ovarian abscess

2.   Mucinous cystadenoma or cystadenocarcinoma

3.   Cystic teratoma (rare)

Isointense T1, Isointense T2

1.   Fibroma

K-38   Common Adnexal Masses in Women by Signal (Cont'd)

Isointense T1, Mild Hyperintense T2 (Solid Lesions)

1. Solid ovarian neoplasm

2. Endometriosis with hyperacute or acute hemorrhage

3. Hemorrhagic ovarian cyst with acute or hyperacute hemorrhage

4. Krukenberg tumor[§]

5. Metastasis from endometrial carcinoma

---

* Hyperintensity layers dependently on T1 and nondependently on T2 for hemorrhagic cysts and endometriosis.

† Fluid-fluid level shows hyperintensity nondependent on T1 (fat) and dependent on T2 (water).

‡ Punctate signal hyperintensity is wheel-like or peripherally located about the ovary surface.

§ The most common causes of Krukenberg tumor are metastatic colon cancer and gastric carcinoma.

K-39   Adnexal Lesions on MR

1. Cyst: Homogeneous T1 hypointensity, T2 hyperintensity

2. Dermoid: Hyperintense T1, iso- to hyperintense T2, fluid-fluid levels with hyperintense fat nondependent on T1 and hypointense water dependent on T1

3. Endometrioma: Homogeneous T1 hyperintensity and T2 hypo- to hyperintensity *

4. Tubo-ovarian abscess: Tubular or ovoid intermediate T1, hyperintense T2

5. Fibroma: Intermediate T1 and T2 signal

6. Theca lutein cysts: Inhomogeneous T1 hyperintensity and T2 hyperintensity, circumferential serpiginous periadnexal flow void due to hypervascularity

7. Stein-Leventhal syndrome: Wheel-like peripheral punctate T1 hypointensity and T2 hyperintensity

* T2 signal depends on age of hemorrhage, with more recent events being more hypointense.

K-40   Pearls in the Diagnosis of Uterine Adenomyomatosis

1. Women of reproductive age most frequently affected

2. Clinical dysmenorrhea and menorrhagia, progressive

3. Treatment: Hysterectomy, not dilatation and curettage

4. Signal

    a. Heterotopic endometrium and myometrium with myometrial hyperplasia

    b. Punctate foci of T2 hyperintensity surrounded by marked functional zone hypointensity (80%)

    c. Hyperintensity of punctate foci on T1 (20%)

5. Endometrial tissue is of the basalis type, and therefore, not hormonally responsive in adenomyomatosis

6. Endometriosis tissue is of the functionalis type and therefore is hormonally responsive

K-41 Müllerian Duct Anomalies & MR Findings *

Class and Type | **MR Findings**

I. Segmental agenesis/hypoplasia
  A. Vaginal
  B. Cervical
  C. Fundal
  D. Tubal
  E. Combined

Agenesis: No identifiable organ or small amorphous tissue remnant. Hypoplasia: uterus–small for age, maintains adult body/cervix ratio of 2:1, reduced inter-cornual distance (<2 cm), low signal on T2 with poor zonal differentiation, endometrial/myometrial width reduced

II. Unicornuate
  A1. Rudimentary horn w/ endometrium
    a. Communicating w/ main uterine cavity
    b. Not communicating w/ main uterine cavity
  A2. Rudimentary horn w/o endometrium
  B. No rudimentary horn

Banana-shaped uterus, normal width of endometrium and myometrium, endometrial:myometrial ratio preserved

III. Didelphys

Double, separate uterus, cervix and upper vagina; each uterine cavity of normal volume; endometrium and myometrium of normal width; endometrial:myometrial ratio normal

IV: Bicornuate
  A. Complete
  B. Partial
  C. Arcuate

Uterine fundus concave or flattened outward; two horns visible with increased intercornual distance (>4 cm), septum–high signal intensity myometrium on T2 at level of fundus; high signal intensity myometrium or low signal intensity fibrous tissue at level of lower uterine segment

V: Septate
  A. Complete
  B. Incomplete

Uterine fundus convex outward, normal intercornual distance (2-4 cm), each uterine cavity reduced in volume, endometrial/myometrial width and ratio normal, septum–low signal on T1 & T2

* Carrington MB, Hricak H, Nuruddin RN, et al. Müllerian Duct Anomalies: MR Imaging Evaluation. Radiology 176:715, 1990.

K-42   True & False Lumen in Aortic Dissection

1. Flow is slower in the false lumen; therefore, flow phenomena are more common
2. Clot or thrombus is more common in the false lumen
3. Great vessels communicate with the true lumen
4. False lumen often larger than true lumen
5. False lumen more often posterior to true lumen

CATEGORY L: IMAGES & PREDICAMENTS

CATEGORY L: IMAGES & PREDICAMENTS

Section 1: Contraindications

L-1   Carotid Clamps

Severe Deflection: Do Not Scan

Poppen-Blaylock (stainless steel)

Mild Deflection: Considered Safe, Avoid MR if Possible

Crutchfield

Kindt

Salibi

Selverstone

Nominal Deflection: Safe to Scan

Tantalum

L-2   Aneurysm Clips

Undeflected: Safe

Gastrointestinal anastomosis clip (Autosuture SGIA [SS])

Heifetz (Elgiloy)

Hemoclip #10 (316L SS)

Hemoclip (Tantalum)

Ligaclip #6 (316L SS)

Ligaclip (Tantalum)

Olivecrona

Stevens (50-4190, Silver alloy)

Surgiclip Auto Suture S M 9.5 (SS)

Sugita (Elgiloy)

Vari-angle McFadden (MP 35 N)

Yasargil (all)

Minimal Deflection: Avoid MR

Drake DR 20

Scoville (EN 58 J)

Moderate Deflection: Do Not Scan

Drake (301 SS)

Drake (DR 16, DR 14, DR 24)

Housepian

Mayfield (304 SS)

Mayfield (301 SS)

McFadden (301 SS)

Pivot (17-7PH)

L-2   Aneurysm Clips (Cont'd)

Marked Deflection: Do Not Scan

Downs multipositional (17-7PH)

Heifetz (17-7PH)

Kapp straight and curved (404-SS)

Kapp straight and curved (405-SS)

Sundt-Kees (17-7PH)

Sundt-Kees (301 SS)

Vari-angle (17-7PH)

Vari-angle Micro (17-7 PM SS)

Vari-angle Spring (17-7 PM SS)

L-3   Cardiac Valves

Marked Deflection: Do Not Scan

Starr-Edwards, Model Pre 6000

Deflected: Safe

Beall

Bjork-Shiley (universal spherical)

Bjork-Shiley (Model MBC)

Bjork-Shiley (Model 25 MBRC 11030)

Carpentier-Edwards (Model 2650)

Carpentier-Edwards (porcine)

Hall-Kaster (Model A 7700)

Hancock I (porcine)

Hancock II (porcine)

Hancock extracorporeal (Model 242R)

Hancock extracorporeal (M4365-33)

Ionescu-Shiley

Lillehi-Kaster (Model 300 S)

Lillehi-Kaster (Model 5009)

Medtronic Hall

Medtronic Hall (Model A7700-D-16)

Omnicarbon (Model 3523T029)

Omniscience (Model 6522)

St. Jude (A101)

St. Jude (M101)

Smeloff-Cutter

Starr-Edwards (Model 1260)

Starr-Edwards (Model 2320)

L-3   Cardiac Valves (Cont'd)

Undeflected: Safe

Bjork-Shiley (convex/concave)

Hancock-Vascor (Model 505)

Starr-Edwards (Model 2400)

L-4   Intravascular Stents, Coils & Filters

Undeflected: Safe

Amplatz retrievable IVC filter

Cragg nitinol spiral IVC filter

Greenfield IVC filter

Maas helical IVC filter

Maas helical endovascular stent

Mobin-Uddin umbrella IVC filter

Mildly Deflected: Safe

Gianturco embolization coil*

Gianturco zig-zag stent*

Greenfield filter (stainless steel)

New retrievable IVC filter*

Palmaz endovascular stent*

Markedly Deflected: Reportedly Safe, Avoid MR if Possible

Gianturco Bird's Nest IVC filter*

Gunther retrievable IVC filter*

* Ferromagnetic coils, filters and stents typically become firmly incorporated into the vessel wall several weeks following placement making it highly unlikely that they will become dislodged by magnetic forces.

L-5   Prosthetic Ear Implants*

Undeflected: Safe

Cody tact

House-type incus prosthesis

McGee stainless steel piston

Reuter drain tube

Richards House-type wire loop

Richards-McGee Piston

Richards Plasti-pore with Armstrong style platinum ribbon

Richards-Schuknecht Teflon wire

Richards Trapeze platinum ribbon

Schuknecht Gelfoam and wire prosthesis, Armstrong-style

Shea stainless steel and Teflon wire prosthesis

Xomed stapes prosthesis Robinson-style

Marked Deflection: Do Not Scan

Cochlear implant (3M/House)

Cochlear implant (3M/Vienna)

McGee piston stapes prosthesis

* Only undeflected ear implants are recommended for scanning.

L-6   Penile Prostheses*

Undeflected: Safe

AMS Malleable 600 (American Medical Systems, Minnetonka, MN)

AMS Malleable 700 CX Inflatable (American Medical Systems, Minnetonka, MN)

Flexi-Flate (Surgitek, Medical Engineering Corp., Racine, WI)

Flexi-Rod Standard (Surgitek, Medical Engineering Corp., Racine, WI)

Flexi-Rod II Firm (Surgitek, Medical Engineering Corp., Racine, WI)

Jonas (Dacomed Corp., Minneapolis, MN)

Mentor Flexible (Mentor Corp., Minneapolis, MN)

Mentor Inflatable (Mentor Corp., Minneapolis, MN)

Deflected: Do Not Scan

OmniPhase (Dacomed Corp., Minneapolis, MN)

* Only undeflected prostheses are recommended for scanning.

L-7   Cervical Spine Braces

Ferrous Components: Avoid Scanning

EXO adjustable collar

Guilford cervical orthosis

S.O.M.I. cervical orthosis

Image Quality Unacceptable: Avoid Scanning if Possible*

EXO adjustable collar

Guilford cervical orthosis

S.O.M.I. cervical orthosis

Image Quality Acceptable*

Bremer halo cervical orthosis

Modified Guilford orthosis

Modified PMT cervical orthosis

MR-compatible Bremer orthosis

Philadelphia collar

PMT halo cervical orthosis

* Safely scanned at all field strengths up to 1.5T.

L-8   Dental Materials*

Undeflected: Safe

Acrylic/polyvinyl crown

Aluminum crown

Brace band (SS)

Dental amalgam

Gold crowns

Microfilled resin

Silver points

Permanent crown (amalgam)

Mild to Moderate Deflection: Safe

Linkplus pin

Orthodontic bands (all types)

Stainless steel crown

Zinc phosphate cement

Severe Deflection: Safe

Para post

TMS pin

   * Modified from Hinshaw DB, Holshouser BA, Engstrom HIM, et al. Dental Material Artifacts on MR Images. Radiology 166:778, 1988.

L-9 Metallic Otologic Implants *

Undeflected and Safe

1. Austin tytan piston (titanium)
2. Berger "V" bobbin ventilation tube (titanium)
3. Ehmke hook stapes prosthesis (platinum)
4. House single loop (SS)
5. House single loop (tantalum)
6. House double loop (SS)
7. House-type wire loop stapes prosthesis (316L SS)
8. House-type SS piston and wire (SS)
9. McGee piston stapes prosthesis (316L SS)
10. McGee piston stapes prosthesis (platinum/316L SS)
11. McGee Shepherd's Crook stapes prosthesis (316L SS)
12. Plasti-pore piston (316L SS/plasti-pore material)
13. Platinum ribbon loop stapes prosthesis (platinum)
14. Reuter bobbin ventilation tube (316L SS)
15. Richards piston stapes prosthesis (platinum/fluoroplastic)
16. Richards bucket handle stapes prosthesis (316L SS)
17. Robinson-Moon offset stapes prosthesis (SS)
18. Robinson-Moon-Lippy offset stapes prosthesis (SS)
19. Robinson incus replacement prosthesis (SS)
20. Ronis piston stapes prosthesis (316L SS/fluoroplastic)
21. Schea cup piston stapes prosthesis (platinum/fluoroplastic)
22. Scheer piston stapes prosthesis (316L SS/fluoroplastic)
23. Schuknecht tef-wire incus attachment (SS)
24. Schuknecht tef-wire malleus attachment (SS)
25. Schuknecht piston stapes prosthesis (3126L SS/fluoroplastic)
26. Sheehy incus replacement (SS)
27. Sheehy-type incus replacement strut (316L SS)

L-9   **Metallic Otologic Implants (Cont'd)**

28.   Spoon bobbin ventilation tube (316L SS)

29.   Tantalum wire loop (tantalum)

30.   Tef-platinum piston (platinum)

31.   Trapeze ribbon loop stapes prosthesis (platinum)

32.   Williams microclip (316L SS)

33.   Xomed stapes (SS)

* From Shellock FG, Schatz CJ. Metallic Otologic Implants: In Vitro Assessment of Ferromagnetism
  at 1.5 T. AJNR 12:280, 1991.

L-10   Miscellaneous Devices

Undeflected: Safe

Artificial urinary sphincter AMS 800

Central venous catheters

Coronary artery washer/ markers for bypass

Dentures (nonmagnetic type)

Dural venous sinus clips

Forceps (titanium)

Hakim valve and pump

Holter-Rickam Reservoir

Harrington rods

Intraocular lens implant (Binkhorst, iridocapsular lens, titanium loop)

Intraocular lens implant (Worst, platinum clip lens)

Metallic clips and sutures (see L-3); remove skin staples if possible

Metallic craniotomy steel plate

Omaya Reservoir

Orthopedic joint, extremity prosthesis, screws, nails and plates

Pessaries and intrauterine devices (Copper-7 and Lippes Loop)

Port-a-cath access ports

Radioactive seed implants and applicators

Sternotomy wires and wire sutures

Swan-Ganz catheters

Tantalum and steel wire mesh

Tantalum powder

Ventriculoatrial and ventriculoperitoneal shunts and Accu-Flow shunt connectors (all)

Weck's clip

L-10   Miscellaneous Devices (Cont'd)

Deflected: Safe

Contraceptive diaphragm, Koroflex

Contraceptive diaphragm, Flat Spring

Contraceptive diaphragm, All Flex

Hickman port

Q-Port

L-11   Devices Contraindicated in the MR Scanner

Aneurysm clips (selected items, see L-2)

BBs

Cardiac valves (selected items, see L-3)

Cardiac pacemakers

Cerebral ventricular shunt tube connector (type unknown)

Cochlear implants (3M House or Vienna only, see L-5)

Insulin pump

Neurostimulator (TENS unit)

Ocular shrapnel, imbedded

Penile prosthesis (Omniphase only, see L-6)

Holter monitor or defibrillator (permanent)

Respirator

Stents or vascular filters (selected items, see L-4)

Tissue expander with magnetic port

Western European retinal tack

CATEGORY L: IMAGES & PREDICAMENTS

Section 2: Contrast   Page

L-12   Factors Influencing Vascular Signal Gain

Slow flow

Laminar flow

Long repetition time

Short echo time

Thick sections (weak gradients)

Flow in plane or tangent to a plane of section

Flow along the Y axis (weaker gradient)

Use of even echoes (40/80, 20/40, etc.)

Larger flip angles

Partial saturation

Single slice gradient echo techniques

Low field imaging

L-13   Factors Increasing Vascular Signal Loss

Fast flow

Turbulent flow

Short repetition time

Long echo time

Thin sections (strong gradients)

Perpendicular flow

Flow along the X axis (stronger gradient)

Use of odd echoes

Smaller flip angles

Spin echo sequences

Multislice spin echo techniques

High field imaging

L-14   Factors Governing Black Blood or Bright Blood

Black Blood

Presaturation

Phase dispersion

Time-of-flight effects

Bright Blood

Slice entry phenomenon

Pseudogating to diastole

Intentional diastolic gating

Even echo rephasing

Flow compensation or gradient motion rephasing

Gradient echo imaging

L-15   Paramagnetic Ions

Transition Metals

Titanium (Ti^{3+})

Nickel (Ni^{2+})

Iron (Fe^{3+})

Vanadium (V^{4+})

Cobalt (Co^{3+})

Chromium (Cr^{3+})

Manganese (Mn^{2+})

Copper (Cu^{2+})

Lanthanide Series

Praseodymium (Pr^{3+})

Gadolinium (Gd^{3+})

Europium (Eu^{3+})

Dysprosium (Dy^{3+})

Actinide

Protactinium (Pa^{4+})

Nitroxide-Stable Free Radicals (NSFRs)

Radicals

Pyrolidine

Piperdine

Molecular oxygen (O_2)

L-16   Classes of MR Contrast Agents & Their Signal Effects

T1 Shortening (Paramagnetic): Hyperintense T1 Signal with Enhancement

Gadolinium-DTPA[a]

Gadolinium-DOTA

Gadolinium-albumin

Ferric ammonium citrate (Geritol)[a]

Manganese-DPDP (Enhances normal liver)

T2 Shortening (Superparamagnetic): Hypointense T1 and T2 Signal at Enhancement Sites

Magnetite microspheres[b]

Fat-containing Agents: T1 Hyperintensity (Not as Pronounced as Paramagnetic Species)

Mineral oil[a]

Milk shake[a]

Nonproton Agents: T1 and T2 Hypointensity

Perfluorohydrocarbons (perfluorohexylbromide)

Fluosol

Effervescent[a]

Diamagnetic Agent: Hypointensity on T1 and T2

Kaolin (Kaopectate)[a]

Barium sulfate

a   *Used as a bowel contrast agent*
b   *Uptake by the reticuloendothelial system*

L-17   Guidelines in the United States (FDA) for Magnetic Field, Time-Bearing Gradient & RF Exposure

1.   Static magnetic field: 2 Tesla
2.   Time varying magnetic field ΔB/Δt: 3 Tesla per second
3.   Radiofrequency specific absorption rating (SAR): 0.4 watts per kilogram (whole body) or 2.0 watts per kilogram (per gram of tissue)

L-18   Recommendations for Pregnancy

1.   Avoid routine scanning in the first trimester of pregnancy
2.   When a maternal indication requires ionizing radiation for diagnosis, MR is preferable if it has the contrast and spatial resolution to make the diagnosis
3.   Second and third trimester imaging may be performed for maternal or fetal indications and should be substituted for any imaging procedure utilizing ionizing radiation when possible

L-19   **Hypointensity or Black Signal on Gradient Echo**

1. Susceptibility effects or artifacts
2. Hemorrhage: Intracellular methemoglobin, deoxyhemoglobin or hemosiderin
3. Ferritin
4. Calcification
5. Air
6. Turbulent or shear flow
7. Contrast agents (superparamagnetic compounds or high concentrations of paramagnetic compounds)
8. Mucoid concretion

L-20   Types of Magnetic Behavior

1. Ferromagnetism

    a. Unpaired electrons

    b. Interacting domains (unpaired electron spins permanently aligned by positive exchange forces)

    c. Positive susceptibility*

2. Superparamagnetism

    a. Electrons unpaired

    b. Noninteracting domains (thermodynamically independent)

    c. Positive susceptibility

3. Paramagnetism

    a. Electrons unpaired

    b. Noninteracting permanent moments (independent action of molecular magnetic moments)

    c. Positive susceptibility

4. Diamagnetism

    a. Electrons paired

    b. No permanent spin moment

    c. Independent of external factors (except some metal systems)

    d. Negative susceptibility; therefore, negative induced magnetization

* Susceptibility: Induced magnetization in a substance placed within a magnetic field is additive to that of the applied field. The ratio of induced magnetization to the applied field is that substance's susceptibility. This is a measure of the extent to which a substance is susceptible to external magnetization.

L-21   Summary of Fast Scan Imaging Methods

Utilization of Short Repetition Time

Gradient echo

1.   Spoiled FLASH
2.   Spoiled GRASS
3.   Steady state FLASH
4.   FISP
5.   FLASH
6.   GRASS
7.   Fast or C-fast

Spin Echo with Optimized Flip Angle

1.   Flame
2.   Multiplanar GRASS
3.   RF-driven equilibrium sequence
4.   QUICK STEP
5.   Steady state free precession

Decrease the Number of Views (Y Steps)

Reduce acquisition matrix

1.   Asymmetric field of view
2.   Half-Fourier imaging
3.   Half-excitation imaging (or quarter-excitation imaging)
4.   Conjugate synthesis
5.   Strip scanning

L-21   Summary of Fast Scan Imaging Methods (Cont'd)

Acquire Views (Y Steps) More Rapidly
1. Hybrid
2. Short shot/echo planar
3. STEAM
4. RARE

Decrease Number of Excitations
1. Single excitation imaging

L-22   Evaluating the Need for Contrast

Should Always be Used

Central Nervous System

1. Primary brain tumors
2. Metastatic disease
3. Seizures
4. Inflammatory disease
5. Postoperative brain
6. Recurrent tumor versus scar
7. Acoustic neuroma (also evaluation of deafness)
8. Pituitary adenoma
9. Differentiation of microvascular from macrovascular infarction
10. Selected cases of complex vascular disease

Spine

1. Differentiation of recurrent disc versus scar or granulation tissue
2. Spinal cord neoplasm
3. Any case of myelopathy
4. Inflammatory cord disease, particularly myelitis or multiple sclerosis

Contrast May be of Assistance (Intravenous or Intra-articular)

1. Differentiation of synovitis from other causes of joint effusion or capsulosynovial thickening when given intravenously
2. Selected cases of liver disease or lesions requiring further qualification when diagnosis is not clear with noncontrast intravenous MR
3. Intra-articular administration
   a. Diagnosis of meniscal tear in previously oversewn meniscus
   b. Diagnosis of small complete rotator cuff tear or labral tear with equivocal noncontrast MR

CATEGORY L: IMAGES & PREDICAMENTS

Section 3: Artifacts   Page

L-23   Image Ghosting

System Causes of Ghosting
1.   Eddy currents
2.   60 Hz noise

Patient Causes of Ghosting
1.   Patient motion
2.   Mild peristalsis
3.   Involuntary swallowing, coughing, sneezing or eye movement
4.   Variation in heart rate during gating
5.   Cerebrospinal fluid pulsation
6.   Respiration

L-24   Artifact by Etiology

Patient
1.   Pulsatile blood flow ghosting
2.   Respiratory blurring or ghosting
3.   Patient motion, coughing, blinking, or swallowing

Main Magnet
1.   Geometric distortion
2.   Main magnetic field distortion or inhomogeneity

Acquisition-related
1.   Wraparound or aliasing artifact
2.   Ringing artifact
3.   Chemical shift
4.   IR boundary artifact

L-25   Artifact by Appearance

Wraparound or Aliasing

1.   Due to coil selection, too small for image body part

Oblique Stripes

1.   Loss of data or anomalous data

Blurred Image

1.   Partial volume averaging due to large slice thickness

2.   Excessive eddy current

3.   Lack of sharpness due to coughing, blinking, or other patient motion

Center Line

1.   Residual transverse magnetization due to excessively long readout, weak spoiler gradient or superimposition of RF pulses

Center Point

1.   DC current offset

Chemical Shift

1.   Difference in Larmor frequencies of fat and water produce pixel shift predominant in the X direction

Signal Variation Between Odd & Even Images Resulting in Altered Contrast & Signal-to-Noise

1.   Crosstalk secondary to lack of slice gap between slices, especially with multiecho imaging

Discrete Lines Perpendicular to the Frequency Encoded Axis

1.   RF noise or interference from outside sources

2.   Crosstalk due to poorly formed or configured RF pulses

L-25   Artifact by Appearance (Cont'd)

Geometric Distortion with or without Signal Loss

1.   Susceptibility artifact with tissues or substances adjacent to one another with varying susceptibility

No Image

1.   Poor patient centering or failure of center frequency check
2.   Poor shimming

Ghosting

1.   Variation in signal due to patient motion, respiration, coughing, sneezing, peristalsis, blinking or cardiac or vascular pulsation
2.   Transmitter or gradient instability
3.   Eddy currents

Excessive Image Noise

1.   Faulty electronics or failed preamplifier
2.   Poor choice of sequence parameters
3.   Poor coil selection
4.   Poor eddy current compensation
5.   Poor coil tuning

L-26   Solutions for Artifacts

Wraparound

1. Oversampling utilizing no phase wraparound or extended fields of view
2. Use band pass filtering in the X direction
3. Use presaturation techniques
4. Intentionally increase field of view
5. Call service engineer

Image Blurring

1. Reduce slice thickness, field of view or image matrix
2. Call service engineer for excessive eddy currents

Center Line (A Line Running Through the Center of the Image)

1. Increase spoiler gradient strength
2. Shorten readout
3. Alternate RF pulse phase

Center Point (A Point Positioned in the Center of the Image)

1. Alternate the phase of RF pulse

Chemical Shift

1. Increase the readout gradient
2. Reduce the field of view (which reduces artifact relative to pixel size)
3. Utilize fat saturation or spectroscopic fat subtraction techniques

Crosstalk Artifact (Contrast and Signal Noise Reduction)

1. Increase interslice gap
2. Optimize RF sync pulses for better slice profile
3. Utilize pulsing sequences such as gradient echo single slice acquisition that complete a single slice excitation before going on to the next slice

L-26   Solutions for Artifacts (Cont'd)

Parallel Line Artifact (Parallel Lines Perpendicular to Frequency Encoding Axis)

1. Check integrity of RF shielding
2. Check for outside sources of RF interference
3. Check stability of power supply

Geometric or Aspect Ratio Distortion

1. Shorten echo time
2. Increase readout gradient
3. Use spin echo instead of gradient echo
4. Use single echo instead of multiecho
5. Move external or internal metal objects
6. Check the magnetic environment
7. Check shim power supply

Susceptibility Artifact (Signal Void Between Tissues of Differing Susceptibilities)

1. Shorten the echo time
2. Increase the readout gradient
3. Use spin echo instead of gradient echo
4. Use single echo instead of multiecho
5. Remove external or internal metal objects

Image Ghosting

1. Reduce patient motion with sedation, prone positioning, coaxing or internal magnet mirrors
2. Reduce respiratory motion by prone positioning or central or respiratory ordered phase encoding
3. Reduce cardiac pulsation artifacts with peripheral pulse gating or ECG gating
4. Reduce peristaltic ghosting with glucagon or fasting the night before an exam
5. Average out ghosting artifacts with increased number of repetitions
6. Service engineer for excessive eddy currents or gradient or transmitter instability

L-26   Solutions for Artifacts (Cont'd)

Absent Image

1. Check patient centering and center frequency function when prescanning
2. Tighten all coil connections
3. Check preamplifier and amplifier function or call service engineer

Excessive Image Noise

1. Make sure patient's body is not touching the magnet sides or pad the side of the patient, separating him or her from the bore
2. Use thicker slice, larger pixel size or larger field of view
3. Change receiver or surface coil
4. Have service engineer check amplifier or preamplifier and eddy current compensation
5. Check coil connections and coil tuning mechanism or manually tuned receivers
6. Examine patient for occult metal objects, dental plate, earrings, makeup, etc.
7. Consider single echo long TR/short TE sequences

L-27   Reducing Motion Artifact

Reduces Image Blurring

1. Breath-holding
2. ECG or peripheral pulse gating
3. Respiratory gating

Reduces Image Ghosting

1. Breath-holding
2. Signal averaging
3. Presaturation
4. Gradient motion rephasing
5. Respiratory or central ordered phase encoding (ROPE, COPE)
6. Short-time inversion recovery sequence (STIR)
7. ECG gating
8. Respiratory gating
9. Glucagon
10. Prone positioning

L-28   Reducing Motion Artifact in Abdominal Imaging

1.   Respiratory or central ordered phase encoding
2.   Respiratory gating (increase scan time by two- to three-fold)
3.   Cardiac gating (increased set-up and scan time)
4.   Peripheral pulse gating (increased set-up and scan time)
5.   Glucagon administration (side effects, invasive)
6.   Flow compensation or gradient rephasing (decreased minimum echo time without increase in scan time)
7.   Prone positioning (can perform following abdominal surgery)
8.   Short TR/short TE imaging (can only get a small number of sections for each series)
9.   Multiple averages or excitations (averages out noise due to motion with some increase in scan time)
10.   Breath-holding (requires proper sequences and patient cooperation)
11.   Presaturation pulses (useful for creating black blood, particularly on single-echo sequences, but may decrease number of allowable slices per given TR)
12.   Short-time inversion recovery (some lengthy pulsing sequences null the signal fat and limit the number of slices for a given TR)
13.   Surface coil (reduces coherent image noise outside the field of view but results in image shading and limited signal depth of penetration)

L-29   Artifacts Due to External Fixation Devices *

Composition	Artifact
Graphite	None-minimal
Titanium	Minimal
Aluminum	Mild-moderate
Stainless steel	Moderate-severe

* From Berquist TH. MRI of the Musculoskeletal System, p63. New York, Raven Press, 1990.

CATEGORY L: IMAGES & PREDICAMENTS

L-30   Pearls & Rules of Thumb for MR Scanning

(Read this gamut before selecting scanning parameters or protocols)

1. Avoid scan times > 10-12 minutes

2. For T1, one or two averages, and for T2, two or four averages

3. Flow compensating gradients should be used for T2 or T2-appearing images (white blood), while presaturation is reserved for T1 images (black blood)

4. T2 spin echo images should be avoided in the spine, except for myelopathy

5. T2 spin echo images should be avoided in joint assessment unless one is evaluating soft tissues, ligaments, or tendons

6. Avoid section thickness under 5-7 mm when scanning with the body coil

7. Use the smallest coil and FOV that will image the area of interest

8. Indications for CEMR in spine: Neoplasm, inflammation/demyelination, disc vs. scar, arachnoiditis, occult infarct

9. When evaluating radiculopathy, use T2 fast scan images instead of T2 spin echo

10. To confirm meniscus tears or osteochondral injury, use T2 fast scan images instead of T2 spin echo in the knee

11. One may substitute T1 fast scan imaging for T1 spin echo for most applications

12. Variable (low) bandwidth is used in the brain only; it improves image signal with no scan time penalty

13. T2 axial cross-sections are advisable when assessing soft tissue and extremity masses

14. After a great deal of experience, pure T1 or T1 pre- and post-contrast imaging may (and should) be used in the IACs, sella, knee, neck, TMJ, heart and aorta

15. T2-appearing fast scan images are used in the TMJ, heart and aorta only if cine MR is desirable

16. Oblique images are utilized in assessment of spine discs (oblique axial), TMJ (oblique sagittal), heart (oblique sagittal and coronal), aorta (oblique sagittal), orbit (oblique sagittal and axial), shoulder (oblique coronal and sagittal) and wrist (oblique axial)

17. When using T1 imaging, utilize the shortest echo time available

L-30   Pearls & Rules of Thumb for MR Scanning (Cont'd)

18.   T2 fast scan imaging is a wide latitude technique utilizing short echo time, low flip angle (< 20 degrees) and moderate repetition time (20-500 msec)

19.   For T1 use a longer TR on high field units (500-800 msec) than on low field units (300-500 msec) since T1 is a field-dependent phenomenon and contrast is optimized in these ranges

20.   A scout sequence is a set-up sequence
   a.   Utilize the shortest TR, TE and number of excitations
   b.   The scan plane is the operator's choice
   c.   The scout can sometimes be used as a diagnostic sequence (a T1 centered on the spinous processes can be used as both a scout image and a diagnostic T1 sagittal sequence)

21.   *If T2 hybrid echo planar (fast spin echo) techniques are available, the following may be substituted for T2 spin echo in the brain, spine and extremities*
   a.   TR: 4000-6000 msec
   b.   TE effective: 100 msec
   c.   Echo train length: 8
   d.   Optional fat suppression in the extremities and spine

L-31   Pre- & Post-Contrast T1 Neuro Imaging

1. Sella

2. IAC

3. Brain: Inflammation, cortical infarct, primary or metastatic neoplasm, seizures with positive EEG

4. Posterior fossa: Inflammation; infarct with negative noncontrast MR, primary or metastatic neoplasm

5. Spine: Intramedullary primary or metastatic neoplasm, myelopathy with negative noncontrast MR, cord inflammation, disc vs. scar, demyelination, arachnoiditis

L-32   General Scanning Protocols

Head

2 DFT Slice (mm)................5.0
3 DFT Slice (mm)................3.0-5.0
Matrix ....192 or 256
FOV (cm) 24
Sequence.............................N(h), T2
Key Planes[a]........................Axial, coronal
Other....................................F comp, T1C+ neoplasm, inflammation, cortical infarction, etc.

Sella

2 DFT Slice (mm)................3.0
3 DFT Slice (mm)................1.0-1.5
Matrix ....192 or 256
FOV (cm) 16-18
Sequence.............................T1C+ and T1C- [b]
Key Planes[a]........................Coronal, sagittal
Other....................................T2 optional

IAC

2 DFT Slice (mm)................3.0
3 DFT Slice (mm)................1.5
Matrix ....192 or 256
FOV (cm) 20
Sequence.............................T1C+, T1C-
Key Planes[a]........................Coronal, axial
Other....................................F comp axial T2 recommended, T1C+ for tumor, inflammation, etc.

Posterior Fossa-Skull Base

2 DFT Slice (mm)................5.0
3 DFT Slice (mm)................3.0-4.0
Matrix ....192 or 256
FOV (cm) 22
Sequence.............................N(h), T2, T1
Key Planes[a]........................Coronal, axial
Other....................................Flow comp on T2 and T2* images, presaturation on T1, axial obliques

L-32   General Scanning Protocols (Cont'd)

Cervical Spine

2 DFT Slice (mm)	4.0-5.0
3 DFT Slice (mm)	1.0-2.0
Matrix	192 or 256
FOV (cm)	22
Sequence	T1, T2F
Key Planes[a]	Sagittal, axial
Other	See posterior fossa above, use spin echo T2 and T1C+, and T1C-

Thoracic Spine

2 DFT Slice (mm)	5.0
3 DFT Slice (mm)	3.0-4.0
Matrix	192 or 256
FOV (cm)	32-38
Sequence	T1, T2F[c]
Key Planes[a]	Sagittal, axial oblique
Other	See lumbar spine below

Lumbar Spine

2 DFT Slice (mm)	5.0
3 DFT Slice (mm)	3.0
Matrix	192 or 256
FOV (cm)	24
Sequence	T1, T2F
Key Planes[a]	Sagittal, axial
Other	T1 instead of or with T2F for myelopathy, neoplasia or post-op spine

Hip

2 DFT Slice (mm)	5.0-7.0
3 DFT Slice (mm)	4.0-5.0
Matrix	192
FOV (cm)	24
Sequence	T1, T2F
Key Planes[a]	Coronal, axial
Other	

L-32   General Scanning Protocols (Cont'd)

Knee

2 DFT Slice (mm)................4.0
3 DFT Slice (mm)................1.5-2.0
Matrix 192
FOV (cm) 14-18
Sequence............................T1, T2F
Key Planes[a]........................Sagittal, coronal
Other...................................N(h) and T2 sagittal for cruciates, N(h) and T2 coronal for collaterals

Patella

2 DFT Slice (mm)................4.0
3 DFT Slice (mm)................2.0
Matrix 192
FOV (cm) 14
Sequence............................T1, T2F
Key Planes[a]........................Axial
Other...................................

Shoulder

2 DFT Slice (mm)................4.0-5.0
3 DFT Slice (mm)................3.0-4.0
Matrix 192
FOV (cm) 16-20
Sequence............................T1, N(h), T2
Key Planes[a]........................Sagittal, coronal
Other...................................Use sagittal and coronal obliques

Labrum

2 DFT Slice (mm)................4.0
3 DFT Slice (mm)................2.0
Matrix 192
FOV (cm) 16
Sequence............................T1, T2F
Key Planes[a]........................Axial
Other...................................

L-32   General Scanning Protocols (Cont'd)

Wrist

2 DFT Slice (mm)	4.0
3 DFT Slice (mm)	1.0-2.0
Matrix	192
FOV (cm)	10
Sequence	T1, T2F
Key Planes[a]	Coronal, axial
Other	Use axial obliques

Foot, Ankle

2 DFT Slice (mm)	4.0-5.0
3 DFT Slice (mm)	4.0
Matrix	192
FOV (cm)	16
Sequence	T1, T2F
Key Planes[a]	Coronal, sagittal
Other	

a *Does not include scout.*
b *T1C+ and T1C- = contrast-enhanced T1 and noncontrast-enhanced T1.*
c *T2F = T2-appearing fast scan and gradient echo imaging.*

L-33   Field of View Selections

Coil Size from Smallest to Largest

1. Finger: Less than or equal to 8 cm
2. Hand or wrist: 10-12 cm
3. Ankle or foot: 12-16 cm
4. Elbow: 14 cm
5. Knee: 14-18 cm
6. Forearm and upper arm: 16 cm
7. Shoulder: 16-18 cm
8. Sella: 16-18 cm
9. Anterior neck: 16-20 cm
10. Calf or lower leg: 18 cm
11. Thigh and hip: 18-24 cm
12. Internal auditory canals: 20 cm
13. Posterior fossa: 20-22 cm
14. Skull base: 20-22 cm
15. Brain: 20-24 cm
16. Cervical spine: 20-24 cm
17. Lumbar spine: 22-24 cm
18. Thoracic spine: 32-38 cm
19. Bilateral hips and/or pelvis: 26-34 cm
20. Abdomen: 32-40 cm

L-34   Scan Time

Increase

Prolonged TR
Increased Y matrix
Increased averages or excitations
Large flip angle
3 DFT - slice number (increase)
Multislice gradient echo -
    slice number (increase)

Decrease

Short TR
Decreased Y matrix
Decreased averages or excitations
Small flip angle
3 DFT - slice number (decrease)
Multislice gradient echo -
    slice number (decrease)

L-35   Signal to Noise

Increase

Prolonged repetition time
Short echo time
Single echo
Decreased matrix
Increased slice thickness with gap
Increased averages or excitations
Surface coil
3 DFT
Large FOV
Large flip angle
High field strength

Decrease

Short repetition time
Long echo time
Multiple echo
Increased matrix
Decreased slice thickness without gap
Decreased averages or excitations
Whole volume coil
2 DFT
Small FOV
Small flip angle
Low field strength

L-36   Spatial Resolution (SR)

Increase SR

Decreased FOV
Decreased slice thickness
3 DFT
Surface coil
Increased matrix size

Decrease SR

Increased FOV
Increased slice thickness
2 DFT
Whole volume coil
Decreased matrix size

L-37   Available Slice Number

Increase	Decrease
Increased TR	Decreased TR
Decreased TE	Increased TE
3 DFT	2 DFT
No flow compensation	Flow compensation
No presaturation	Presaturation
No gating	Gating
Spin echo	Gradient echo
Single echo	Multiple echo

L-38   T1 & T2 Contrast Effects

T1-Appearing Images

Short TR + Short TE = Spin echo
Spoiled fast scan techniques
Partial saturation technique
Large flip angle

T2-Appearing Images

Long TR + Long TE = Spin echo
Gradient echo techniques
Steady state free precession
Small flip angle

CATEGORY L: IMAGES & PREDICAMENTS

Section 5: MR Versus CT   Page

L-39   Imaging the Supratentorial Brain

MR Preferred

1. Primary and metastatic neoplasia
2. Congenital anomalies
3. De- and dysmyelination
4. Sella and pituitary disease
5. Arteriovenous malformation and aneurysm
6. Vasculitis
7. Inflammatory disease in HIV patients
8. Infarction or inflammatory disease or abscess with negative CT
9. Complex or advanced neurodegenerative disease and/or dementia
10. Extra-axial trauma (subdural or epidural) with negative CT

Nuclear SPECT and Positron Emission Tomography (PET) Preferred

1. Grading of intracranial brain tumors
2. Tumor versus radiation necrosis
3. Neurodegenerative dementia
4. Localization of partial complex temporal lobe epilepsy

CT Preferred

1. Stroke
2. Intracranial abscess
3. Acute intracranial trauma
4. Skull fracture

L-40   Imaging the Posterior Fossa & Skull Base

MR Preferred

1. Virtually all applications, in view of its superior contrast and absence of beam hardening artifacts like those seen on CT
2. Temporal lobes
3. Sella
4. Internal auditory canals (7th and 8th nerve complexes)

CT Preferred

1. Primary skull base bone disease, including otospongiosis or otosclerosis, Paget's disease
2. Middle ear and otomastoid inflammation
3. Skull base tumors
4. Skull base fractures
5. Craniocervical junction bony anomalies

L-41 **Imaging the Spine**

MR Preferred
1. Primary and secondary or metastatic neoplasm
2. Vertebral column metastasis
3. Trauma with associated myelopathy
4. Any cause of myelopathy
5. Most cases of simple disc herniation
6. Postoperative disc recurrence
7. Discitis and (inflammatory cord) myelitis
8. Vascular malformation
9. Congenital anomalies
10. Arachnoiditis
11. Spinal stenosis involving multiple levels (more than 3) extensively in conjunction with CT
12. Any acute spine disease in pregnancy
13. Spinal block from metastatic disease, mass or any process

CT Preferred
1. Bony foraminal or central canal stenosis with less than 3 segments involved; MR may be combined with CT in lieu of CT myelography *
2. Lumbar disc disease in patients past the childbearing years with acute radiculopathy localized to one level
3. Disc disease when MR is contraindicated
4. Bony spine trauma
5. Facet arthropathy or arthritis
6. Primary bone neoplasms and primary bone anomalies

L-41   Imaging the Spine (Cont'd)

Myelography Preferred

1. Selected and difficult cases of canal stenosis and foraminal bony stenosis in the cervicothoracic and lumbar regions
2. Cases where MR is contraindicated
3. Definite radiculopathy with negative MR

Bone & SPECT Scintigraphy Preferred

1. Adjunct and screening for spinal metastatic disease
2. Assessment of extent and levels of arthritic involvement
3. Diagnosis of stress injury, low grade compression injury of the vertebral column and spondylolysis in cases where CT or plain film are negative (use SPECT - it is not uncommon for SPECT to be positive with CT, planar bone scan and conventional radiographs negative)

If plain film shows evidence of prominent bony disease at a few segmental levels, CT may be the first diagnostic algorithm in the lumbar spine. If there is extensive bone disease, MR should be used to localize the worst levels, then MR combined with CT. CT may be used to qualify bony foraminal encroachment in the cervical region after MR excludes soft disease. Soft disc disease or acute symptoms strongly favor the use of MR over CT, especially in the cervical region. For foraminal bone disease or central bony canal stenosis, use only plain films & CT in the cervical and lumbar regions.

L-42   Imaging the Orbits

MR Preferred

1. Conal or globe neoplasms or masses
2. Vascular abnormalities
3. Ophthalmopathy versus orbital pseudotumor
4. Retinal hemorrhage or subretinal effusion
5. Sudden blindness
6. Cortical blindness or optic pathway disease
7. Optic neuritis
8. Phakomatoses
9. Suprasellar chiasmatic disease
10. Retrochiasmatic optic pathway disease

CT Preferred

1. Infectious cellulitis or abscess
2. Orbital trauma and blowout fracture
3. Foreign body

L-43   Imaging the Head & Neck

MR Preferred
1. Oropharyngeal and nasopharyngeal neoplasm
2. Neck masses or adenopathy
3. Salivary gland tumor
4. Hypopharyngeal mass or neoplasm
5. Parathyroid adenoma (with negative ultrasound)
6. Characterization of unusual sonographic thyroid mass
7. Characterization of neck cysts (with equivocal ultrasound)
8. Sensorineural hearing loss
9. Tic douloureux
10. Bell's palsy

CT Preferred
1. Laryngeal mass, paralysis or staging of laryngeal carcinoma
2. Initial diagnosis of neck cellulitis, phlegmon and peritonsillar abscess
3. Primary facial bone and jaw masses
4. Dental-associated masses (with conventional radiography)
5. Screening sinus disease
6. Bony head and neck trauma
7. External and middle ear anomalies and inflammatory disease
8. Primary skull base and bony neoplasms

L-44   Orthopedic Imaging

MR Preferred

1. Avascular necrosis
2. Primary tumors and metastatic disease (with conventional radiography)
3. Osteochondral defects, osteochondritis dissecans and osteoarthritis (with conventional radiography)
4. Lymphoma and multiple myeloma (with conventional radiography)
5. Occult joint effusion
6. Osteomyelitis and septic arthritis (with conventional radiography)
7. Tendinous, ligamentous and rotator cuff complex injury or tear
8. Shoulder impingement syndrome
9. Carpal tunnel syndrome of the wrist and any associated neural impingement syndrome
10. Shoulder labral disease
11. Meniscus tear
12. All soft tissue masses
13. Staging of fractures about the knee joint
14. Peri- and intra-articular soft tissue masses
15. Primary synovial disease
16. Triangular fibrocartilage tear of the wrist

L-45   Imaging the Abdomen

MR Preferred

1.   Mesenteric and portal vein thrombosis
2.   Hepatocellular carcinoma
3.   Hepatic metastatic disease with negative CT or with history of iodinated contrast reaction
4.   Intravascular staging of advanced renal cell carcinoma
5.   Vascular invasion or compression by neoplasm
6.   Confirmation of cavernous hemangioma of the liver
7.   Differentiation of regenerating nodules from hepatoma
8.   Confirmation of fatty liver metamorphosis or infiltration suspected on equivocal CT
9.   Abdominal aortic dissection or occlusion
10. Retroperitoneal fibrosis, malignant versus benign
11. Differentiation of low grade from high grade adrenal masses
12. Splenic mass characterization with equivocal CT
13. Abdominal screening for pheochromocytoma

CT Preferred

1.   Initial liver evaluation for metastatic disease
2.   Staging of intra-abdominal primary metastatic carcinoma, including abdominal adenopathy and peritoneal disease
3.   Initial evaluation of abdominal trauma and visceral injury
4.   Abdominal inflammatory disease (diverticulitis, appendicitis, ischemic bowel, cholangitis, and intra-abdominal abscess)
5.   Gallbladder disease (CT as adjunct with ultrasound and hepatobiliary scintigraphy as initial primary evaluators)
6.   Staging of lymphoma (Hodgkin's and non-Hodgkin's)

L-46   Imaging the Male Pelvis

MR Preferred

1. Localized pelvic staging of prostate carcinoma and bladder carcinoma (with endorectal coil) and initial evaluation of pelvic soft tissue mass of unknown origin

2. Initial evaluation of pelvic bony metastases

3. Staging and local extent of rectal carcinoma

4. Distinction of recurrent rectal carcinoma versus postoperative or radiation change (PET a preferred substitute to distinguish fibrosis or radiation change versus recurrent neoplasm)

5. Postoperative perineal abscess and fistula

CT Preferred

1. Inflammatory disease, including diverticulitis, appendicitis, prostatitis and pelvic abscess

2. Evaluation of ascites

3. Initial evaluation of pelvic trauma or hemorrhage

4. Initial evaluation of the testicles and scrotum is best undertaken with ultrasound with or without nuclear scintigraphy for testicular torsion

L-47   Imaging the Female Pelvis

MR Preferred

1.   Initial localized staging of uterine, cervical, vaginal, urethral and bladder carcinoma with or without endorectal or phased array coil
2.   Differentiation of adnexal versus uterine mass with equivocal ultrasound
3.   Occult pelvic pain with negative CT or ultrasound
4.   Urethral fistula formation

CT Preferred

1.   Initial evaluation of all pelvic inflammatory disease and pelvic fluid collections
2.   Pelvic trauma

L-48   Imaging the Chest

MR Preferred

1.   Fibrosing mediastinitis
2.   Caval thrombosis and superior vena caval compression syndrome
3.   Characterization of mediastinal masses only as adjunct to CT
4.   Staging of tracheal neoplasms
5.   Evaluation of dissecting and nondissecting aortic aneurysms
6.   Differentiation of hilar mass versus vascular pseudomass
7.   Main pulmonary artery compression or thrombosis

CT Preferred

1.   Primary or metastatic lung carcinoma
2.   Pleural disease
3.   Lung inflammation and pneumonia, abscess, empyema
4.   Initial evaluation of mediastinal masses/adenopathy

L-49   Imaging the Cardiovascular System

MR Preferred

1. Simple and complex congenital heart disease
2. Constrictive pericarditis
3. Cardiac and pericardial masses
4. Verification of equivocal or bizarre echocardiogram
5. Primary myocardial neoplasm
6. Differentiation of ventricular tumor from ventricular thrombus

Magnetic Resonance Angiography Preferred

1. Screen for carotid bifurcation disease and vertebrobasilar insufficiency
2. Screen for intracranial aneurysm, arteriovenous malformation or arterial or veno-occlusive disease in conjunction with conventional cut film angiography
3. Evaluation of pulmonary embolus when iodinated contrast is absolutely contraindicated
4. Evaluation of mesenteric vein thrombosis, including cava, portal vein and superior mesenteric vein

L-50   MR Angiography Imaging Techniques

2D Time-of-Flight (2DTF)

Advantages

1. Sensitivity to slow flow
2. Relatively short scan times
3. Lack of saturation effects
4. Multiple projections, including subvolumes

Disadvantages

1. Thrombus or other short T2 substance may simulate flow
2. Patient motion artifact
3. Insensitivity to in-plane flow
4. Relatively long echo time

3D Time-of-Flight (3DTF)

Advantages

1. Short scan times
2. High spatial resolution
3. Very short echo times
4. Reprojection and subvolume images possible

Disadvantages

1. Thrombus or other short T1 substance may simulate flow
2. Insensitivity to slow flow
3. Saturation effects
4. Field distortion artifacts such as air-bone susceptibility gradients

L-50   MR Angiography Imaging Techniques (Cont'd)

2D Phase Contrast (2DTF)

Advantages

1.   Short acquisition time

2.   Variable velocity encoding, allowing imaging of slow or fast flow

3.   Directional flow images

4.   Excellent background suppression

Disadvantages

1.   No reprojection images

2.   Large voxel size

3.   Relatively long echo times

3D Phase Contrast (3DPC)

Advantages

1.   Variable velocity encoding, allowing imaging of slow or fast flow

2.   Excellent background suppression

3.   Minimized saturation effects

4.   Small voxel size

5.   Directional flow information

6.   Reprojection and subvolume images possible

Disadvantages

1.   Long acquisition time

2.   Relatively long echo times

L-50   MR Angiography Imaging Techniques (Cont'd)

Cine Phase Contrast

Advantages

1. Variable velocity encoding, allowing imaging of cerebrospinal fluid, venous or arterial flow
2. Quantitative flow measurement
3. Time-resolved information
4. Hemodynamic flow information

Disadvantages

1. Loss of signal intensity with overlapping vessels
2. Large voxel size

* Adapted from Huston J and Ehman RL. Comparison of Time-of-Flight and Phase-Contrast MR Neuroangiographic Techniques. RadioGraphics 3:18, 1993.